Recent Advances in

Gastroenterology
11

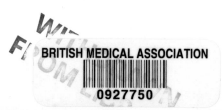

Recent Advances in

Gastroenterology
11

Edited by

Chris Probert MD FRCP FHEA

Professor of Gastroenterology
Clinical Science at South Bristol
University of Bristol and
University Hospitals of Bristol
Bristol, UK

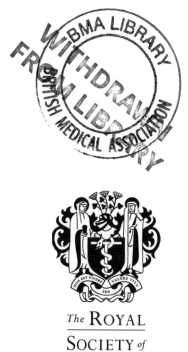

The ROYAL
SOCIETY *of*
MEDICINE
PRESS *Limited*

Published by the Royal Society of Medicine Press Ltd
1 Wimpole Street, London W1G 0AE, UK
Tel: +44 (0)20 7290 2921
Fax: +44 (0)20 7290 2929
Email: publishing@rsm.ac.uk
Website: www.rsmpress.co.uk

British Library Cataloguing in Publication Data
A catalogue record for this book is available from the British Library
ISBN 978–1–85315–710–3

Distribution in Europe and Rest of World:

Marston Book Services Ltd
PO Box 269, Abingdon
Oxon OX14 4YN, UK
Tel: +44 (0)1235 465500
Fax: +44 (0)1235 465555
Email: direct.order@marston.co.uk

Distribution in the USA and Canada:

Royal Society of Medicine Press Ltd
c/o BookMasters Inc
30 Amberwood Parkway
Ashland, OH 44805, USA
Tel: +1 800 247 6553/+1 800 266 5564
Fax: +1 419 281 6883
Email: order@bookmasters.com

Distribution in Australia and New Zealand:

Elsevier Australia
30-52 Smidmore Street
Marrickville NSW 2204, Australia
Tel: +61 2 9517 8999
Fax: +61 2 9517 2249
Email: service@elsevier.com.au

Editorial services and typesetting by GM & BA Haddock, Ford, Midlothian, UK

Printed in India by Replika Press Pvt. Ltd.

Contents

Contributors

Lachlan Ayres MBChB MRCP(UK)
Clinical Fellow in Gastroenterology, Department of Gastroenterology, The Great Western Hospital, Swindon, UK

Hugh Barr MD(Dist) ChM FRCS FRCSE FHEA
Professor and Consultant Upper Gastrointestinal Surgeon, Department of Upper Gastrointestinal Surgery and Biophotonics Research Unit, Gloucestershire Royal Hospital, Gloucester, UK

Rachel Bradley MB ChB MRCP MSc
Consultant Physician and Geriatrician at University Hospitals Bristol, Bristol; and St Martins Continence Promotion Unit, Bath and Bristol General Hospital, Bristol, UK

Ronald Bremner MB ChB BSc(Med Sci) DM MRCPCH
Specialist Registrar, Department of Paediatric Gastroenterology, Bristol Royal Hospital for Children, Bristol, UK

Mark P. Callaway MRCP FRCR
Consultant Gastrointestinal Radiologist, Bristol Royal Infirmary, Bristol, UK

Peter Collins BMSc MBChB MD MRCP(UK)
Consultant Hepatologist, Department of Digestive Disease, Bristol Royal Infirmary, University Hospital Bristol NHS Foundation Trust, Bristol, UK

Tom J. Creed MD MRCP
Consultant Gastroenterologist, University Hospitals of Bristol, Bristol, UK

Fiona H. Gordon MA MD MBBChir FRCP
Consultant Hepatologist, Bristal Royal Infirmary, Bristol, UK

Catherine Kendall MSc PhD MIPEM
Royal Society Dorothy Hodgkin Research Fellow, Biophotonics Research Unit, Gloucestershire Royal Hospital, Gloucester, UK

Katherine J Mabey BS(Hons), BSc(Hons)
Clinical Gastrointestinal Physiologist, Bristol Royal Infirmary, Bristol, UK

C. Anne McCune BSc MBBS MRCP MD
Consultant Gastrenterologist and Hepatologist, Clinical Effectiveness Lead, Medicine, Bristol Royal Infirmary, Bristol, UK

Anne E. Mills AGIP MIIR DipReflex
Clinical Gastrointestinal Physiologist, Bristol Royal Infirmary, Bristol, UK

Simon J.W. Monkhouse MA MBBChir(Hons) MRCS
Spelialist Registrar in General Surgery, Southmead Hospital, Bristol, UK

Justin D.T. Morgan MB BCh MD PGCME FRCS
Consultant General, Endocrine and Transplant Surgeon, Southmead Hospital, Bristol, UK

Sally A. Norton MB ChB MD FRCS(Ed)
Consultant General, Laparoscopic and Upper GI Surgeon, Southmead Hospital, Bristol, UK

Richard Parker MB ChB
Clinical Fellow, Department of Hepatology, Bristol Royal Infirmary, Bristol, UK

Chris Probert MD FRCP FHEA
Professor of Gastroenterology, Clinical Science at South Bristol, University of Bristol and University Hospitals of Bristol, Bristol, UK

Pramila Ramani MBBS PhD FRCPath
Consultant, Department of Paediatric Histopathology, Bristol Royal Hospital for Children, Bristol, UK

Bhupinder K. Sandhu MBBS MD FRCP FRCPCH
Professor, Department of Paediatric Gastroenterology, Bristol Royal Hospital for Children, Bristol, UK

Geeta Shetty DM MRCS
Research Fellow and Specialist Registrar, Department of Upper Gastrointestinal Surgery and Biophotonics Research Unit, Gloucestershire Royal Hospital, Gloucester, UK

John E. Smithson MD FRCP (for correspondence)
Consultant Gastroenterologist, Department of Gastroenterology, University Hospitals Bristol, Bristol, UK.

Robin Spiller MD(Cantab) MSc(Lond) FRCP
Professor of Gastroenterology, Wolfson Digestive Diseases Centre, University Hospital, Nottingham, UK

Christine H. Spray MB ChB MRCP FRCPCH
Consultant, Department of Paediatric Gastroenterology, Bristol Royal Hospital for Children, Bristol, UK

Nicholas Stone MSc MSc PhD MBA MIPEM CSci
National Institute of Health Senior Research Fellow, Biophotonics Research Unit, Gloucestershire Royal Hospital, Gloucester, UK

Wolf W.W. Woltersdorf MD MRCP FRCPath
Consultant Chemical Pathologist and Head of U-STAR Research Medical Director of Avon Diagnostic Laboratories Ltd, Department of Laboratory Medicine, University Hospitals Bristol, Bristol, UK

Preface

Recent Advances in Gastroenterology provides a series of articles to update doctors in the latest developments in gastroenterology and hepatology. The book has been written primarily for the gastroenterologist in training, general medical trainees and general practitioners developing specialty clinics. However, as consultants have become focussed on subspecialty interests, I hope this book will help them to gain insights into areas of work outside their day-to-day practice.

It is over a decade since gastroenterology and hepatology was last covered in this format and much has changed. As a result, I have had to be highly selective in the topics reviewed. The 12 chapters each cover areas that I find exciting, inflammatory bowel disease; challenging, the assessment of NAFLD; or stimulating, such as the insights into Hepatitis E. I am sure that some readers will feel that I have overlooked some important topics, but a balance had to be struck between depth and breadth.

I am grateful to the authors for the hard work and timely delivery of their chapters. I appreciate their forbearance with my attempts to edit their contributions.

I am grateful to RSM Press for inviting me to lead this manuscript and to Gill Haddock for carefully compiling the work. Finally, I thank family and friends to their help and tolerance during its realization.

Chris Probert MD FRCP FHEA
Professor of Gastroenterology
Clinical Science at South Bristol
University Hospital at Bristol
Bristol, UK

Christine H. Spray Ronald Bremner
Bhupinder K. Sandhu Pramila Ramani

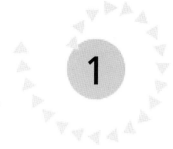

Eosinophilic oesophagitis: an emerging entity

Small numbers of eosinophils are present normally in the gut as part of the host's natural defence, although rarely in the oesophagus. Until recently, the presence of eosinophils in the oesophagus was thought to be related to either gastro-oesophageal reflux disease (GORD) or allergy. However, as far back as 1978, Landres *et al.*[1] reported a case of food impaction associated with a dense eosinophilic infiltrate of the oesophageal mucosa called eosinophilic oesophagitis and was considered to be a separate entity to GORD. Over the last decade, eosinophilic oesophagitis has been increasingly recognised with increasing numbers of cases reported both in children and adults world-wide and is the most common of the eosinophilic gastrointestinal disorders.

DEFINITION

Eosinophilic oesophagitis is a histological diagnosis where eosinophilic infiltration of the oesophagus is greater than 15 epithelial eosinophils per high-power field (magnification ×400) in association with symptoms of oesophageal dysfunction such as reflux-like symptoms especially dysphagia and food impaction that are unresponsive to treatment with proton pump inhibitors (PPIs) and other causes of eosinophilia have been excluded.[2]

Christine H. Spray MB ChB MRCP FRCPCH (for correspondence)
Consultant, Department of Paediatric Gastroenterology, Bristol Royal Hospital for Children, Upper Maudlin Street, Bristol BS2 8LY, UK. E-mail: christine.spray@UHBristol.nhs.uk

Ronald Bremner MB ChB BSc(Med Sci) DM MRCPCH
Specialist Registrar, Dept Paediatric Gastroenterology, Bristol Royal Hospital for Children, Bristol, UK

Bhupinder K. Sandhu MBBS MD FRCP FRCPCH
Professor, Department of Paediatric Gastroenterology, Bristol Royal Hospital for Children, Bristol, UK

Pramila Ramani MBBS PhD FRCPath
Consultant, Department of Paediatric Histopathology, Bristol Royal Hospital for Children, Bristol, UK

EPIDEMIOLOGY

Eosinophilic oesophagitis is seen world-wide and increasing numbers of cases have been reported from Europe, the US, South America, Asia and Australia.[3,4] It is more common in boys, being reported to be between 66–91% male preponderance in published series and often associated with atopy.[5,6] A retrospective analysis of children in West Virginia calculated the prevalence to be less than 1:10,000,[7] although the prevalence appears to be increasing. A population-based study in a mid-western community in the US identified a 4-fold increase over a 4-year period from 2000 to 2003 reaching a prevalence of 4.3 per 10,000 children at the end of 2003.[8] The authors also found a familial pattern raising the possibility of either a genetic predisposition or exposure to an unknown environmental factor. The authors suggested the incidence for eosinophilic oesophagitis was perhaps higher than those for other well-recognised paediatric conditions such as Crohn's disease. Another study reported that 9.3% of children presenting to a tertiary gastrointestinal unit, between 1993 and 1995, with oesophageal eosinophilia were given a diagnosis of eosinophilic oesophagitis.[9] In Australia, an increase from 0.05/10,000 to 0.89/10,000 in a paediatric population was seen over a 10-year period. This study also identified an increase in severity of inflammation.[3,8] This may reflect an increasing awareness of the utility of mucosal biopsies for histology as a routine in both children and adults undergoing endoscopy even if macroscopic appearances of the oesophagus is normal. Up to one-third of patients with severe eosinophilic oesophagitis may have normal appearance of the oesophagus at endoscopy.[9] This applies particularly to those patients unresponsive to acid suppression and with normal pH-monitoring results. This may also explain why eosinophilic oesophagitis is thought to be more common in children than adults. In a population-based study, up to 1% of Swedish adults had oesophageal eosinophilic infiltration, 54% of whom did not have significant symptoms.[10] Alternatively, it may be a true increase in the prevalence, as has been documented with other diseases associated with atopy over recent decades.

CLINICAL FEATURES

The presenting symptoms of eosinophilic oesophagitis are variable. Most children have symptoms suggestive of GORD (50–80%) or food impaction (20–50%).[6,9,11] Symptoms are typically age-dependent with non-specific symptoms such as vomiting, nausea, food refusal, abdominal pain and failure-to-thrive in infants and younger children. Older children and adults commonly present with dysphagia and food impaction but not odynophagia.[12] The clinical course is characterised by either relapse and remission or persistent symptoms.[13] Several studies have implicated allergic predisposition to either food or aero-allergens. In one paediatric study, 60% of children were found to have food allergies[9] and about half paediatric and adult patients with eosinophilic oesophagitis have been found to have other allergic symptoms such as eczema and asthma.[14] Blood eosinophilia may be seen in approximately 30% of adults and 60% of children and increased IgE levels in 55% of adults and 40–73% of children.[15] Neither symptoms nor eosinophilia respond to anti-reflux treatment with PPIs.

The differential diagnosis includes other causes of intestinal eosinophilic infiltration including: infection (helminthic, parasitic), inflammatory bowel disease, coeliac disease, GORD, eosinophilic gastroenteritis, collagen vascular diseases, or hyper-eosinophilic syndromes.[16] There is no documented association with malignancy or progression to systemic hypereosinophilia, but the chronic inflammation could lead to permanent structural or functional abnormality.

Diagnosis is by endoscopy and biopsy. Barium radiology may demonstrate strictures, often reflecting the ringed oesophageal narrowing seen at endoscopy.[17] Manometric studies may demonstrate spasticity, hypercontractility, and abnormal peristalsis.[18] These investigations are not diagnostic, as findings are non-specific. Oesophageal pH monitoring may be normal or show alkaline reflux.[6]

Endoscopy findings

Endoscopic appearances may be normal in one-third of children despite severe histological changes.[9] In adults, features include ringed oesophagus (55%), oesophageal strictures (38%), linear furrows (33%), narrow oesophagus (10%) and normal (7%).[19] The 'crêpe paper mucosa' description reflects the fragility of the oesophageal lining and its furrowed appearance.[20] When there are multiple concentric rings, the oesophagus is described as 'feline' or 'tracheal' (Figs 1 and 2). It is speculated that the release of histamine, eosinophilic chemotactic factor or platelet activating factor by the mast cells in the oesophageal wall in response to allergens could lead to ring formation. These substances stimulate eosinophils to release toxic proteins which, in turn,

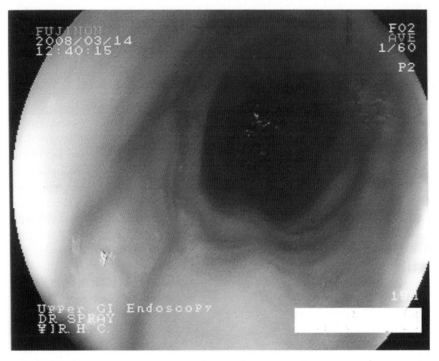

Fig. 1 Endoscopic appearances of oesophagus showing concentric mucosal rings and linear furrowing characteristics of eosinophilic oesophagitis.

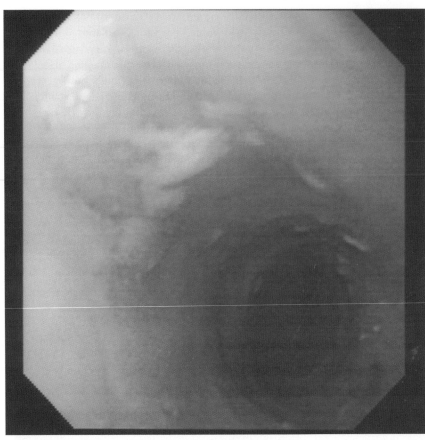

Fig. 2 Typical endoscopic appearance of plaques/exudates seen in eosinophilic oesophagitis.

stimulate activation of acetyl choline causing contraction of muscle fibres in muscularis mucosa resulting in oesophageal rings.[21] Multiple white papules that mimic fungal infections, but correlate with eosinophilic micro-abscesses in the mucosa on histology, may be seen.[22] Strictures have been reported in children and adults.[23] Endoscopic complications including mucosal laceration and perforation are more common in adults with eosinophilic oesophagitis, and are more likely in those with more severe histological changes and stricture dilatation.[20] Because normal endoscopic appearances are common, routinely obtaining mucosal biopsies is essential particularly in patients with classical symptoms of dysphagia and food impaction. Oesophageal biopsies should be taken from both proximal and distal oesophagus when considering eosinophilic oesophagitis as a diagnosis.[24]

Endoscopic ultrasonography shows a significant increase in oesophageal wall thickness in eosinophilic oesophagitis[25] suggesting that the deeper muscular layers of the oesophageal wall as well as the superficial mucosa may also be affected.

Histopathology
The diagnosis is often suggested by the clinical presentation and the endoscopic appearance, but is confirmed by the histological features. The

proximal oesophagus is often involved, as opposed to the oesophagitis in GORD where distal changes are typical.[26] Because eosinophilic oesophagitis can be present in the presence of normal endoscopic appearances, routine biopsies are essential as part of a full evaluation. Histological examination of the proximal oesophagus may, therefore, improve diagnostic accuracy.

Eosinophils are infrequent in the oesophagus without gastrointestinal pathology, with rarely more than one eosinophil per high-power field. A recent consensus of a minimum of 15 eosinophils per high-power field has been reached as the pathological criterion.[2] Eosinophilic oesophagitis is characterised by an increase in intra-epithelial eosinophils seen along the length of the oesophagus.[27]

Other helpful, but non-diagnostic, features are the superficial distribution of eosinophils, particularly on the juxtaluminal aspect. Micro-abscess formation, comprising pockets of at least four or more eosinophils grouped together are seen in many cases (Figs 3 and 4). Eosinophilic micro-abscesses are more likely when eosinophilic infiltrates are more severe.[27] Numerous degranulating eosinophils are usually evident. Other typical features are the marked epithelial hyperplasia including basal zone hyperplasia, intercellular oedema and severe papillary elongation, which are more marked than in GORD.[27] Ulceration is generally not a feature. Eosinophils are present in the lamina propria and muscularis propria, although these are not usually included in most oesophageal biopsies,[27] and sub-epithelial fibrosis is related to histological severity in children.[28] Gastric and duodenal biopsies generally show a normal number of eosinophils.

It is important to fix the biopsies in formalin-based fixatives, because Bouin's preservative can make identification of eosinophils difficult.[24] While a minimum of five biopsy samples is necessary to achieve 100% sensitivity in adults,[26] the precise number of biopsy samples necessary to achieve this degree of accuracy in diagnosis in children has not been reported.

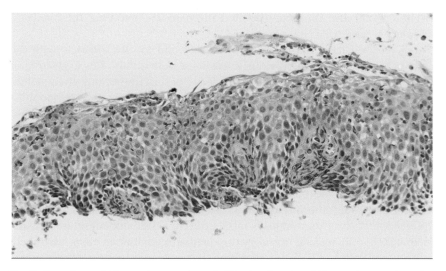

Fig. 3 Oesophageal biopsy shows a dense infiltrate of eosinophils, concentrated on the superficial (luminal) side. Note the surface exudates of eosinophils, a histological correlate of whitish patches seen on endoscopy (×200).

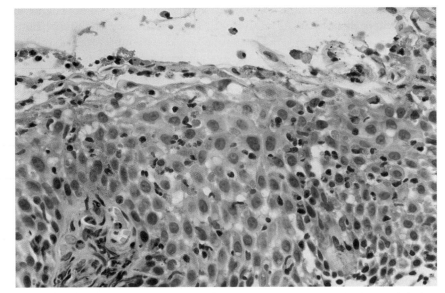

Fig. 4 Oesophageal biopsy shows an increased number of eosinophils plus epithelial hyperplasia (×400).

Allergy testing

Specific IgE-based serology, allergen skin prick or patch testing is positive in up to 80% of patients with eosinophilic oesophagitis.[29] Triggers detected by skin response testing are most commonly egg, milk and wheat. A paucity of new diagnoses in North American children in the winter suggests a possible link with aero-antigens in allergic eosinophilic oesophagitis.[30]

Pathophysiology

The exact pathogenesis is unclear, and most likely it is a complex interplay of environmental and immune-mediated mechanisms involving IgE-mediated and the helper T-cell (Th2) pathways.[31]

IgE released from mast cells, systemically and locally, interacts with the aero- or food allergens in previously sensitised individuals. This leads to mast cell degranulation followed by the release of histamine and chemokines, including eotaxin, cytokines such as interleukin (IL)-5, and eosinophilic chemotactic factors.[32] These induce eosinophil migration and degranulation.

Non-IgE-mediated immune response comprises a Th2-type immune response and local or systemic Th2 overproduction.[33] It plays a key role in eosinophil recruitment, which involves multiple steps, including eosinophil proliferation, transmigration from the bone marrow into the circulation, activation within the bloodstream, adhesion to the vascular endothelium, diapedesis through the vascular wall into the tissue and migration toward the epithelium. Each of these steps is influenced by a different subset of cytokine mediators. An increasing numbers of potential mediators is being identified, with up-regulation of IL-5 and interferon (IFN)-γ seen in biopsies from patients with eosinophilic oesophagitis.[34]

IL-5 is the key cytokine responsible for the proliferation, maturation, release, migration of eosinophils from the bone marrow and the activation of eosinophils.[35] IL-5 is also expressed by eosinophils, and increased levels of IL-5 are seen in oesophageal biopsies. The role of IL-5 as an important mediator is shown by the improvement in the clinical and/or pathological features seen after anti IL-5 treatment, which probably counteracts both the systemic as well as the local effects of IL-5.[36]

Another important cytokine involved in the pathogenesis of eosinophilic oesophagitis is IL-13, which also regulates several other eosinophil functions.[37] For example, the adhesion, rolling and diapedesis of eosinophils from the vascular spaces into the mucosa is facilitated by induction of cell surface adhesion molecules such as VLA-4 and vascular cell adhesion molecule-1 (VCAM-1) on the surface of eosinophils and endothelial surfaces, respectively. IL-13 activates eosinophils to release leukotriene and platelet-activating factor. IL-13 also induces the expression of the chemokine eotaxin-3, which is up-regulated 50-fold in oesophageal biopsies.[38]

Eotaxins are important chemo-attractants in recruiting eotaxin-3 receptor (chemokine receptor CCR3)-bearing eosinophils, mast cells and subsets of macrophages.[39] In a recent study, using microarray expression profile analysis, Blanchard et al.[40] identified eotaxin-3 as the most highly-induced gene in a cohort of patients with eosinophilic oesophagitis compared to its expression level in healthy individuals. A single nucleotide polymorphism in the human eotaxin-3 gene was associated with disease susceptibility. Furthermore, mice deficient in CCR3 were protected from experimental eosinophilic oesophagitis. Higher levels of eotaxin-3 gene expression are seen in the mucosa in eosinophilic oesophagitis compared to GORD.[41]

The importance of eotaxin-1 and IL-5 in the pathogenesis of eosinophilic oesophagitis has been validated using IL-5 and eotaxin-1 gene-targeted mice. In this study, mice challenged with IL-13 (a cytokine proven to induce eosinophilic oesophagitis in wild-type mice) showed a significant decrease in the oesophageal eosinophilic infiltrate in both IL-5 and eotaxin-1 deficient mice when compared with wild-type mice.[37]

TGF-β1 also makes an important contribution to the pathogenesis of eosinophilic oesophagitis by inducing epithelial proliferation, increased vascular density and vascular activation by up-regulating VCAM-1. It is also implicated in the formation of strictures as it stimulates fibrosis, collagen formation, smooth muscle hyperplasia and the loss of elasticity of oesophageal wall.[42]

Eosinophils release a variety of products, including growth factors, such as TGF and VEGF, and oesophageal granule proteins such as eosinophil basic protein (EBP), eosinophil peroxidase (EPO), eosinophil cationic protein (ECP) and eosinophil-derived neurotoxin (EDN).[43] These share pro-inflammatory properties and cause tissue damage via their cytotoxic activity. Eosinophils also generate large amounts of three lipid mediators – leukotriene C4 that is metabolised to leukotrienes LTD4 and LTE4. These increase eosinophil trafficking, vascular permeability and stimulate smooth muscle contraction.

GENETICS

There is a familial association with eosinophilic oesophagitis, with 1 in 12 children having a first-degree relative affected.[8] Male predisposition suggests a possible link to the X-chromosome, where genes coding for two of the IL-13 receptor chains are found. A single-nucleotide polymorphism of the eotaxin-3 gene has been linked to eosinophilic diseases.[40]

TREATMENT

Therapeutic choices include elimination diets, corticosteroids, leukotriene inhibitors and immunomodulators. Full assessment with endoscopy and allergy testing guides therapy. Assessment of treatment response should not only include symptomatic control but also document the effect on inflammation with repeat mucosal biopsies.

Dietary manipulation

Food allergy is a potential trigger or exacerbating factor in eosinophilic oesophagitis. Several paediatric trials have found that elimination diets guided by allergy test results or complete food allergen exclusion with elemental diets are effective in up to 90% of cases[44] Elemental diets have been used for a 6–8-week period, followed by staged food re-introduction guided by skin prick or patch testing results. The mean time to symptomatic improvement was 8.5 days in one series.[44] Relapse is common after food re-introduction, and repeat periods with a dietary restriction may be required. There are no large-scale studies of allergen-exclusion diets in adults, and poor tolerance and taste may limit its use. One small case series suggested exclusion of a single allergen (wheat) in sensitised adults was ineffective.[45]

Medical therapy

Anti-reflux therapy is ineffective.[46]

In a retrospective cohort of 20 children with persistent symptoms, systemic corticosteroid therapy with 1.5 mg/kg methylprednisolone in two divided doses a day for 4 weeks reduced symptoms and improved histological appearance in 19 cases.[47] Within a year, 10 had relapsed, although only two required repeat treatment courses.

Azathioprine or 6-mercaptopurine has been found effective to maintain remission and reduce steroid burden in steroid-dependent adults.[48] The powerful immunosuppressive effect of the thiopurines and the lack of extensive evidence-base for their use mean that they should be reserved for only the most severely affected.

The arachidonic acid metabolites play an important role in inflammation and the leukotrienes are mediators of mast cell and eosinophil degranulation. An open-label study of Montelukast (10 mg daily), a leukotriene D4 receptor antagonist used in asthma treatment, in 8 adults with eosinophilic oesophagitis showed symptomatic improvement in 6 without change in histological severity.[49] Relapse was common on discontinuing treatment. An open-label study of 8 children showed similar results (5–10 mg daily).[50] This therapy has not been evaluated in a randomised, controlled trial.

Topical steroid therapy

Local application aims to reduce the systemic side-effects of corticosteroids. A randomised trial of 36 children over 3 months showed histological improvement in 50% with swallowed fluticasone (440 µg [2 puffs] twice daily) compared to 9% with placebo.[51] Improvement in vomiting was more likely in the treatment group (67% versus 27%). In an open-label study, 19 of 21 adults with dysphagia improved after swallowed fluticasone (220 µg twice daily for 6 weeks), with repeat treatment required in 4 of 17 after 1 year.[52] In a randomised trial over 3 months with a 4-week induction and a dose-tapering regimen over 8-weeks, swallowed fluticasone matched oral prednisolone for remission rate and time-to-relapse with improvement in 94% ofsubjects.[53] Within 6 months, 45% of subjects had relapsed. Systemic side-effects were noted in 40% with prednisolone, and oral candidiasis occurred in 15% with fluticasone. An open study of a viscous preparation of budesonide (twice daily oral budesonide suspension 500 µg mixed with sucrose for 3 months) showed improved symptoms in 80% and induced statistically significant histological improvement, without detectable effect on early morning cortisol, in a cohort of 20 children with neurodevelopmental problems who were unable to use an inhaler.[54]

Biological therapy

In view of the central role of IL-5 in eosinophil trafficking and activation, an anti-IL-5 monoclonal antibody therapy (mepolizumab, 750 mg) is under evaluation for eosinophilic oesophagitis. Initial data from open label studies suggested both symptomatic, quality-of-life and histological improvement after a total of three, monthly intravenous infusions.[36] The long-term safety profile of this therapy is currently unknown and is of concern particularly in view of the possible association of another biological compound, infliximab, used in the treatment of Crohn's disease and the rare, but fatal, hepatosplenic T-cell lymphoma.[55] Future targets for therapy could include eotaxin, chemokine receptors or IL-13.

Management of strictures

Case-series reports illustrate that dilatation of oesophageal strictures in eosinophilic oesophagitis is effective in treatment-resistant cases with a variable, but often prolonged, effect.[13] However, because of the associated mucosal fragility, mucosal tears and oesophageal rupture are more likely, especially with food bolus removal with rigid endoscopes and dilation procedures.[56]

Key points for clinical practice

- Eosinophilic oesophagitis is a newly described and emerging clinicopathological disease distinct from gastro-oesophageal reflux disease characterised by upper gastrointestinal symptoms unresponsive to treatment with proton pump inhibitors.

- Eosinophilic oesophagitis is a common condition in both adults and children but more common in males.

- Eosinophilic oesophagitis should be considered a possible diagnosis in patients presenting with dysphagia and food impaction.

(continued)

Key points for clinical practice (continued)

• Endoscopy can identify classical appearances of eosinophilic oesophagitis but may be normal in up to one-third of children and oesophageal biopsies are necessary both proximal and distally.

• Eosinophilic oesophagitis is a histological diagnosis with 15 or more eosinophils per high-power field in any one oesophageal biopsy specimen.

• Natural history of eosinophilic oesophagitis is unknown but oesophageal strictures may develop.

• Allergic triggers should be identified in patients with eosinophilic oesophagitis.

• Various treatments are available including elemental and elimination diets as well as oral/inhaled steroids, Montelukast and biologicals but larger multicentred studies are needed.

• Genetic predisposition has been postulated and may direct future treatments.

References

1. Landres RT, Kuster GG, Strum WB. Eosinophilic esophagitis in a patient with vigorous achalasia. *Gastroenterology* 1978; **74**: 1298–1301.
2. Furuta GT, Forbes D, Boey C, *et al*. Eosinophilic Gastrointestinal Diseases. Third FISPGHAN Working Group Report. *J Pediatr Gastroenterol Nutr* 2007; **47**: 234–238.
3. Cherian S, Smith NM, Forbes DA. Rapidly increasing prevalence of eosinophilic oesophagitis in Western Australia. *Arch Dis Child* 2006; **91**: 1000–1004.
4. Nielsen RG, Husby S. Eosinophilic oesophagitis: epidemiology, clinical aspects, and association to allergy. *J Pediatr Gastroenterol Nutr* 2007; **45**: 281–289.
5. Cheung KM, Oliver MR, Cameron DJ, Catto-Smith AG, Chow CW. Esophageal eosinophilia in children with dysphagia. *J Pediatr Gastroenterol Nutr* 2003; **37**: 498–503.
6. Sant'Anna AM, Rolland S, Fournet JC, Yazbeck S, Drouin E. Eosinophilic esophagitis in children: symptoms, histology and pH probe results. *J Pediatr Gastroenterol Nutr* 2004; **39**: 373–377.
7. Gill R, Durst P, Rewalt M, Elitsur Y. Eosinophilic esophagitis disease in children from West Virginia: a review of the last decade (1995–2004). *Am J Gastroenterol* 2007; **102**: 2281–2285.
8. Noel RJ, Putnam PE, Rothenberg ME. Eosinophilic esophagitis. *N Engl J Med* 2004; **351**: 940–941.
9. Liacouras CA, Spergel JM, Ruchelli E *et al*. Eosinophilic esophagitis: a 10-year experience in 381 children. *Clin Gastroenterol Hepatol* 2005; **3**: 1198–1206.
10. Ronkainen J, Talley NJ, Aro P *et al*. Prevalence of oesophageal eosinophils and eosinophilic oesophagitis in adults: the population-based Kalixanda study. *Gut* 2007; **56**: 615–620.
11. Orenstein SR, Shalaby TM, Di LC *et al*. The spectrum of pediatric eosinophilic esophagitis beyond infancy: a clinical series of 30 children. *Am J Gastroenterol* 2000; **95**: 1422–1430.
12. Muller S, Puhl S, Vieth M, Stolte M. Analysis of symptoms and endoscopic findings in 117 patients with histological diagnoses of eosinophilic esophagitis. *Endoscopy* 2007; **39**: 339–344.
13. Straumann A, Spichtin HP, Grize L, Bucher KA, Beglinger C, Simon HU. Natural history of primary eosinophilic esophagitis: a follow-up of 30 adult patients for up to 11.5 years. *Gastroenterology* 2003; **125**: 1660–1669.

14. Fox VL, Nurko S, Furuta GT. Eosinophilic esophagitis: it's not just kid's stuff. *Gastrointest Endosc* 2002; **56**: 260–270.
15. Sgouros SN, Bergele C, Mantides A. Eosinophilic esophagitis in adults: a systematic review. *Eur J Gastroenterol Hepatol* 2006; **18**: 211–217.
16. Rothenberg ME. Eosinophilic gastrointestinal disorders (EGID). *J Allergy Clin Immunol* 2004; **113**: 11–28.
17. Zimmerman SL, Levine MS, Rubesin SE *et al*. Idiopathic eosinophilic esophagitis in adults: the ringed esophagus. *Radiology* 2005; **236**: 159–165.
18. Lucendo AJ, Castillo P, Martin-Chavarri S *et al*. Manometric findings in adult eosinophilic oesophagitis: a study of 12 cases. *Eur J Gastroenterol Hepatol* 2007; **19**: 417–424.
19. Pasha SF, DiBaise JK, Kim HJ *et al*. Patient characteristics, clinical, endoscopic, and histologic findings in adult eosinophilic esophagitis: a case series and systematic review of the medical literature. *Dis Esophagus* 2007; **20**: 311–319.
20. Straumann A, Rossi L, Simon HU, Heer P, Spichtin HP, Beglinger C. Fragility of the esophageal mucosa: a pathognomonic endoscopic sign of primary eosinophilic esophagitis? *Gastrointest Endosc* 2003; **57**: 407–412.
21. Leung JW, Mann NS. Pathogenesis of esophageal rings in eosinophilic esophagitis. *Med Hypotheses* 2005; **64**: 520–523.
22. Straumann A, Spichtin HP, Bucher KA, Heer P, Simon HU. Eosinophilic esophagitis: red on microscopy, white on endoscopy. *Digestion* 2004; **70**: 109–116.
23. Aceves SS, Newbury RO, Dohil R, Schwimmer J, Bastian JF. Distinguishing eosinophilic esophagitis in pediatric patients: clinical, endoscopic, and histologic features of an emerging disorder. *J Clin Gastroenterol* 2007; **41**: 252–256.
24. Furuta GT, Liacouras CA, Collins MH *et al*. Eosinophilic esophagitis in children and adults: a systematic review and consensus recommendations for diagnosis and treatment. *Gastroenterology* 2007; **133**: 1342–1363.
25. Fox VL, Nurko S, Teitelbaum JE, Badizadegan K, Furuta GT. High-resolution EUS in children with eosinophilic 'allergic' esophagitis. *Gastrointest Endosc* 2003; **57**: 30–36.
26. Gonsalves N, Policarpio-Nicolas M, Zhang Q, Rao MS, Hirano I. Histopathologic variability and endoscopic correlates in adults with eosinophilic esophagitis. *Gastrointest Endosc* 2006; **64**: 313–319.
27. Collins MH. Histopathologic features of eosinophilic esophagitis. *Gastrointest Endosc Clin North Am* 2008; **18**: 59–71.
28. Chehade M, Sampson HA, Morotti RA, Magid MS. Esophageal subepithelial fibrosis in children with eosinophilic esophagitis. *J Pediatr Gastroenterol Nutr* 2007; **45**: 319–328.
29. Spergel JM, Brown-Whitehorn T, Beausoleil JL, Shuker M, Liacouras CA. Predictive values for skin prick test and atopy patch test for eosinophilic esophagitis. *J Allergy Clin Immunol* 2007; **119**: 509–511.
30. Wang FY, Gupta SK, Fitzgerald JF. Is there a seasonal variation in the incidence or intensity of allergic eosinophilic esophagitis in newly diagnosed children? *J Clin Gastroenterol* 2007; **41**: 451–453.
31. Swoger JM, Weiler CR, Arora AS. Eosinophilic esophagitis: is it all allergies? *Mayo Clin Proc* 2007; **82**: 1541–1549.
32. Kirsch R, Bokhary R, Marcon MA, Cutz E. Activated mucosal mast cells differentiate eosinophilic (allergic) esophagitis from gastroesophageal reflux disease. *J Pediatr Gastroenterol Nutr* 2007; **44**: 20–26.
33. Blanchard C, Rothenberg ME. Basic pathogenesis of eosinophilic esophagitis. *Gastrointest Endosc Clin North Am* 2008; **18**: 133–143.
34. Gupta SK, Fitzgerald JF, Kondratyuk T, HogenEsch H. Cytokine expression in normal and inflamed esophageal mucosa: a study into the pathogenesis of allergic eosinophilic esophagitis. *J Pediatr Gastroenterol Nutr* 2006; **42**: 22–26.
35. Mishra A, Hogan SP, Brandt EB, Rothenberg ME. IL-5 promotes eosinophil trafficking to the esophagus. *J Immunol* 2002; **168**: 2464–2469.
36. Stein ML, Collins MH, Villanueva JM *et al*. Anti-IL-5 (mepolizumab) therapy for eosinophilic esophagitis. *J Allergy Clin Immunol* 2006; **118**: 1312–1319.
37. Mishra A, Rothenberg ME. Intratracheal IL-13 induces eosinophilic esophagitis by an IL-5, eotaxin-1, and STAT6-dependent mechanism. *Gastroenterology* 2003; **125**: 1419–1427.

38. Blanchard C, Mingler MK, Vicario M *et al.* IL-13 involvement in eosinophilic esophagitis: transcriptome analysis and reversibility with glucocorticoids. *J Allergy Clin Immunol* 2007; **120**: 1292–1300.

39. Bullock JZ, Villanueva JM, Blanchard C *et al.* Interplay of adaptive Th2 immunity with eotaxin-3/c-C chemokine receptor 3 in eosinophilic esophagitis. *J Pediatr Gastroenterol Nutr* 2007; **45**: 22–31.

40. Blanchard C, Wang N, Stringer KF *et al.* Eotaxin-3 and a uniquely conserved gene-expression profile in eosinophilic esophagitis. *J Clin Invest* 2006; **116**: 536–547.

41. Bhattacharya B, Carlsten J, Sabo E *et al.* Increased expression of eotaxin-3 distinguishes between eosinophilic esophagitis and gastroesophageal reflux disease. *Hum Pathol* 2007; **38**: 1744–1753.

42. Aceves SS, Newbury RO, Dohil R, Bastian JF, Broide DH. Esophageal remodeling in pediatric eosinophilic esophagitis. *J Allergy Clin Immunol* 2007; **119**: 206–212.

43. Hogan SP, Rosenberg HF, Moqbel R *et al.* Eosinophils: biological properties and role in health and disease. *Clin Exp Allergy* 2008; **38**: 709–750.

44. Spergel JM. Eosinophilic esophagitis in adults and children: evidence for a food allergy component in many patients. *Curr Opin Allergy Clin Immunol* 2007; **7**: 274–278.

45. Simon D, Straumann A, Wenk A, Spichtin H, Simon HU, Braathen LR. Eosinophilic esophagitis in adults–no clinical relevance of wheat and rye sensitizations. *Allergy* 2006; **61**: 1480–1483.

46. Ruchelli E, Wenner W, Voytek T, Brown K, Liacouras C. Severity of esophageal eosinophilia predicts response to conventional gastroesophageal reflux therapy. *Pediatr Dev Pathol* 1999; **2**: 15–18.

47. Liacouras CA, Wenner WJ, Brown K, Ruchelli E. Primary eosinophilic esophagitis in children: successful treatment with oral corticosteroids. *J Pediatr Gastroenterol Nutr* 1998; **26**: 380–385.

48. Netzer P, Gschossmann JM, Straumann A, Sendensky A, Weimann R, Schoepfer AM. Corticosteroid-dependent eosinophilic oesophagitis: azathioprine and 6-mercaptopurine can induce and maintain long-term remission. *Eur J Gastroenterol Hepatol* 2007; **19**: 865–869.

49. Attwood SE, Lewis CJ, Bronder CS, Morris CD, Armstrong GR, Whittam J. Eosinophilic oesophagitis: a novel treatment using Montelukast. *Gut* 2003; **52**: 181–185.

50. Vanderhoof JA, Young RJ, Hanner TL, Kettlehut B. Montelukast: use in pediatric patients with eosinophilic gastrointestinal disease. *J Pediatr Gastroenterol Nutr* 2003; **36**: 293–294.

51. Konikoff MR, Noel RJ, Blanchard C *et al.* A randomized, double-blind, placebo-controlled trial of fluticasone propionate for pediatric eosinophilic esophagitis. *Gastroenterology* 2006; **131**: 1381–1391.

52. Arora AS, Perrault J, Smyrk TC. Topical corticosteroid treatment of dysphagia due to eosinophilic esophagitis in adults. *Mayo Clin Proc* 2003; **78**: 830–835.

53. Schaefer ET, Fitzgerald JF, Molleston JP *et al.* Comparison of oral prednisone and topical fluticasone in the treatment of eosinophilic esophagitis: a randomized trial in children. *Clin Gastroenterol Hepatol* 2008; **6**: 165–173.

54. Aceves SS, Dohil R, Newbury RO, Bastian JF. Topical viscous budesonide suspension for treatment of eosinophilic esophagitis. *J Allergy Clin Immunol* 2005; **116**: 705–706.

55. Mackey AC, Green L, Liang LC, Dinndorf P, Avigan M. Hepatosplenic T cell lymphoma associated with infliximab use in young patients treated for inflammatory bowel disease. *J Pediatr Gastroenterol Nutr* 2007; **44**: 265–267.

56. Cohen MS, Kaufman AB, Palazzo JP, Nevin D, Dimarino Jr AJ, Cohen S. An audit of endoscopic complications in adult eosinophilic esophagitis. *Clin Gastroenterol Hepatol* 2007; **5**: 1149–1153.

Hugh Barr Geeta Shetty
Nicholas Stone Catherine Kendall

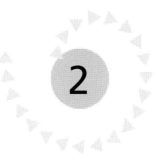

2

Barrett's oesophagus – how should I treat it?

Columnar-lined oesophagus (Barrett's oesophagus) was first described by Norman Rupert Barrett in 1950.[1] He noted the association with oesophageal inflammation and ulceration. His suggestion was that this was due to a congenital short oesophagus with an intrathoracic stomach. Allison and Johnstone[2] demonstrated that the columnar epithelium was proximal to the lower oesophageal sphincter, thereby establishing that the condition was clearly an oesophageal problem. This was confirmed by Lortat-Jakob,[3] who described 'endobrachyoesophagus' with shortening of the oesophageal mucosa but not the muscular tube. Bremner *et al.*[4] clearly demonstrated regeneration of columnar cells in the distal oesophagus in an experimental model of chronic gastro-oesophageal reflux disease. It is now clear that Barrett's oesophagus is an acquired condition in humans.[4] Although the eponymous name for columnar-lined oesophagus is Barrett's oesophagus, the first description may be more properly ascribed to Tileston[5] in 1906 who described peptic ulceration in the distal oesophageal mucosa.

Hugh Barr MD(Dist) ChM FRCS FRCSE FHEA (for correspondence)
Professor and Consultant Upper Gastrointestinal Surgeon, Department of Upper Gastrointestinal Surgery and Biophotonics Research Unit, Cranfield Health, Gloucestershire Royal Hospital, Great Western Road, Gloucester GL1 3NN, UK
E-mail: hugh.barr@glos.nhs.uk

Geeta Shetty DM MRCS
Research Fellow and Specialist Registrar, Department of Upper Gastrointestinal Surgery and Biophotonics Research Unit, Cranfield Health, Gloucestershire Royal Hospital, Great Western Road, Gloucester GL1 3NN, UK

Nicholas Stone MSc PhD MBA MIPEM
National Institute of Health Senior Research Fellow, Biophotonics Research Unit, Cranfield Health, Gloucestershire Royal Hospital, Great Western Road, Gloucester GL1 3NN, UK

Catherine Kendall MSc PhD MIPEM
Royal Society Dorothy Hodgkin Research Fellow, Biophotonics Research Unit, Cranfield Health, Gloucestershire Royal Hospital, Great Western Road, Gloucester GL1 3NN, UK

All types of columnar epithelium, including junctional (cardiac), fundic and specialised (intestinal) types, can be found in Barrett's oesophagus. It is thought that only the intestinal type gives rise to its most worrying complication of carcinoma. Some have suggested that the complete definition of Barrett's oesophagus requires the presence of intestinal metaplasia on biopsy. This is challenged because the detection of this metaplastic change depends on the intensive nature of the biopsy regimen. The current recommendation is that Barrett's oesophagus diagnosis is not dependent on the demonstration of intestinalisation.[6]

Barrett's oesophagus is of profound interest because of the increased potential for neoplastic degeneration through dysplasia into adenocarcinoma. This is particularly pertinent, since there is both a current and dramatic rise in the incidence of oesophageal adenocarcinoma centred on the UK (5–8.7 per 100,000). This is more than double the incidence in the US (3.7 per 100.000), where adenocarcinoma has risen 5-fold over three decades. This epidemic is very localised and is not evident in Asia, where squamous cell cancer remains the predominant oesophageal malignancy. The largest rises of up to 30% per year, are seen in West European white men, a rise not mirrored in Eastern Europe.[7,8]

More worryingly, the incidence is tracked very closely by the mortality of oesophageal adenocarcinoma. The prognosis from this cancer is universally dreadful. The median survival has hardly changed over the past few decades. The survival was 0.75 years between 1973–1977 and more recently has barely altered to 0.9 years between 1993–1999. This insubstantial change suggests that it may not be as a result of earlier detection and better treatment, but could be accounted for by improved reporting and detection bias.[9]

WHAT IS BARRETT'S OESOPHAGUS?

The original, and now classical, definition requires the presence of a circumferential oesophageal segment lined by columnar epithelium anywhere from 30 mm to as much as the whole oesophagus. However, any length chosen as a diagnostic criterion is necessarily arbitrary and the gastro-oesophageal transition is anatomically poorly delineated. It is often divided into short (< 30 mm) and long segment (> 30 mm) depending on the abnormal appearing oesophageal lining identified by endoscopic examination.

The more appropriate and accurate definition, and full and correct diagnosis, depends on close and detailed pathological and endoscopic correlation.[10] The precise terminology for Barrett's oesophagus is 'the condition in which the distal oesophagus is lined by a variable length of columnar epithelium'. This statement, although simple, requires very careful application. It is important to identify what is the lower oesophagus. Unfortunately, during endoscopy, the precise boundaries can be easily mistaken[11] and the distinction of the oesophagus, hiatus hernia and the cardia of the stomach may be very difficult. There is also a major difficulty for pathologists because there is no clear and defining histological characteristic. The gastric cardia is lined by columnar cardiac or junctional epithelium, but there is no pathological consensus on what is the cardia. At endoscopy, it is vitally important not to over inflate the oesophagus and thus to identify the upper part of the gastric folds as clearly stomach.

It is important to recognise that cardia type epithelium can extend into the oesophagus, but is this normal or a variant of Barrett's oesophagus? The one clear diagnostic feature, often not seen in standard sized endoscopic biopsies, is the presence of a submucosal oesophageal gland duct.[12]

CLASSIFICATION OF NEOPLASTIC DEGENERATION

The mechanisms of neoplastic transition from metaplasia, into dysplasia, and finally to invasive neoplastic degeneration are subject of intense investigation.[13] The pathological definition of dysplasia is as 'an unequivocal neoplastic alteration of the gastrointestinal epithelium which has the potential to progress to invasive malignancy that remains confined within the basement membrane of the gland within which it arose'. There is general agreement on the classification of neoplastic change in the gastrointestinal mucosa. The system has five categories: (i) negative for dysplasia; (ii) indefinite for dysplasia; (iii) low-grade dysplasia; (iv) high-grade dysplasia; and, finally, (v) invasive carcinoma.[14] However, clinicians and pathologist continue to be concerned about their ability to achieve consistent and accurate diagnosis for neoplastic change in Barrett's oesophagus using the published criteria.

Montgomery *et al.*[15] identified some clear categories for the grading of dysplasia, including: (i) the absence of surface maturation; (ii) architectural changes at low-magnification; and (iii) neoplastic cytological features. The latter is often emphasised by Japanese pathologists as being highly important. The confounding factors that cause difficulty are mostly related to the presence of inflammation, which troubles histopathologists greatly. Lesions classified as negative for dysplasia display surface maturation, an intact lamina propria with normal glandular structure and ratio, with little inflammation. Indefinite for dysplasia is characterised by preservation of architectural ratio of glands to lamina propria, surface maturation, with nuclear alterations that are not particularly prominent, and tends to be complicated by inflammation. Low-

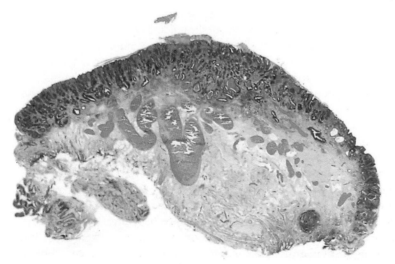

Fig. 1 Histopathology of dysplastic Barrett's oesophagus removed by endoscopic mucosal resection. The majority of the specimen is of high-grade dysplasia.

grade dysplasia lesions lose surface maturation but retain nuclear polarity, display nuclear alterations, have minimal glandular crowding, and lack inflammation. In high-grade dysplasia, surface maturation is lost, glands become crowded (over-running the lamina propria), nuclear alterations become striking (Fig. 1), and abundant inflammation is not typical, although may be present.[15–17] The outcome of patients with histological diagnosis of dysplasia may indicate the rate of progression, natural history of these conditions and the true malignant potential. In one series, four of 22 patients with a diagnosis of indefinite for dysplasia progressed to invasive cancer (median progression-free survival was 62 months). Also, four of 25 patients with low-grade dysplasia, progressed (median progression-free survival was 60 months). Whereas 20 of 33 patients with high-grade dysplasia progressed to cancer (median progression-free survival was 8 months).[15,16] However, there is contradictory data in which the rate of progression of patients with high-grade dysplasia to cancer was far less aggressive. The cumulative cancer incidence of patients, with a histological diagnosis of high-grade dysplasia, over 5 years was only 9%, with only 12 of 75 (16%) patients developing cancer during 13.9 years of surveillance. This study adopted a very aggressive approach to the diagnosis of synchronous cancer with 3-monthly endoscopic biopsy in the first year before the patient was categorised as having only high-grade dysplasia.[18]

AETIOLOGY AND GASTRO-OESOPHAGEAL REFLUX DISEASE

It is now established that there is a relationship between symptomatic heartburn due to gastro-oesophageal reflux disease, Barrett's oesophagus and oesophageal adenocarcinoma. This is best demonstrated in the nation-wide Swedish case-controlled study, which demonstrated an odds ratio of 7.7 of oesophageal adenocarcinoma for patients with a history of reflux symptoms. There was a very convincing dose-response relationship for those with severe long-standing (> 20 years) reflux who were 43.5 times more likely to develop cancer than the control group.[19,20] There is also a clear relationship with body mass index (BMI), with increasing risk with increasing BMI.

In addition, recent reports have shown that the prevalence of Barrett's oesophagus in asymptomatic patients is greater than in patients with clinical gastro-oesophageal reflux disease. Yet, it remains unclear why some patients with severe oesophagitis do not develop Barrett's oesophagus, whereas, patients with minimal or no symptoms develop Barrett's change. It has been demonstrated that there is a high incidence of hiatus hernia in Barrett's patients and there is a significant correlation with the duration of reflux. There was no association found with *Helicobacter pylori* infection.[21] Many questions remain unanswered and are the subject of intense investigation. Similarly, a genetic predisposition for the development of Barrett's oesophagus has been suggested; however, the proof remains elusive. Some groups have attempted to study the heritability as presumptive evidence of a genetic contribution to the disease. There is a curious predominance in whites males. Family cohort studies have shown that Barrett's oesophagus does indeed occur in family groups more frequently than would be expected by chance. Some families show an autosomal dominant pattern of inheritance with nearly complete penetrance. Other reports have shown that the incidence of Barrett's oesophagus is approximately 20%, and that the incidence of gastro-oesophageal reflux disease is approximately 40% among relatives. One group has reported that about 50% of the affected family members are indeed first-degree relatives.[22] Although shared dietary or environmental factors in these families could play a role, the earlier age of onset of Barrett's oesophagus in some families suggests the influence of genetic factors. The molecular progression to cancer remains an interesting and challenging problem. A variety of molecular genetic changes have been correlated with the metaplasia to dysplasia and onto carcinoma sequence. Some studies have suggested that one of the earliest molecular events is the selection and propagation of specific metaplastic clones within the specialised intestinal metaplasia. The clonality of the disease remains a subject of debate. This is followed by loss of cell cycle check points and genomic instability which contributes to the slow clonal expansion and increases cellular proliferation. There is also inhibition of apoptosis, which occurs in a proportion of cells with high-grade dysplasia and is a relatively late event. Invasive cancer may be preceded by alteration of cell adhesion, whereas subsequent cumulative genetic errors may result in the generation of multiple clones of transformed cells, thereby expanding the population of altered cells with both an angiogenic and metastatic potential. An important study with prospective data of lesions biopsied at sequential endoscopies show that alterations in p53, p16 and CDKN2A occur at early stages in the neoplastic progression. It has been demonstrated that there is loss of cyclin D1 over-expression and losses of the APC, Rb and DCC loci. The overall genetic heterogeneity is demonstrated by aneuploidy and abnormal methylation resulting in stepwise changes in differentiation, proliferation, and apoptosis, allowing disease progression under selective pressure. In high-grade dysplasia, there is a high prevalence of p53 mutations. They are found in approximately 60% of patients. A similar rate is found in patients with adenocarcinoma. Abnormalities in expression of the epidermal growth factor family and cell adhesion molecules, especially cadherin/catenin complexes, may occur early in neoplastic transformation.[25,26]

TREATMENT

REFLUX CONTROL AND ACID SUPPRESSION – MEDICAL

It is highly likely that patients with symptomatic reflux disease will be receiving acid suppressive and usually proton pump inhibitor therapy at an early stage. These drugs are highly effective for both acid suppression and symptomatic relief. In addition, they lower the total volume of duodenogastric and oesophageal refluxate. Gastro-oesophageal reflux is a chronic condition that usually needs long-term maintenance therapy. Proton pump inhibitors will heal oesophagitis and will lead to a significant improvement in the overall quality of life. The vital question remains as to whether they can have an effect on Barrett's oesophagus and prevent the progression of the disease to dysplasia and adenocarcinoma. There is now some molecular evidence that full and effective acid suppression favours cellular differentiation and decreases excessive proliferation. This may have the overall effect of stabilising the epithelium with the possibility of chemoprevention of cancer.[27] In addition, there is also some clinical evidence that with continuous treatment with full acid suppression, certain histological parameters of Barrett's oesophagus are improved. There is also a limited decrease in the length of the Barrett's segment with an increase in the number and extent of squamous islands. There is also a reduction in the proportion of sulphomucin-rich intestinal metaplasia. A randomised, double-blind study has confirmed that profound acid suppression with a proton pump inhibitor, leading to elimination of acid reflux, induces a possible and partial regression of the columnar-lined segment.[28]

REFLUX CONTROL – SURGERY

There is clear evidence that surgery will control reflux more completely than medical therapy. It will prevent all constituents of the refluxate from entering the oesophagus, in particular the contents of the duodenum including bile. These agents are not suppressed by proton pump therapy. There is, therefore, the possibility that surgery may be more effective at preventing the neoplastic degeneration. These issues have been addressed by retrospective analysis. A very important epidemiological study of gastric and oesophageal cancer after anti-reflux surgery was conducted in Sweden. This study included 10,000 patients (anti-reflux surgery) and a further 67,000 patients with gastro-oesophageal reflux disease who were treated medically.[29] The findings were that the incidence of cancer of the oesophagus and cardia was elevated in both study groups (standardised incidence ratio of 6.3 for oesophageal and 2.4 for gastric carcinoma in patients with gastro-oesophageal reflux, and 14.1 and 5.3, respectively, after surgery for reflux) compared with the rest of the population. These data confirmed a previous report of a very marked association between symptoms of gastro-oesophageal reflux disease and the development of adenocarcinoma of the oesophagus. The striking and remarkable finding of a stronger association of this cancer with the surgically treated patients may be a phenomenon more related to the fact that patients with very severe reflux are more likely to have a surgical option offered to them. It is somewhat counterintuitive to assume that it is as a result of the anti-reflux surgery. Further data from the US examined a total of 4678 patient-years of follow-up after anti-reflux surgery for gastro-oesophageal reflux disease. There was a reduced cancer rate of 3.8 per 1000 patient-years in patients treated with surgery, compared to 5.3 per 1000 patient-years after medical therapy. Despite there being a clear 30% reduction in the rate of cancer development following surgery, in this meta-analysis the results did not achieve statistical significance.[30]

ASPIRIN AND NON-STEROIDAL ANTI-INFLAMMATORY DRUGS

Large, case-control/cohort studies have shown that aspirin and other non-steroidal anti-inflammatory drugs (NSAIDs) appear to have a protective effect on the development of all forms of oesophageal cancer. The meta-analysis found over a 30% reduction in adenocarcinoma in patients, who had been exposed to aspirin or NSAID therapy. Similarly, a large cohort study, the National Health and Nutrition Examination Survey I of over 14,000 people in the US, followed for 12–16 years, demonstrated that the relative risk of oesophageal cancer was 0.1 for occasional aspirin users compared to people who never used it.[31–33] The mechanisms of this protective effect are under investigation. Gastro-oesophageal refluxate produces an intense inflammatory reaction and the degeneration to cancer is driven by this process. Inflammation is mediated through cyclooxygenase and prostaglandins, which are over expressed in the columnar-lined oesophagus. These enzymes could mediate neoplastic transformation since they cause an alteration in gene function, they inhibit the ability of the metaplasia to repair and eradicate genetic error. Aspirin, NSAIDs and the cyclooxygenase-2 inhibitors are important and powerful suppressors of these processes and could, therefore, act as chemoprotective agents. Inhibition of cyclooxygenase normalises cell proliferation, and is a powerful suppressor of cancer in experimental systems. There is now clear rationale to explore chemoprevention cancer strategies using aspirin and proton pump inhibitor therapy. Currently, Cancer Research UK and National Cancer Research Network in the UK are conducting a large randomised trial on chemoprevention – the Aspirin and Esomeprazole: Chemoprevention Trial (AspECT).

SURVEILLANCE OF BARRETT'S OESOPHAGUS

The minimum biopsy protocol for a segment of Barrett's oesophagus should be of any visible abnormality and also in each quadrant at 2-cm intervals.

A large meta-analysis identified a cancer conversion incidence rate of 0.76% (95% CI, 0.56–1.0%) per year.[34] There was no evidence of funnel plot asymmetry suggesting these data are not due to publication bias. Furthermore, meta-analysis of papers from the UK suggests the cancer conversion rate is greater at approximately 1% per year (95% CI, 0.67–1.39%). This correlates with the UK having the highest incidence of oesophageal adenocarcinoma in the world. Since the prognosis for symptomatic oesophageal adenocarcinoma is so poor, the development of surveillance programmes has to be considered. Guidelines recommend that patients with Barrett's oesophagus should have upper gastrointestinal endoscopy every 2–3 years to detect oesophageal adenocarcinoma at an early stage when the prognosis is much more favourable.[6] The value of surveillance is still subject to considerable debate and remains of unproven worth. There are some observational data to suggest that patients enrolled in surveillance programmes have oesophageal cancer detected at an earlier stage than non-surveillance detected cancers and have a better actuarial survival. These are very weak data in epidemiological terms, however, as patients attending surveillance programmes are very different from patients presenting with advanced oesophageal adenocarcinoma and the positive results could be due to any one of a number of different forms of bias. A better method is to compare directly patients with prospectively identified Barrett's oesophagus that attend and do not attend for surveillance. There is only one paper that has reported this design and this did not find any benefit of surveillance in 409 Barrett's oesophagus patients.[34] There is anecdotal data that cancer may be detected at an earlier stage. There is also evidence to suggest that patients with Barrett's oesophagus have either a normal life expectancy or if it is reduced, this is attributable to other diseases and not mortality from oesophageal adenocarcinoma.[35] The most appropriate method of evaluating whether surveillance reduces oesophageal adenocarcinoma and overall mortality is through a randomised controlled trial. This is now funded by the National Health Service Health Technology Agency as the Barrett's Oesophagus Surveillance Study (BOSS).

MANAGEMENT OF DYSPLASIA

INDEFINITE OR LOW-GRADE DYSPLASIA

The diagnosis of dysplasia is challenging and the use of the indefinite grade is important since certainty can be difficult. This is the rationale for allowing indefinite and low-grade to be considered together. It is suggested that there is a period of high-dose proton pump inhibitor therapy for a period of 8–12 weeks. When there is histological improvement, 6-monthly surveillance with repeat biopsy is necessary until at least two consecutive endoscopic biopsies reveal no dysplasia. The patient should then enter 2-yearly surveillance. If there is no improvement, 6-monthly endoscopic surveillance on proton pump therapy should continue.

HIGH-GRADE DYSPLASIA

Since the diagnosis of high-grade dysplasia (Fig. 2) results in more radical interventions, it must be confirmed by at least one other expert pathologist. Full clinical and pathological discussion of these patients is essential. It is important when doubt remains, and for confirmation, to repeat the endoscopy with a rigorous biopsy protocol including diagnostic endoscopic mucosal resection. This latter step is vital when there is a concern regarding intramucosal or invasive cancer for full staging. It has previously been recommended that the detection of high-grade dysplasia is an indication to end surveillance and proceed to surgical excision. Others have clearly demonstrated that surveillance with strict adherence to biopsy protocols can

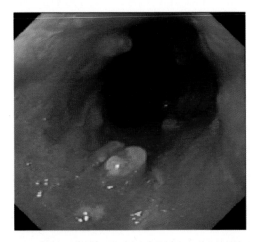

Fig. 2 Endoscopic appearance of high-grade dysplasia in Barrett's oesophagus.

differentiate dysplasia from intramucosal cancer.[18] There is also the problem that many patients are reluctant to consider radical life-threatening surgery when asymptomatic. There are many patients who are too great an operative risk to be considered for radical resection. It is important that minimally invasive oesophagectomy may adjust the criteria. The development of endoscopic ablative therapy and endoscopic mucosal resection allows minimally invasive options to be offered to patients with persistent high-grade dysplasia or mucosal neoplastic disease.

Endoscopic mucosal ablation and resection
Prior to endoscopic mucosal resection, a high-resolution endoscopy should be performed to detect and map the extent of the lesion. Recent technological advances can detect early superficial neoplastic changes. Autofluorescence imaging increasing the yield of early neoplasia nearly 2-fold when compared with high-resolution endoscopy. The problem is the confusion caused by inflammation and patients should have been on proton pump inhibitor therapy. The associated high false-positive rate of autofluorescence (81%) was reduced to 26% when combined with narrow band imaging.[36] Endoscopic mucosal resection has the advantage of removing the mucosa and the upper submucosa for histological staging. Three techniques are possible: (i) a lift-and-cut technique following submucosal injection of saline under the lesion; (ii) the suck-and-cut method; or (iii) the band to create a pseudopolyp and cut. All involve diathermy snare removal following the production of an artificial polyp. The first method involves direct injection to allow a cushion of saline to allow safe snare removal. The second simply sucks the mucosa into a cap (Fig. 3) followed by diathermy removal. The third technique requires aspiration of the mucosa into a variceal bander, ligation with a band or tie and subsequent snare removal. The most suitable lesions are < 20 mm in diameter, being well or moderately differentiated carcinomas (grading G1/G2) or areas of focal high-grade dysplasia. The endoscopic macroscopic appearance should be types I (polypoid), IIa (flat raised), IIb (flat at mucosal level), and IIc (slightly depressed). Lesions that are greater in size, ulcerated (type III), poorly

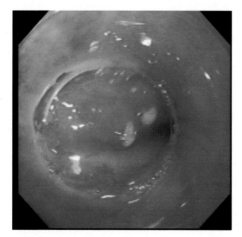

Fig. 3 Area of high-grade dysplasia being sucked into mucosal resection cap prior to removal by endoscopic mucosal resection.

differentiated or infiltrating the mucosa can be treated if the patient is unsuitable or unwilling for other therapy but has high-risk of recurrence. The management of multifocal areas of high-grade dysplasia may be technically difficult requiring multiple interventions and photodynamic therapy may need to be considered. There are now very substantial case series over many years demonstrating that endoscopic mucosal resection for the eradication of early cancers is highly effective. Patients with early Barrett's cancer and dysplasia have a calculated 5-year survival of 98%.[37]

Thermal ablation and photodynamic therapy

Endoscopic destruction of the superficial mucosa in a non-selective fashion is possible using a laser, multipolar electrocoagulation or argon beam plasma coagulation. Barrett's columnar metaplastic tissue is slightly thicker than normal squamous mucosa. Full-thickness or deep damage risks immediate or delayed perforation with the consequences of mediastinitis, peritonitis and death. Damage that does not penetrate to the external surface, yet reaches the muscle causing damage could result in healing by fibrosis and stricture formation. Limitation of the depth of thermal destruction may be important to allow regeneration with squamous rather than columnar cells. The type of epithelium that re-grows is, in part, determined by the depth of injury. In order to ensure squamous regeneration, some of the superficial squamous lined ducts of the oesophageal mucus glands must survive.

Photodynamic therapy is based on the systemic administration of photosensitising agents that are retained with some selectivity in malignant tissue. When exposed to appropriate wavelength laser light, a cytotoxic reaction occurs causing cellular destruction. The strongest evidence for mucosal ablation comes from the 5-year follow-up of the randomised, multicentre, multinational, pathology-blinded trial of photodynamic therapy to eradicate high-grade dysplasia. Photodynamic therapy was significantly more effective at eradicating high-grade dysplasia than omeprazole only (77% versus 39%) and reduced by half the likelihood of developing cancer with a significantly longer time to progression in the photodynamic therapy group.[38] It may be necessary to repeat ablation at intervals and the patients should remain in life-long surveillance. A further randomised trial compared thermal ablation with argon plasma coagulation against surveillance in 40 patients after surgical reflux control. There was a significant reversal of Barrett's oesophagus in those patient treated by ablation (63% versus 15%).[39]

Comparative studies of photodynamic therapy and argon plasma coagulation have differing results. One showed no significant difference in efficacy between the two treatments, whereas others have shown that argon plasma coagulation is more effective than photodynamic therapy with aminolaevulinic acid.[39,40] Photodynamic therapy was more effective in eradicating dysplasia at 12 months (67% versus 77%). A randomised, partially-blinded trial assessed argon plasma coagulation and multipolar electrocoagulation; the latter required less sessions and complete ablation occurred in 88% compared with 81% (argon plasma coagulation).[41] A detailed cost-effectiveness analysis of the management of high-grade dysplasia has been modelled (no strategy, oesophagectomy, endoscopic photodynamic therapy and endoscopic surveillance). Photodynamic therapy was the most effective yielding 15.5 discounted quality adjusted life years compared to 15.0 for surveillance and 14.9 for oesophagectomy.[42]

CONCLUSIONS

Gastro-oesophageal reflux disease is the precursor to oesophageal adenocarcinoma. Early detection and treatment may have profound affects on the incidence of this cancer. These issues are being addressed in large, national, clinical trials which will inform the strategy for future management.

Key points for clinical practice

- Reflux oesophagitis is associated with the development of oesophageal adenocarcinoma. There is a clear dose response with severity of reflux and increased incidence.

- The incidence of oesophageal adenocarcinoma continues to rise and current treatment has had little effect on survival over the past three decades.

- The major other risk factors are male sex, white races, obesity and residence in the UK.

- Family clustering does occur but no clear genetic predisposition has been demonstrated.

- Treatment and control of reflux either medically or surgically has not yet demonstrated a clinical effect in reducing risks of progression to cancer. Both are highly effective in symptomatic control.

- The diagnosis of Barrett's oesophagus requires very careful endoscopic and histological assessment and correlation.

- The diagnosis and recognition of dysplasia remains an endoscopic and histopathological challenge.

- Enhanced endoscopic systems are being developed to detect very early changes in the mucosa of the oesophagus.

- Modern endoscopic resectional and ablation techniques are proving to be highly effective in the management of high-grade dysplasia and preventing the development of invasive cancer.

- Patients should be entered into the current randomised trials designed to answer these questions, Aspirin and Esomeprazole Chemoprevention Trial (AspECT) and Barrett's Oesophagus Surveillance Study (BOSS).

References

1. Barrett NR. Chronic peptic ulcer of the oesophagus and 'oesophagitis'. *Br J Surg* 1950; **38**: 175–182.
2. Allison PR, Johnstone AS. The oesophagus lined with gastric mucous membrane. *Thorax* 1953; **8**: 87–110.

25

3. Lortat-Jacob JL. L'endobrachy-oesophage. *Ann Chir* 1957; **11**: 1247–1252.
4. Bremner CG, Lynch VP, Ellis FH. Barrett's esophagus: congenital or acquired? An experimental study of esophageal mucosal regeneration in the dog. *Surgery* 1978; **68**: 209–216.
5. Tileston W. Peptic ulcer of the oesophagus. *Am J Sci* 1906; **132**: 240–242.
6. Report of Working Party of the British Society of Gastroenterology. *Guidelines for the diagnosis and management of Barrett's columnar-lined oesophagus.* 2005 <http://www.bsg.org.uk>.
7. Shaheen NJ. The changing epidemiology of esophageal adenocarcinoma. *Semin Gastrointest Dis* 2003; **14**: 112–127.
8. el Serag. The epidemic of esophageal adenocarcinoma. *Gastroenterol Endosc Clin North Am* 2002; **31**: 21–44.
9. Mason AC, Eloubeidi MA, el Serag. Temporal trends in survival of patients with esophageal adenocarcinoma 1973–1997. *Gastroenterology* 2001; **122**: A30.
10. Attwood SEA, Morris CD. Who defines Barrett's oesophagus: endoscopist or pathologist. *Eur J Gastroenterol* 2001; **13**: 97–99.
11. Falk GW. Barrett's esophagus. *Gastroenterology* 2002; **122**: 1569–1591.
12. Shepherd NA. Dysplasia in Barrett's oesophagus. *Acta Endosc* 2000; **30**: 123–132.
13. Jankowski JA, Harrison RF, Perry I, Balkwill F, Tselepis C. Barrett's metaplasia. *Lancet* 2000; **356**: 2079–2085.
14. Schlemper RJ, Riddell RH, Kato Y *et al.* The Vienna classification of gastrointestinal epithelial neoplasia. *Gut* 2000; **47**: 251–255.
15. Montgomery E, Bronner MP, Goldblum JR *et al.* Reproducibility of the diagnosis of dysplasia in Barrett's oesophagus: a reaffirmation. *Hum Pathol* 2001; **32**: 368–378.
16. Montgomery E, Goldblum JR, Greenson JK *et al.* Dysplasia as a predictive marker for invasive carcinoma in Barrett's esophagus: a follow-up study based on 138 case from a diagnostic variability study. *Hum Pathol* 2001; **32**: 379–388.
17. Montgomery E. Is there a way for pathologists to decrease interobserver variability in the diagnosis of dysplasia? *Arch Pathol Lab Med* 2004; **129**: 174–176.
18. Schnell TG, Sontag SJ, Chejfec G *et al.* Long-term non-surgical management of Barrett's esophagus with high-grade dysplasia. *Gastroenterology* 2001; **120**: 1607–1619.
19. Lagergren J, Bergstrom R, Lindgren A, Nyren O. Symptomatic gastroesophageal reflux as a risk factor for esophageal adenocarcinoma. *N Engl J Med* 1999; **340**: 825–831.
20. Solaymani M, Logan RFA, West J *et al.* Risk of oesophageal cancer in Barrett's oesophagus and gastro-oesophageal reflux. *Gut* 2003; **53**: 1070–1074.
21. Toruner M, Soykan I, Ensari A, Kuzu I, Yurdaydin C, Oxden A. Barrett's esophagus: prevalence and its relationship with dyspeptic symptoms. *Gastroenterol Hepatol* 2004; **19**: 535–540.
22. Chak A, Lee T, Kinnard MF, Brock W *et al.* Familial aggregation of Barrett's oesophagus, oesophageal adenocarcinoma and oesophagogastric junctional adenocarcinoma in Caucasian adults. *Gut* 2001; **51**: 323–328.
23. Reid BJ, Levine DS, Longton G, Blount PL, Rabinovitch PS. Predictors of progression to cancer in Barrett's esophagus: baseline histology and flow cytometry identify low- and high-risk patient subsets. *Am J Gastroenterol* 2000; **95**: 1669–1676.
24. Rabinovitch PS, Longton G, Blount PL, Levine DS, Reid BJ. Predictors of progression in Barrett's esophagus III: baseline flow cytometric variables. *Am J Gastroenterol* 2001; **96**: 3071–3083.
25. Bailey T, Biddleston L, Shepherd N, Barr H, Warner P, Jankowski J. Altered cadherin/catenin complexes in the dysplasia-adenocarcinoma sequence: correlation with disease progression and dedifferentiation. *Am J Pathol* 1998; **152**: 135–144.
26. Hall PA, Woodman AC, Campbell SJ, Shepherd NA. Expression of the p53 homologue p63alpha and deltaNp63alpha in the neoplastic sequence of Barrett's oesophagus: correlation with morphology and p53 protein. *Gut* 2001; **49**: 618–623.
27. Ouata-Lascar R, Fitzgerald RC, Triadafilopoulos G. Differentiation and proliferation in Barrett's esophagus and the effects of acid suppression. *Gastroenterology* 1999; **117**: 327–335.
28. Peters FTM, Ganesh S, Kuipers EJ *et al.* Endoscopic regression of Barrett's oesophagus during omeprazole treatment; a randomised double blind study. *Gut* 1994; **45**: 489–494.

29. Ye W, Chow WH, Lagergren J, Yin L, Nyren O. Risk of adenocarcinoma of the esophagus and gastric cardia in patients with gastroesophageal reflux disease and after antireflux surgery. *Gastroenterology* 2001; **121**: 1506–1508.

30. Corey KE, Schmitz SM, Shaheen NJ. Does a surgical antireflux procedure decrease the incidence of esophageal adenocarcinoma in Barrett's esophagus? *Am J Gastroenterol* 2003; **98**: 2390–2394.

31. Corley DA, Kerlikowske K, Verma R *et al*. Protective association of aspirin/NSAIDs and esophageal cancer. A systematic review and meta-analysis. *Gastroenterology* 2003; **124**: 47–56.

32. Funkhouser EM, Sharp GB. Aspirin and reduced risk of esophageal carcinoma. *Cancer* 1995; **76**: 116–119.

33. Buttar NS, Wang KK, Leontovic O *et al*. Chemoprevention of esophageal adenocarcinoma by COX-2 inhibitors in an animal model of Barrett's esophagus. *Gastroenterology* 2002; **122**: 1101–1112.

34. Macdonald CE, Wicks AC, Playford RJ. Final results from 10 year cohort of patients undergoing surveillance for Barrett's oesophagus: observational study. *BMJ* 2000; **321**: 1252–1255.

35. Anderson LA, Murray LJ, Murphy SJ *et al*. Mortality in Barrett's oesophagus: results from a population based study. *Gut* 2003; **52**: 1081–1084.

36. Curvers WL, Sigh R, Wong-Kee Song L-M *et al*. Endoscopic trimodal imaging for detection of early neoplasia in Barrett's oesophagus: a multi-centre feasibility study using high-resolution endoscopy, autofluorescence imaging and narrow band imaging incorporated in one endoscopy system. *Gut* 2008; **57**: 167–172.

37. Lopes CV, Hela M, Pesenti C *et al*, Circumferential endoscopic resection of Barrett's esophagus with high-grade dysplasia or early adenocarcinoma. *Surg Endosc* 2007; **21**: 820–824.

38. Overholt BF, Wang KK, Burdick JS *et al*. Five-year efficacy and safety of photodynamic therapy with Photofrin in Barrett's high-grade dysplasia. *Gastrointest Endosc* 2007; **66**: 460–468.

39. Ackroyd R, Tam W, Schoeman M *et al*. Prospective randomised controlled trial of argon plasma coagulation ablation vs. endoscopic surveillance of patients with Barrett's after anti-reflux surgery. *Gastrointest Endosc* 2004; **59**: 1–7.

40. Ragunath K, Krasner N, Raman VS *et al*. Endoscopic ablation of dysplastic Barrett's oesophagus comparing argon plasma coagulation and photodynamic therapy: a randomised prospective trial assessing efficacy and cost-effectiveness. *Scand J Gastroenterol* 2005; **40**: 750–758.

41. Dulai GS, Jensen DM, Cortina G *et al*. Randomised trial of argon plasma coagulation versus multipolar electrocoagulation for ablation of Barrett's oesophagus. *Gastrointest Endosc* 2005; **61**: 232–240.

42. Shaheen NJ, Inadomi JM, Overholt BF *et al*. What is the best management strategy for high-grade dysplasia in Barrett's oesophagus? A cost-effectiveness analysis. *Gut* 2004; **53**: 1736–1744.

Anne E. Mills Katherine Mabey

3

Gastrointestinal physiology

Specialist gastrointestinal investigations were formerly performed by research registrars for their fellowship theses, learning the practical aspect, and to improve measurement technique. However, as the diagnostic usefulness has become more of a necessity, over the past 15 years, units have been established in hospitals run by medical technicians or endoscopy nurses. The service is now delivered by registered gastrointestinal physiologists who train in parallel to cardiophysiologists, neurophysiologists and respiratory physiologists, all sent on a 4-year block release Bachelor of Science in Clinical Physiology degree with specialist modules for each discipline.

The role of the gastrointestinal physiologist has advanced significantly over the years. Previously, precise clinical measurement would be performed, providing consultants with an objective and unbiased report; however, it is now a requirement to think on a more physiologically holistic and diagnostic level, providing an overall insight into the results achieved, and also to estimate percentage success of likely surgery or treatment. As a result, gastrointestinal physiologists are often required to attend case-study meetings, along with other healthcare professionals, to discuss appropriate treatment for patients.

A more recent development has been the new UK National Institute for Health and Clinical Excellence (NICE) *Clinical Guidelines for Faecal Incontinence*,[1] which outlines the importance of biofeedback therapy as an intervention before referral for surgery. In addition to urge and passive faecal incontinence, these guidelines cover obstructive defaecation with incontinence and slow transit constipation with overflow incontinence. This has markedly

Anne E. Mills AGIP MIIR DipReflex (for correspondence)
Clinical Gastrointestinal Physiologist, Physiology – Queens Day Unit, Level 4 Queens Building, Bristol Royal Infirmary, Bristol BS2 9HW. E-mail: anne.mills@UHBristol.nhs.uk

Katherine J. Mabey BS(Hons), BSc(Hons)
Clinical Gastrointestinal Physiologist, Bristol Royal Infirmary, Bristol, UK
E-mail: katherine.mabey@UHBristol.nhs.uk

increased the likelihood of referrals directly from general practitioners (GPs), as well as from consultant physicians and surgeons prior to surgery and to enhance surgical success. In some cases, this has had implications in changes for primary care trust funding of Local Delivery Plans (LDPs) and Service Level Agreements (SLAs) for gastrointestinal physiology units.

Referrals for gastrointestinal investigation arise from several different levels in the patient pathway. GPs may refer patients directly for specialist investigations, biofeedback therapy and breath tests prior to referring to consultant surgeons or physicians; however, in general, the largest portion of referrals are from consultants to obtain diagnostic information before considering surgery or treatment, and then, if surgery does not seem appropriate, for conservative treatment, and for biofeedback therapy.

This chapter discusses which patients should be referred to the gastrointestinal physiology unit, which tests might be performed and how they are interpreted. Finally, the role of the unit in therapy, in biofeedback and hypnotherapy, is discussed.

WHO TO REFER AND WHEN

The conditions and symptoms for which a patient would be referred to a gastrointestinal physiology unit for investigation or therapy are many and varied; mostly typical of certain medical disorders but also occasionally atypical and idiopathic.

Upper gastrointestinal referral

Manometry
The indications for an upper gastrointestinal referral to the department would be patients with dysphagia. This may be a primary or secondary oesophageal dysmotility in association with a systemic disease, for example, systemic sclerosis. Patients have usually had a previous investigation, such as endoscopy and/or barium swallow to eliminate strictures, carcinomas, diverticuli and other structural abnormalities.

Achalasia can only be diagnosed by oesophageal manometry although a dilated oesophagus can be seen on the endoscopy and barium swallow. Clinically, the patients normally complain of chest pain at the apex of the sternum, and dysphagia to solids and liquids with associated regurgitation of oesophageal contents, which can be seconds or hours after eating. However, there may be more atypical symptoms which can often seem similar to reflux symptoms. Patients with achalasia also have progressive weight loss and may have respiratory symptoms, which are secondary to the dysmotility. The exact aetiology of achalasia is not known but is thought to result from degeneration of the oesophageal myenteric plexus although early in the condition there is an infiltrate of eosinophils, mast cells and T-cells and loss of inhibitory postganglionic neurons from the Auerbach plexus. This may have initially occurred in response to an environmental or viral infection.

Diffuse oesophageal spasm can also be diagnosed by oesophageal manometry sometimes during a static manometry study, but more gainfully over a 24-h study; this can be difficult to detect due to the intermittent nature.

Clinically, patients complain of angina-like chest pain which can radiate down the arms and up into the neck, and they may also have symptoms of dysphagia and regurgitation. Most patients should have received a full cardiac testing to exclude a cardiovascular cause for their symptoms. Diagnosis of the cause of chest pain can be difficult owing to the close anatomical relationship between the heart and the oesophagus, especially if the patient is asymptomatic during the study.[2] However, there is a greater likelihood with 24-h ambulatory manometry in detecting hypertensive contractions and prolonged multipeaked contractions of diffuse oesophageal spasm although the diagnostic yield is quite small.[3]

Non-specific oesophageal motility disorders can be defined by the oesophageal contraction amplitudes and the resting lower oesophageal sphincter pressure. Manifestations of these disorders can be both hypertensive and hypotensive oesophageal contraction amplitudes as well as lower oesophageal sphincter pressures.

Oesophageal pH monitoring

Gastro-oesophageal reflux disease (GORD) manifests itself clinically as oesophageal symptoms of retrosternal burning, acid regurgitation, extra-oesophageal symptoms such as chest pain, asthma, chronic coughs and laryngitis, and there may be complications such as ulcers, strictures and Barrett's oesophagus.[4] Patients with failure to respond to acid suppressant therapy or those being considered for antireflux surgery, should be referred for 24-h oesophageal pH monitoring and manometry. This also includes patients who have failed to respond to antireflux surgery and are still symptomatic.

Electrogastrography

Electrogastrography (EGG) is the cutaneous recording of gastric electrical activity, and although some gastrointestinal investigation units can offer this service, it is primarily used for research purposes to investigate gastric motility. It is principally indicated for patients where a diagnosis of idiopathic or diabetic gastroparesis is warranted. Patients normally present with nausea, vomiting, post-prandial fullness and abdominal bloating. Surface electrodes are placed on the skin over the epigastrium and the gastric motility is measured for an hour, during which time the patient is required to keep as still as possible. A diagnosis of bradygastria or tachygastria may be obtained by the analysis of the gastric cycles ($n = 3/\text{min}$), any deviations from this figure helping to identify these conditions.

Breath tests to detect gastrointestinal disorders

Gastrointestinal physiology departments can offer [^{13}C]-urea breath tests to detect active *Helicobacter pylori* infection after the patient has tested positive on serology or with a CLO test: they may also be performed to gauge the effectiveness of the triple eradication treatment. Test kits are used in the main, as there are few clinical departments with their own [^{13}C]-gas analyser.

Small bowel bacterial overgrowth, lactose intolerance, fructose malabsorption and orocaecal transit times are investigated by hydrogen breath test. Gastrointestinal physiology departments may offer this test for malabsorption of different sugars but generally the conditions above are the most requested. These are simple tests but time consuming, lasting 3—5 h. Although few tests prove to be positive, they do assist diagnosis through elimination.

Lower gastrointestinal referrals

Referrals for investigations of lower gastrointestinal maladies by anorectal physiology studies are patients with functional bowel disorders such as:

1. Faecal incontinence – both urge (external anal sphincter [EAS] impairment or neuropathy) and passive (internal anal sphincter [IAS] impairment or neuropathy).

2. Constipation, which may be due to infrequent bowel movements, hard stool consistency, loss of rectal call-to-stool, difficulty evacuating, or general slow intestinal transit.

3. Obstructive defaecation, which may be caused by rectal mucosal prolapse, internal or full thickness, rectocoeles, posterior tilting of vagina or uterus, paradoxical sphincter or puborectalis contraction, sphincter or puborectalis non-relaxation.

4. Other conditions in which the sphincter anatomy is important such as anal fissures, haemorrhoids and peri-anal abscesses and fistulas.

5. Pre-operative assessment prior to surgery – for example closure of loop ileostomies, sphincterotomies, sphincter repairs following trauma or obstetric injuries.

The outcomes of anorectal physiology are to: (i) assess sphincter and rectal function; (ii) determine whether any impairment is contributing to the conditions outlined; and (iii) determine if conservative treatment, such as biofeedback therapy, is required. Such outcomes may better benefit the patient or increase the successful outcome of surgery.

Patients with functional problems which do not warrant a surgical intervention, may also be directly referred for biofeedback therapy and bowel habit advice.

HOW INVESTIGATIONS ARE PERFORMED

As each gastrointestinal investigation unit has developed individually according to equipment acquired and funding, the need for standardising clinical measurement has evolved. The fore-runner of the Association of Gastrointestinal Physiologists (AGIP), the Clinical Measurement Committee, established standards for basic technique, and guidelines are in the process of being put in place to be made available nationally. However, each unit will differ depending on the equipment available, how it has developed, and its own set of approved written protocols. Though technique may vary from unit to unit, the basics are fundamentally the same.

The importance of history-taking

As clinicians have increasingly less time to take a detailed history of patient symptoms, the role of the gastrointestinal physiologist has been to obtain an objective description by the patient. For instance, 'indigestion' may cover acid

THE BRISTOL STOOL FORM SCALE

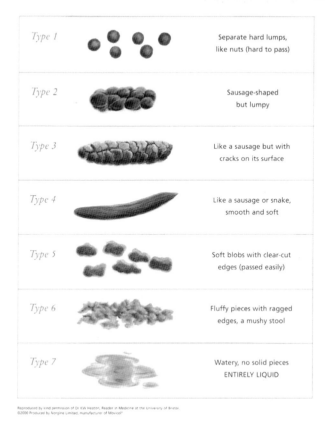

Type 1	Separate hard lumps, like nuts (hard to pass)
Type 2	Sausage-shaped but lumpy
Type 3	Like a sausage but with cracks on its surface
Type 4	Like a sausage or snake, smooth and soft
Type 5	Soft blobs with clear-cut edges (passed easily)
Type 6	Fluffy pieces with ragged edges, a mushy stool
Type 7	Watery, no solid pieces ENTIRELY LIQUID

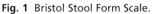

Reproduced by kind permission of Dr KW Heaton, Reader in Medicine at the University of Bristol.
©2000 Produced by Norgine Limited, manufacturer of Movicol®

Fig. 1 Bristol Stool Form Scale.

reflux, acid regurgitation, trapped wind, epigastric pain and bloating, excessive belching, upper abdominal pain and bloating, and chest pain. In lower gastrointestinal problems, patients' view of degree of faecal incontinence and how it affects them, may range from slight smearing on underclothes that might distress them to great extent, or gross urge incontinent episodes to which they have adjusted their life-style and managed to cope with, perhaps because they have accepted faecal incontinence as part of ageing.

Therefore, in upper gastrointestinal history-taking, description, length, frequency of symptoms such as 'indigestion' or 'heartburn' and their associations to diet, meal-times, supine or upright position better illuminates the outcome of investigations, especially for the 24-h studies. In notating lower gastrointestinal symptoms, many of the following factors are taken into account: frequency of bowel movement; degree of call-to-stool or urgency; stool consistency (Fig. 1); degree and frequency of any faecal incontinence; abdominal or anorectal symptoms of discomfort; effects of micturition, menstruation, sexual intercourse, and medications for other medical problems.

Upper gastrointestinal measurement

Oesophageal investigation looks at two basic aspects: (i) oesophageal motility, both static and ambulatory – upper and lower oesophageal sphincter function measured manometrically; and (ii) reflux (acid or non-acid) by measurement of pH or intraluminal impedance.

Oesophageal manometry

Some units use water-perfused catheters as standard for static oesophageal manometry, but we find it more convenient to use a solid-state catheter. These are comprised of thin film resistive strain gauge sensors sensing pressure changes and creating electrical signals (Gaeltec Ltd). Our preference over water-perfused catheters is partly because of ease of intubation, but also because we routinely carry out manometry combined with pH measurement over 24 h and it negates the necessity of having to intubate a patient twice. Another advantage is that ambulatory manometry can be carried out over 24 h to determine oesophageal motility over a patient's normal day in comparison to over a short period under laboratory conditions.

Clinical measurement of oesophageal motility requires a station or continuous pull-through to calculate the high pressure zone of the lower oesophageal sphincter in relation to gastric pressure. The catheters with three or more transducers are passed *per nares*, the patient is unsedated, but persuaded to swallow water through a straw to position it. This requires highly-developed motivational skills by the physiologist to re-assure and encourage. A recent development, in some centres, is the use of hypnosis to relax the patient beforehand, in particular for those individuals with either fear of interruption of breathing or a strong gag reflex.

The Bristol Unit will be currently training one physiologist in hypnosis not only to facilitate oesophageal intubation but also with patients with symptoms of irritable bowel syndrome, especially those exacerbated by stress, and also with patients who are suffering idiopathic gastrointestinal pain. This could also be helpful in patients undergoing endoscopy and save the trusts money spent on sedation and hospital bed recovery space.

Intubation continues until all transducers are in the stomach, and the pull-through is then performed marking each 0.5 cm or 1 cm level, noting the respiratory changes. The point at which respiration changes from a positive deflection on inhalation in the stomach to a negative pressure on inhalation denotes the passage through the diaphragm into the oesophagus. The lower oesophageal sphincter (LOS) pressure is calculated as the highest basal pressure at the end exhalation point, minus the gastric pressure (Fig. 2). It is also possible to measure the sphincter length, length of the gastric and oesophageal portions of the sphincter and the position of the respiratory inversion point, though this is more for research purposes than as a diagnostic aid.

To investigate the motility of the oesophagus, the catheter is taped to the nose so that the lowest transducer in the oesophagus is 5 cm above the LOS, then two more at 10 cm and 15 cm above the LOS effectively covering distal, mid and upper oesophageal contraction amplitudes on swallowing. Once in position, the patient is asked to swallow at least 10 consecutive 5-ml aliquots of water, so that mean averages of amplitudes at these three different positions in the oesophagus can be determined, swallow types and presence or absence of peristalsis. Velocity and contraction length can also be calculated if required.

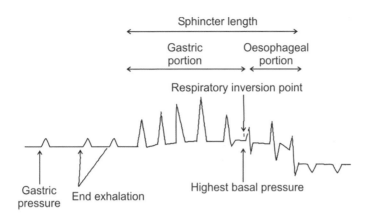

Fig. 2 Changes in intraluminal pressures on station pull-through.

In the Bristol Unit, the catheter utilised has five transducers, one in or around the upper oesophageal sphincter (UOS) to detect swallow initiation, three in the oesophagus, and one in the stomach. In this way, inadvertent dry swallows can be detected, or any effects on contraction amplitudes by common cavity events (*e.g.* belching, talking or laughing). Also measured are standard solid food swallows, having carefully researched into the size of a standard mouthful of bread (1/9th of a slice of white bread). However, if bread cannot be swallowed, or in the case of patients due to undergo gastric banding (who will be advised not to eat bread postoperatively), then instant mashed potato is used.

More recently, a high resolution manometry[5,6] system has been developed; the catheter has 36 pressure sensors spaced at 1-cm intervals extending the length of the oesophagus. The advantage is that the discomfort of a pull-through for the patient is eliminated, lower oesophageal sphincter pressure is automatically calculated and motility of the whole oesophagus is evident on the monitor, pressures depicted as varying range of colour, or pressures whichever is preferred by the operator. The disadvantage is that this system can not be used on an ambulatory basis.

24-h oesophageal manometry
The Bristol Unit, in contrast to others, routinely carries out manometry, oesophageal and gastric, in conjunction with pH measurement throughout the whole 24-h. We assert that pH solely is only half the story, and that, by combining pH studies with manometry, we can show if acid reflux is brought on by common cavity events such as persistent belching, and also whether coughing induces a reflux event, or vice versa.[7,8] We can also see exaggerated respiratory changes and also vascular or cardiac impressions and if there are any associations with acid reflux. It is also possible to pick up apnoea, aerophagia, and distinguish diffuse oesophageal spasm from common cavity events. With experience, a 24-h manometry study should not take much longer than 10 min to scan for abnormalities.

Analysis of the manometry data is aided by a patient diary of meal-times, supine periods and activity. Most patients can manage to fill in times for these on a simple diary sheet, as well as pressing an event marker for their main symptoms. If they have more than one symptom, they may in addition be required to write down the time they pressed the marker and which symptom it was for.

Measurement of oesophageal pH

This is performed by intubating the patient with a pH catheter, usually antimony but it can also be glass. Most catheters are single-use for infection control. It is positioned so that the detection port is 5 cm above the LOS and able to detect any acid refluxing from the stomach, remaining *in situ* for 24 h attached to an ambulatory recording box. The patient is encouraged to undergo routine daily activities, eating and drinking as normal.

There is some controversy whether the patients should have a restricted or standardised diet, or whether they should continue their usual diet. Some authors suggest that meals should be omitted completely to improve the diagnosis of acid reflux.[9] In general, patients are advised not to drink carbonated beverages as they are acidic. Some departments suggest the avoidance of alcohol which may relax the lower oesophageal sphincter; this may also be effected by stimulant beverages and smoking. A person in normal daily life would not adhere to a bland diet and avoid alcohol, or stimulants. In our unit, we recommend that the patient has a 'normal day', even if this means drinking alcohol, so long as it is recorded on their diary sheet.

Intraluminal impedance

During the course of measurement of oesophageal pH, there have been occasions when the pH of refluxate drops but not below the level of pH 4, the pH at which prolonged exposure (> 4% of 18 h, minimum) may erode the oesophageal lining. There are also patients who, despite proton pump inhibitors, are still suffering from volume reflux, and many patients, both adult and paediatric, with this non-acid reflux seem to experience respiratory problems

Table 1 Impedance measurements for different media

	Ohm × cm (at 1 kHz)
Gastric contents	30–100
Bile	90
Saline solution	100
Saliva	110
Skeletal muscle	250–700
Milk/yoghurt	300
Custard-based dessert/curds	400
Drinking water	1100
Cola	1100
Oesophageal wall	2000
Epidermis	2000–100,000
Air	10,000,000

Included by kind permission from Ardmore Healthcare Ltd (J.L. Stirling presentation, May 2006).

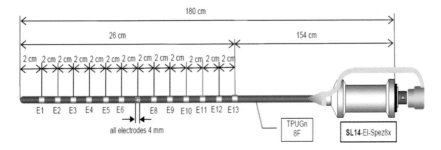

Fig. 3 An impedance catheter. Included by kind permission from Ardmore Healthcare Ltd (J.L. Stirling presentation, May 2006).

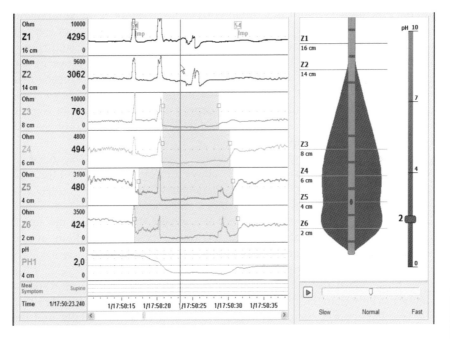

Fig. 4 Trace showing change in impedance during swallowing. Included by kind permission from Ardmore Healthcare Ltd (J.L. Stirling presentation, May 2006).

or unexplained coughing. There are also patients who have problems with bile reflux, aerophagia and belching, ear, nose and throat problems, and pH-metry on its own can not measure the presence of the different refluxing media. To some extent, manometry over 24 h can demonstrate pressure changes that occur with aerophagia and belching but for non-acid reflux it is not always clear.

Impedance was developed to fill this diagnostic gap. It measures the electrical resistance, in Ohms, of a medium by an alternating current (3.2 Hz) between two points, where impedance is the inverse of conductance. For each medium, there is a different impedance measurement, so that it is possible to determine the type of refluxate quite accurately (Table 1).

The catheter used for this purpose usually has 13 metal rings spaced at 1-cm intervals, giving 12 impedance measurements between each pair of rings (Fig. 3).

From changes in impedance, moving proximally to distally or vice versa, and measured in conjunction with pH, the type of bolus can be determined and also the bolus transit time both on swallowing and also on refluxing (Fig. 4). Gastrointestinal physiologists, with practice, should be able to analyse a 24-h recording as easily as a 24-h manometry trace and, as a relatively new technique in the clinical setting, there are workshops for training.

Lower gastrointestinal measurement

Anorectal physiology

Again, the standard techniques for performing anorectal physiology do not alter considerably from unit to unit, although equipment used may be different and the practitioner should be familiar with the local protocol and equipment.

Accurate manometric measurement in many units, as for upper gastrointestinal measurements, is by water-perfused systems. These measure the pressure exerted by a dynamic biological system by resistance to the constant water pressure applied, detected by electrical transducers and registered on a monitor. Constant pressure is applied to a closed water tank either by inert gas pressure such as hydrogen or helium, or by an electric pump. The latter, in most cases, have replaced the need for cylinders of gas and their health and safety implications.

The water, usually degassed and sterile, is perfused at a pressure of 15 pounds per square inch (*i.e.* marginally above atmospheric pressure) through catheters containing 4 or 8 separate channels, so that, at each outlet, any pressure exerted by mucosa only registers at one channel and affects no other. The advantage of having 8 transducers at a remote distance from the actual measurement point is that the 8 channels can be positioned radially at one point, which is useful in measurement of asymmetry of anal sphincters and its role in faecal incontinence.

At present, we use a Mui Scientific water perfusion pump attached to Medtronic Polygram 98. Two types of single-use catheters are normally used. The first has 8 ports, which are radially arranged circumferentially, and the second has 8 ports arranged in a spiral orientation over 5 cm. The latter also has a non-latex balloon attached to the end with a central channel leading to it so that air can be passed into it to conduct rectal sensitivity studies.

Initially, when the patient arrives for the test, a full clinical history is obtained and then the procedure is outlined to the patient. Full written consent is obtained and the patient is asked to remove all clothing from the waist down and to lie in the left lateral position.

The role of a digital examination by a gastrointestinal physiologist as part of anorectal physiology

Before any clinical measurement is carried out, it is imperative that a careful digital examination be performed by the operator. Any external abnormalities are noted, such as haemorrhoids, skin tags, inflammation, excoriation, scarring from operations, abscesses, fistulas or obstetric injuries. Internally, the general sphincter tone is assessed, and if there are any palpable deficits or scar tissue in the anal canal or rectum. In the rectum, the condition of the mucosa, puborectalis, position of anterior or posterior rectal walls, anal cushions are felt; and then the change to both external anal sphincter and puborectalis on squeezing and straining. All observations will be noted, as this will form part of the anorectal physiology report, though it cannot be used solely for gauging anorectal function but lends a general overview which should be backed up by the manometry as well as endo-anal ultrasound and proctogram X-rays.[10]

Station pull-through
The catheter with radial ports is inserted about 6 cm into the rectum with the assistance of aqueous lubricating jelly, and withdrawn 0.5 cm at a time, with pressure measurements taken at each stage. This will build up a pressure profile of the sphincter. Time is allowed for the sphincter to relax after movement of the catheter so that it is as near as possible to the true resting tone of the sphincter. In comparison, the continuous pull-throughs even at as slow a speed as 1 mm/s may tense the anus slightly, despite lubrication. This resting pressure, through the anal canal, incorporates the internal anal sphincter tone and approximately 25% of the external anal sphincter tone.

Continuous pull-through
The catheter is re-inserted and a catheter puller pulls the catheter through the anal canal at a steady rate. This is done with the patient at rest and then repeated with voluntary contraction; the automated computer analysis compares the difference in pressures, percentage asymmetry, position of the high pressure zone, and vector volume, and on the final report produces a 3-D representation.

Resting motility and station squeeze
The catheter is re-inserted a further time, positioned within the high-pressure zone of the anal canal and left *in situ* for a few minutes to observe any significant motility. Presence of any prominent ultraslow waves may be indicative of intermittent low tone and tendency to faecal leakage especially nocturnally when the sphincter is at its most relaxed. Once stable, the patient is asked to squeeze the sphincter for 10 s. From this can be deduced the peak squeeze pressure, and the percentage rate of fatigue after 10 s. Rapid fatigue

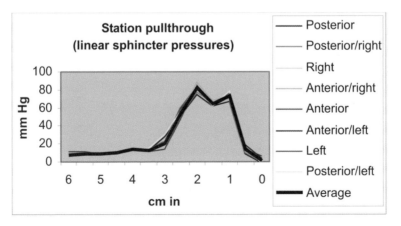

Fig. 5 Sphincter pressures on pull-through.

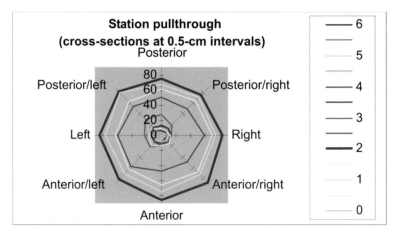

Fig. 6 Cross-section of manometric pressures.

denotes the likelihood of urge faecal incontinence. Analysis of these data is illustrated in the following figures.

Figure 5 shows a station pull-through in the anal canal and illustrates the following: from the 6-cm mark to the 3-cm mark, the catheter is measuring rectal pressure; the anal canal is approximately 2.75 cm in length; the high-pressure zone in this patient is at 1.5 cm into the anal canal and the resting pressure is at 80 mmHg.

The anal canal can also be shown in cross-section (Fig. 6) where any deviation from true symmetry can be determined. Each point relates to one of the perfusion ports on the catheter and the orientation. Selected cross-sections of the anal canal give examples of any asymmetry (Fig. 7). Significant asymmetry (*i.e.* greater than 20%) may indicate sphincter deficits and account for passive faecal incontinence.

When the catheter is positioned in the high-pressure zone, comparison can be made between the resting tone of the anal sphincter, the percentage increase on voluntary contraction can be calculated, and the decrease in pressure (percentage fatigue) over 10 s. Note that the squeeze shown in Figure 8 is moderate with little fatigue. Figure 9 compares data from a patient with local normal values.

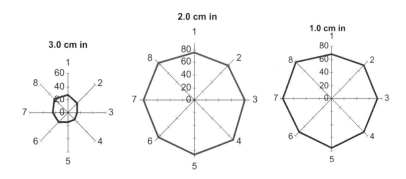

Fig. 7 Selected manometric cross-sections through anal canal.

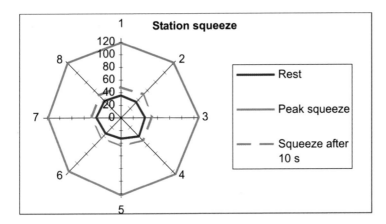

Fig. 8 Station squeeze pressures.

The second part of the procedure uses a catheter with spiral orientation and a non-latex balloon (maximum volume 400 ml): it is inserted into the anorectum with the most distal port at the anal verge so that the ports are positioned throughout the anal canal. If the anal canal is longer than 3.5 cm, the ports are placed in the centre of the high-pressure zone. The patient is asked to cough in order to assess the cough reflex, to squeeze and also to strain. This provides a comparison in pressures but mainly it is to assess whether the sphincter relaxes appropriately on straining. If there is significant increase in pressures, it indicates a tendency to contract the sphincter on straining suggesting that the patient might suffer from difficult or incomplete evacuation; it may also account for history of haemorrhoids, anal fissures or rectal mucosal prolapse.

Recto-anal inhibitory reflex (RAIR) and proctometrogram
The balloon is inflated in the rectum in order to detect the RAIR threshold, the inhibition values (*i.e.* the smallest volume that will induce the relaxation reflex), and the volume at which the sphincter stays relaxed and does not recover to the original resting pressure until after 10 s. If there is no RAIR, Hirschsprung's disease should be considered.

The balloon is then continuously inflated and the patient asked to say when the first sensation, first call-to-stool and maximum tolerated volume are felt.

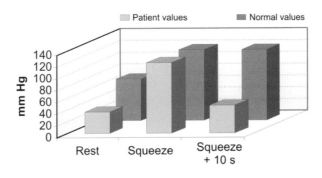

Fig. 9 Station squeeze – comparison of pressures.

This gives an indication of whether the patient will experience normal call-to-stool; low volumes point to a sensitive rectum and account for increased bowel frequency, while high volumes point to an insensitive compliant rectum and explain lack of call-to-stool and infrequent bowel movements. It is also important to compare the measurements obtained to set off the RAIR and those of sensation. Volumes setting off the relaxation reflex which are lower than sensation volumes will explain urgency, or insensible faecal incontinence.

Some neurogastroenterology groups use a barostat to investigate rectal compliance and the role of rectal sensation within irritable bowel syndrome. Studies have shown that a heightened sensitivity may be associated with some of the manifestations of irritable bowel syndrome, although this is mainly used as a research tool and not yet used in routine diagnostics.[11]

Some clinicians dispute whether anorectal physiology carried out on male patients with idiopathic faecal leakage is required at all.[12] In the Bristol unit, rectal balloon tests demonstrate quite often that RAIR can be triggered at low volumes, lower than first sensation. Along with an element of incomplete evacuation on attempting to evacuate because of inadequate sphincter relaxation on straining, or in conjunction with a prominent ultraslow wave resting motility with low-pressure troughs, these symptoms of seepage in men can be explained. In this case, surgery should not be an option, and biofeedback therapy (see below) will be of considerable help.

Percentage sphincter relaxation on straining
In order to detect the presence of anismus, the patient is asked to strain, which is often embarrassing and unnatural for the patient. However, this part of the study can detect if there is an increase in sphincter pressures and whether this is contributing to symptoms of obstructive defaecation and incomplete emptying.

Figure 10 shows the resting pressure in the anal sphincter and the strain pressure. The protocol within our department was changed recently as it was felt that the patients could not effectively bear down without a stimulus, so now RAIR is initiated by inflating the balloon to a volume where sphincter tone is relaxed, and the patient asked to strain again. Figure 10 shows that the

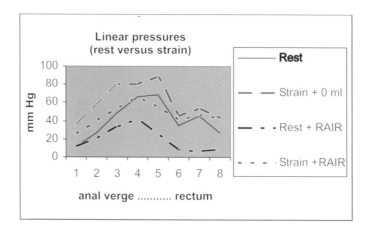

Fig. 10 Sphincter pressures, rest versus strain.

patient contracts the anal sphincter on strain even with the balloon inflated. In normal defaecation, sphincter pressures should reduce and there should be no evidence of contraction. This provides an objective diagnosis helping the understanding of dysfunctional defaecation.[13]

Nerve conduction

Pudendal nerve terminal motor latency (PNTML) measurement as a tool for detecting neuropathic sphincters is still a point of debate between clinicians regarding reliability, but the gastrointestinal physiologist's responsibility is to obtain optimum readings, providing a standard for the unit so that neural function of the anal sphincter can be determined. The pudendal nerve is stimulated with a pulsing current at the ischial tuberosity by a St Mark's electrode and the resultant muscle contraction registered; latency is the time in milliseconds between stimulation and contraction ($n = 2.0$).

In conjunction with PNTML and using the same electrode, anal sensation can also measured. This is performed using gradually increasing stimulation of the anal canal mucosa at 1-cm intervals and the patient response noted, giving a representation of sensation as a factor in continence. It is especially useful in gauging how obstetric deliveries affect anal sensation.[14]

Few units now perform needle electromyography of the anal sphincter to detect muscle fibre action potentials to gauge fibre density, or indeed, jitter, the more accurate judge of on-going sphincter neural impairment as opposed to past neuropathy. This may be because fewer clinicians are carrying this out, and gastrointestinal physiologists are not required to do this as part of their training.

Proctograms

Proctograms are carried out when a patient describes symptoms of obstructive defaecation, and videofluoroscopy of barium paste introduced into the rectum is used to detect any of the following when the patient is asked to bear down and pass the contrast: rectocoeles, mucosal prolapse or intussusception, enterocoeles, relative position of the vagina or prostate, inadequate widening of the anal canal, puborectalis contraction or non-relaxation and insufficient emptying of the contrast. The result of this is of infinite use in the biofeedback therapy and advice given to correct defaecatory dysfunction.

Endo-anal ultrasonography

Some gastrointestinal physiology departments offer endo-anal ultrason-ography in addition to the anorectal physiology service although in the majority of hospitals it is still undertaken by a radiologist.

The normal equipment used is a Bruel and Kjaer Medical Ultrasound machine, but models can vary. A 10-MHz, 360° rotating transducer is covered with a 17-mm hard plastic cone which is attached to a hand-held probe. The probe end is filled with degassed sterile water through a tap on the probe and pushed through a hole on the tip of the probe so that all bubbles are removed. An image of a series of rings is seen on the ultrasound machine to check for any distortion by air bubbles in the cone. The frequency is set at 10 MHz and the multi-imaging frequency at –2.3. This protocol can vary from unit to unit with pieces of equipment.

The probe is coated with ultrasound gel and then a condom placed over the top for infection control. Further ultrasound gel inserted into the anal canal, with the patient lying in left lateral position, knees bent.

First, the puborectalis is visualised and then withdrawn every 0.5 cm in order to examine the entire anal canal. Images are taken of the puborectalis, deep, mid and superficial aspects of anal canal to assess its integrity.

If ultrasonography is compared with anorectal physiology, hypo-echoic appearance denoting sphincter deficits or hyperechoic areas indicating fibrosis, seem to correlate with manometric sphincter deficits and scar tissue impression, respectively, though there is much documented research on this field yet to be completed.

$[^{13}C]$-Urea breath test to detect active H. pylori infection

The patient has to prepare for the test by abstaining from antibiotics for 28 days, withdrawal from proton pump inhibitors and histamine antagonists for 2 weeks and to fast for at least 6 h before the test. The patient is asked to exhale into two labelled test tubes as a baseline sample, given 250 ml of orange juice or citric acid in order to delay gastric emptying and also maximise the surface area to which the labelled urea is exposed. If it is impossible for the patient to stop antacid medication, the patient can be given a more acidic drink (a solution of citric acid, malic acid and tartaric acid) prior to the substrate to mimic a normally acidic stomach environment. The patient is then asked to drink 75 mg $[^{13}C]$-urea solution in water. After 30 min, the second samples of exhaled breath are taken and the kit is sent for analysis by nuclear magnetic resonance spectroscopy.

The test measures the amount of CO_2 in the initial baseline samples and compares this to the amount produced in the test sample. The principle behind the test is that H. pylori produces urease which metabolises the urea to CO_2 and ammonia. The carbon dioxide samples that are produced are compared at T_0 and T_{30}. If there is a difference between the initial $[^{13}C]$-CO_2 and the final $[^{13}C]$-CO_2 of more than 4.00%, the patient is diagnosed as being positive for H. pylori. The specificity of this test is 98.5% with 97.9% sensitivity.[15]

Hydrogen breath tests

The most commonly requested tests are for small bowel bacterial overgrowth, lactose intolerance and orocaecal transit time. Patients have to prepare for this test by avoiding antibiotics for 28 days, and the day before the test, laxatives, fibre-rich foods, smoking and exercise. They are also requested to fast for 12 h. On arrival, the patient has a full clinical history taken then asked to exhale fully into a breath test monitor measuring hydrogen. If the baseline reading is above 10 ppm, the patient will be asked to swill the buccal cavity with chlorohexidine to exclude hydrogen production by oral bacteria. If the reading is adequately low, the patient is given the relevant substrate (50g of substrate dissolved in water and made up to 200 ml) and breath samples are taken every 20 min over 3—5 h depending on the test.

Small bowel bacterial overgrowth is detected by giving the patient glucose as a substrate and a 20 ppm rise of hydrogen above the initial baseline reading. A positive diagnosis is normally deduced within the first 120 min but can occur further on into the test (Fig. 11).

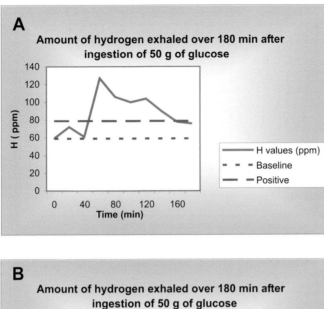

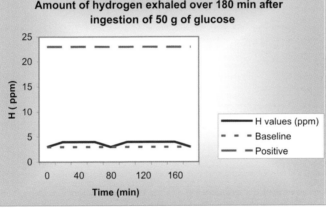

Fig. 11 (A) Positive and (B) negative tests for small bowel bacterial overgrowth.

Lactose intolerance is also detected by a rise of 20 ppm of hydrogen above the baseline but the patient is given lactose as a substrate (Fig. 12). A positive diagnosis of lactase deficiency can manifest itself between 120–250 min depending on transit time of the small bowel. If the initial baseline reading is above 10 ppm and the patient has adhered to all the preparation needed for the test, then small bowel bacterial overgrowth should be excluded because misdiagnosis of sugar malabsorption may occur.[16]

Orocaecal transit time is determined by giving 20 ml of lactulose to the patient as a substrate. Samples of exhaled breath are taken every 20 min and there should be a peak amount of hydrogen produced once most of the lactulose has reached the caecum (Fig. 13).

Fructose malabsorption can also be detected using this procedure, though recent studies have shown that all healthy adults have malabsorption and intolerance with 50 g of fructose and therefore the test amount should be 25 g.[17]

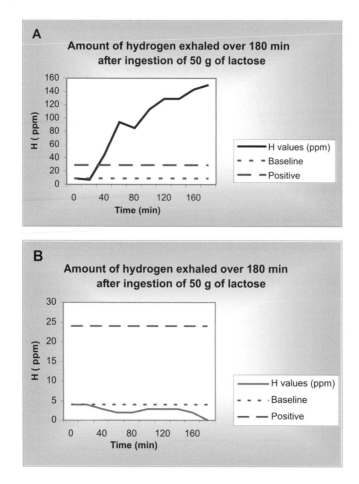

Fig. 12 (A) Positive and (B) negative results for lactase deficiency.

BIOFEEDBACK THERAPY

As the gastrointestinal physiologist's duty towards not just clinical measurement but also correcting anorectal dysfunction has developed, the importance of biofeedback therapy has been augmented. It is recognised that it is essential to correct pelvic floor dysfunction, either as conservative treatment on its own (to avoid the necessity of unnecessary surgery), or to optimise the beneficial outcome of surgical intervention (such as stapled transanal rectal resection [STARR] or rectopexy procedures for rectal prolapse).[18,19]

An example of this is the detection of non-relaxation or paradoxical contraction of the sphincter and/or puborectalis muscle on anorectal physiology. It can be argued that the situation of being asked to bear down as if to pass a bowel movement in the setting of a laboratory is not what would be happening *in vivo*; however, if left uncorrected, there are long-term effects to the patient, such as haemorrhoids, troublesome anal tags, rectal mucosal

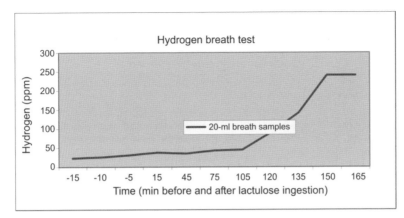

Fig. 13 Lactulose reaches the large intestine at 160 min.

prolapse, constipation and even uterine prolapse, and urinary problems. Ideally, it would be best to refer a patient at the first sign of haemorrhoids, difficulty evacuating, irritable bowel syndrome, constipation or faecal incontinence.

There is a variety of equipment available to show a patient the function of the anal sphincter or pelvic floor. Surface electromyography is probably the most accurate, as it picks up the action potentials fired by the muscle fibres. Whichever method is used, a probe is inserted into the patient's anal canal and connected to some form of visual depiction of the sphincter tone which may be a system of lights, or as a trace on a monitor. We use a water-perfused catheter with linearly arranged ports through the anal canal, which detects manometric changes in pressures when the patient tightens or relaxes the anal sphincter. It also has a rectal balloon (400-ml capacity) so that recto-anal inhibitory reflex and rectal sensation volumes can be demonstrated to the patient, and rectal sensation education can be instigated.

Table 2 shows the different reasons why biofeedback therapy might be carried out and how each affliction may be approached.

In practice, each patient is treated individually for the symptoms they exhibit, taking into account both mental and physical symptoms, and a care plan tailor-made for that particular patient. Success of biofeedback therapy is still being audited; currently, a questionnaire is being developed to be used as an auditing tool. However, as well as the clinical side of education through biofeedback, a large part of the job of the gastrointestinal physiologist is to listen, read in-between the lines, acknowledge the patient's problem, counsel as well as motivate and encourage; and finally provide advice not just regarding sphincter relaxation or strengthening but also life-style changes.

HYPNOTISM

It is acknowledged that some patients can be helped by the deep relaxation and cognitive behavioural therapy that hypnosis can induce. These are patients that have stress-related irritable bowel syndrome or idiopathic abdominal pain, or symptoms that are resistant to conventional changes in diet, improved evacuation techniques,

Table 2 Indications for biofeedback therapy

Indication	Faecal incontinence following trauma or obstetric injuries
Symptoms	Passive or urge faecal incontinence
Anorectal physiology (other studies)	Sphincter asymmetry or defects (backed up by endo-anal ultrasound)
Treatment	Sphincter/puborectalis strengthening exercises (if there is a complete gap exercises will help outcome of sphincter repair but may not prevent faecal incontinence)
Indication	Faecal incontinence following prolonged, breach or difficult child-birth, systemic illnesses such as muscular dystrophy, multiple sclerosis, prolonged constipation and straining at stool
Symptoms	Passive or urge faecal incontinence
Anorectal physiology (other studies)	Fatiguing voluntary sphincter contraction. Volumes required to trigger rectoanal inhibitory reflex (RAIR) lower than first sensation of filling. Low sphincter tone. Neuropathy on electrophysiology
Treatment	Sphincter/puborectalis strengthening exercises. Rectal sensation education with rectal balloon. Sphincter exercises, but may not improve sphincter tone, so help with improving evacuation, so less likelihood of incontinence
Indication	Irritable bowel syndrome, inflammatory bowel diseases, stress, idiopathic abdominal pain or rectal pain
Symptoms	Urgency but no faecal incontinence
Anorectal physiology (other studies)	Loose stool consistency
Treatment	Sphincter/puborectalis strengthening exercises. Dietary advice – increase soluble fibre intake, reduce stimulant beverages. Life-style advice. Relaxation technique. Hypnosis
Indication	Incomplete emptying and difficulty evacuating – patient may be having to resort to suppositories or digital aid to open their bowels but also suffer from faecal leakage
Symptoms	Passive leakage of rectal residue
Anorectal physiology (other studies)	Sphincter/puborectalis contraction or non-relaxation on defaecation. Rectocoeles, mucosal prolapse, uterine prolapse, enterocoeles, vaginal prolapse shown on proctogram X-rays
Treatment	Evacuation technique (includes toileting position, diaphragmatic breathing, avoidance of valsalva manoeuvre, and bracing with transverse abdominal oblique muscles). Sphincter and puborectalis relaxation education
Indication	Obstructive defaecation due to inadequate sphincter non-relaxation
Symptoms	Normal call-to-stool but strains fruitlessly despite normal stool consistency

Table 2 *(continued)* Indications for biofeedback therapy

Anorectal physiology (other studies)	Increase in sphincter pressures on straining, Anal canal not widening on defaecation on proctogram
Treatment	Evacuation technique. Sphincter and puborectalis relaxation education
Indication	Difficulty evacuating and loss of regular call-to-stool
Symptoms	Infrequent call-to-stool and straining fruitlessly, likely to be firmer stool consistency
Anorectal physiology (other studies)	Loss of rectal sensation or high trigger volume. Rectocoeles, mucosal prolapse, uterine prolapse, enterocoeles, vaginal prolapse shown on proctogram X-rays. Transit study markers confined to lower sigmoid colon and rectum
Treatment	Evacuation technique. Sphincter and puborectalis relaxation education. Rectal sensation education with rectal balloon. Regularisation and exercise. Dietary advice – increase of fibre and water intake
Indication	Haemorrhoids, anal fissures, anal pain and bleeding
Symptoms	Difficulty evacuating because of pain, frequent loss of bright red blood on opening bowels
Anorectal physiology (other studies)	Hypertonic anal sphincter, often relaxes over time on measurement, worse with stress. Sphincter and/or puborectalis contraction on straining
Treatment	Relaxation. Diaphragmatic breathing. Hypnosis. Evacuation technique. Sphincter and puborectalis relaxation education
Indication	Slow transit constipation
Symptoms	Long history of loss of regular call-to-stool, with infrequent bowel opening. Difficulty evacuating usually hard pebbly stool. Abdominal pain and bloating
Anorectal physiology (other studies)	History taking prior to anorectal studies. May have sphincter and/or puborectalis contraction on straining. Transit study markers distributed throughout colon
Treatment	Relaxation and exercise. Life-style advice. Regularisation. Diaphragmatic breathing. Hypnosis. Evacuation technique. Sphincter and puborectalis relaxation education. Abdominal massage

and medication. Hypnosis is used in the UK National Health Service as an aid to stress management, pain management (especially in dentistry), and even in some surgical procedures. It is now also being introduced and recognised as a valuable support for biofeedback therapy and to help patients tolerate gastrointestinal procedures such as oesophageal intubation for gastrointestinal physiology investigations and endoscopies. Supporting biofeedback therapy, it helps the patient when in a state of deep relaxation to recognise and visualise the source of their symptoms and to envisage a positive improvement to symptoms, or reduce pain thresholds considerably.[20]

Key points for clinical practice

- The role of gastrointestinal physiologists has increased as training has become standardised nationally in the UK.

- Scope is extending beyond clinical measurement of anorectal function to holistic history-taking and reasoning behind the results obtained, aiding diagnoses and, therefore, treatment.

- It is becoming increasingly evident that functional testing is imperative before major surgery to ensure appropriateness.

- Change in UK NICE guidelines is increasing the trend for biofeedback therapy prior to, or instead of, surgery.

- The requirement to reduce the 18-week referral to treatment waiting times has increased the number of referrals for biofeedback therapy, now regarded as conservative treatment.

- There have been recent advances in equipment to facilitate oesophageal measurement such as intraluminal impedance for non-acid reflux, and high-resolution manometry for static oesophageal function.

- The Bristol gastrointestinal physiology unit advocates combined pH and manometry studies over 24 h as routine.

- Recto-anal inhibitory reflex threshold and inhibition volumes compared with rectal sensation volumes are an aid in rationalisation of patient symptoms.

- Biofeedback therapy includes not only feedback via equipment to educate the patient on evacuation technique, but also counselling, advice on life-style, diet, regularisation of bowel openings, hypnosis, stress management, and relaxation techniques.

- Biofeedback therapy may help patients avoid unnecessary surgery or increase the percentage success rate after surgery such as the stapled transanal rectal resection procedure.

References

1. National Institute for Health and Clinical Excellence. Ref CG17, CG49, CG16 for dyspepsia, faecal incontinence, and irritable bowel syndrome. <http://www.nice.org.uk>..
2. Heatley M, Rose K, Weston C. The heart and the oesophagus: intimate relations. *Postgrad Med J* 2005; **81**: 515–518.
3. Lacima G, Grande L, Pera M, Francino A, Ros E. Utility of ambulatory 24-hour oesophageal pH and motility monitoring in non-cardiac chest pain: report of 90 patient and review of the literature. *Dig Dis Sci* 2003; **48**: 952–961.
4. Corinaldesi R, Salvioli B, Lioce A *et al*. Gastroesophageal reflux disease: clinical and pathophysiological features (Part1). *Clin Ter* 2007; **158**: 77–83.
5. Barham CP, Gotley DC, Fowler A, Mills A, Alderson D. Diffuse oesophageal spasm: diagnosis by ambulatory 24 hour manometry. *Gut* 1997; **41**: 151–155.
6. Barham CP, Alderson D. Gas and liquid reflux during transient lower oesophageal sphincter relaxation. *Gut* 1999; **44**: 897–898.

7. Wo JM, Castell DO. Exclusion of meal periods from ambulatory 24-hour pH monitoring may improve diagnosis of esophageal acid reflux. *Dig Dis Sci* 1994; **39**: 1601–1607.
8. Dobben AC, Terra MP, Deutekom M *et al.* Anal inspection and digital rectal examination compared to anorectal physiology tests and endoanal ultrasonography in evaluating fecal incontinence. *Int J Colorectal Dis* 2007; **22**: 783–790.
9. Fox M, Thumshirn M, Fried M, Schwizer W. Barostat measurement of rectal compliance and capacity. *Dis Colon Rectum* 2006; **49**: 360–370.
10. Titi M, Jenkins JT, Urie A, Molloy RG. Prospective study of the diagnostic evaluation of faecal incontinence and leakage in male patients. *Colorectal Dis* 2007; **9**: 647–652.
11. Agrawal A, Houghton LA, Lea R, Moris J, Reilly B, Whorwell PJ. Bloating and distension in irritable bowel syndrome: the role of visceral sensation. *Gastroenterology* 2008 Mar 8 [Epub ahead of print].
12. Chaliha C, Sultan AH, Emmanuel AV. Normal ranges for anorectal manometry and sensation in women of reproductive age. *Colorectal Dis* 2007; **9**: 839–844.
13. Albert H. Gastro-oesophageal reflux disease in general practice. Utility and acceptability of Infai ^{13}C-urea breath test has been shown. *BMJ* 2002; **324**: 485–486.
14. Nucera G, Gabrielli M, Lupascu A *et al.* Abnormal breath tests to lactose, fructose and sorbitol in irritable bowel syndrome may be explained by small intestinal bacterial overgrowth. *Aliment Pharmacol Ther* 2005; **21**: 1391–1395.
15. European Agency for the Evaluation of Medicinal Products. *Helicobacter Test Infai.* 14 August 1997; Rev.1, 26 May 1998, CPMP/417/97.
16. Rao SS, Attaluri A, Anderson L, Stumbo P. Ability of the normal human small intestine to absorb fructose evaluation by breath testing. *Clin Gastroenterol Hepatol* 2007; **5**: 959–963.
17. Ommer A, Albrecht K, Wenger F, Walz MK. Stapled transanal rectal resection (STARR): a new option in the treatment of obstructive defecation syndrome. *Langenbecks Arch Surg* 2006; **391**: 32–37.
18. National Institute for Health and Clinical Excellence. Interventional Procedure Consultation Document – *Stapled transanal rectal resection for obstructed defaecation syndrome.* <http://www.nice.org.uk>.
19. Bristol Laparoscopic Surgery. *Obstructed defaecation – STARR and PPH* <http://www.bristolsurgery.com>.
20. Roberts L, Wilson S, Singh S, Roalfe A, Greenfield S. Gut-directed hypnotherapy for irritable bowel syndrome: piloting a primary care-based randomised controlled trial. *Br J Gen Pract* 2006; **56**: 115–121.

Lachlan Ayres Peter Collins

Variceal bleeding

In a recent national audit, variceal bleeding accounted for 11% of acute upper gastrointestinal bleeds in the UK.[1] This figure has risen from 6% in 1993 and reflects the rising incidence of cirrhosis. Variceal haemorrhage is a medical emergency requiring prompt multidisciplinary treatment. Although mortality has decreased over the last few years due to improved endoscopic techniques and medical management, it remains high if re-bleeding occurs. The cost of treating a single episode of variceal bleeding is approximately £10,000 and this rises with Childs–Pugh score.[2] The risk of haemorrhage is itself determined by the severity of the underlying liver disease; therefore, the long-term treatment goal of portal hypertension must include preventing the progression of cirrhosis.

In all stages of cirrhosis, the yearly incidence of oesophageal varices is 5–7%, with the incidence of bleeding approximately 25% at 2 years. Bleeding-related mortality is around 20% at 6 weeks.[3]

PATHOPHYSIOLOGY

Alcoholic cirrhosis is the commonest cause of portal hypertension in the UK, although it can develop in cirrhosis of any aetiology and, more rarely, in the absence of cirrhosis. Varices occur usually once the hepatic venous gradient (wedged hepatic vein pressure – hepatic vein pressure) exceeds 10–12 mmHg.

The precise events which trigger variceal rupture are not known. Risk of haemorrhage correlates with portal pressure, varix size, and severity of liver

Lachlan Ayres MBChB MRCP(UK)
Clinical Fellow in Gastroenterology, Department of Gastroenterology, Day Services Unit, The Great Western Hospital, Marlborough Road, Swindon, Wiltshire SN3 6BB, UK
E-mail: lachlanayres@hotmail.com

Peter Collins BMSc MBChB MD MRCP(UK) (for correspondence)
Consultant Hepatologist, Department of Digestive Disease, Bristol Royal Infirmary, University Hospital Bristol NHS Foundation Trust, Marlborough Street, Bristol, Avon BS2 8HW, UK
E-mail: peter.collins@uhbristol.nhs.uk

Table 1 Variceal size

Baveno[4]	Description (BSG)[5]	Endoscopic appearance (BSG)[5]	Grade (BSG)[5]	Description (AASLD)[6]	Endoscopic appearance (AASLD)[6]
< 5 mm	Small	Collapse with air insufflation	1	Small	Minimally elevated veins
	Medium	Not collapsible or occluding lumen	2	Medium	Tortuous veins < one-third of lumen
> 5 mm	Large	Occluding oesophageal lumen	3	Large	Veins > one-third of lumen

disease. Table 1 lists sizing criteria commonly used to record the endoscopic appearances of oesophageal varices. Endotoxin-induced endothelin release increases portal pressure in experimental models,[7] supporting the theory that infection can trigger bleeding. However, infection is not a universal feature of variceal haemorrhage and cannot explain all episodes.

The 'explosion hypothesis' (*i.e.* increased intravariceal pressure secondary to a rapid increase in portal pressure post-prandially or as a response to sepsis causing a varix to rupture) seems a logical premise; however, a recent study demonstrated that cirrhotic patients with a history of variceal haemorrhage demonstrated a lower hepatic venous pressure gradient response to food.[8]

Other contributors to sustaining bleeding include impaired extrinsic clotting pathways (although the experimental evidence is conflicting), reduced platelets and erythrocyte aggregation. Hyperfibrinolysis could also contribute to the risk of haemorrhage; a recent study showed that cirrhotic patients ($n = 8$) had higher basal plasma tissue plasminogen activator activity possibly due to a relative deficiency of plasminogen activator inhibitor.[9] Many contributing factors reflect advanced liver disease, and the causality of individual parameters to variceal rupture has yet to be established.

DETECTION METHODS

The incidence of varices increases with advancing liver disease; 42.7% of Childs–Pugh grade A patients had varices in a US national endoscopic database increasing to 71.9% in grade B/C patients.[10] Current consensus and guidelines, therefore, recommend screening for varices in all patients with cirrhosis.[6,11]

Given the cost implications of performing variceal screening in a population where liver disease is increasing, a non-invasive diagnostic method would be desirable. Further endoscopic assessment could then be more targeted.

ESTIMATING FIBROSIS

The use of ultrasound elastography (Fibroscan) to measure the severity of fibrosis in patients with hepatitis C has been widely validated. In a study involving 165 cirrhotic patients of various causes but mainly hepatitis C, Fibroscan demonstrated good predictive power with respect to the presence of oesophageal varices (AUROC 0.84) and variceal grade ≥ II (AUROC 0.83). This technique is not appropriate for patients with ascites because the low frequency elastic waves do not pass through fluid.[12]

Serum markers of fibrosis have also been assessed: in 146 patients with alcoholic liver disease, a combination of cut-off values for alkaline phosphatase, hyaluronate and prothrombin index had an accuracy of 86% in predicting medium–large varices.[13] Further investigation into whether these tests apply equally to other causes of cirrhosis is required.

FibroTest is a commercial algorithm using several biochemical markers that has been used in the evaluation of cirrhosis. A recent French study of 99 cirrhotic patients demonstrated Fibrotest had greater discriminative power than platelet count or Childs–Pugh score alone in predicting varices of all sizes.[14]

ULTRASOUND AND LABORATORY TESTS

Standard investigations (e.g. ultrasonography and full blood count) may also accurately predict varices and have cost and accessibility advantages over more complicated techniques.

An Italian study involving 266 cirrhotic patients found that portal vein diameter does not correlate with the presence of varices ($P = 0.4$). In fact, patients with portal vein diameter < 12 mm showed a significantly higher prevalence of F1–2 varices and there was an unexpected oscillatory trend of portal vein diameter with respect to the endoscopic findings.[15] The authors concluded that, in the early stages of portal hypertension, varices may actually decompress the portal vein (Fig. 1).

A multicentre validation study of 218 cirrhotic patients found that platelet count (per cubic millimetre)/spleen diameter (millimetre) had a 91.5% sensitivity and 67.0% specificity for diagnosis of varices of any size.[16] Although

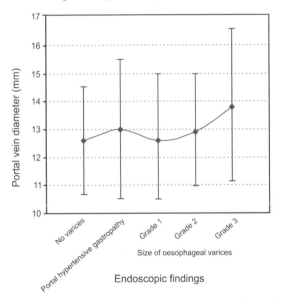

Fig. 1 Mean portal vein diameter and endoscopic findings. Adapted from Zardi et al.[15]

quite accurate, these parameters are imperfect and their isolated use would miss one in ten patients with varices and subject three in ten to an unnecessary gastroscopy. A novel approach may be to substitute relative spleen size; as in clinical practice, borderline splenomegaly in the absence of an obvious cause may often be attributed to body habitus alone.

Although often considered a marker of portal hypertension, a low platelet count alone does not appear to be reliable in predicting varices. Some 15% of patients develop varices when their platelet count is > 150,000 mm^{-3}.[17]

COMPUTED TOMOGRAPHY

In contrast to sonography, most patients being investigated for liver disease will not have a CT scan. There is some evidence that triphasic CT scanning can detect varices. The rate of detection for small varices was around 60%, rising to 92% for larger ones ($\geq$ 3 mm).[18] Additionally, there have been several pilot studies using multidetector CT in the evaluation of the risk of variceal bleeding. A Japanese group[19] have developed a scoring system which correlates significantly with the endoscopic red sign and, therefore, the risk of bleeding but this is unlikely to become established in routine clinical practice.

CAPSULE ENDOSCOPY

Capsule endoscopy is becoming more widely used to investigate occult gastrointestinal bleeding and small bowel disorders. Recently, several publications have compared its accuracy to traditional endoscopy in detecting oesophageal varices. Overall sensitivity for the detection of any grade of varices ranged from 68% to 96%.[20–22] Capsule endoscopy may have significant advantages in terms of patient comfort and avoidance of sedation but more studies are required to investigate cost-effectiveness.

RISK OF BLEEDING

The identification of varices that are likely to bleed is important to ensure the correct management approach. Childs–Pugh score, endoscopic red sign, variceal size and high hepatic venous pressure gradient (HVPG) all correlate with 'high-risk' varices.

HEPATIC VENOUS PRESSURE GRADIENT

The hepatic venous pressure gradient (HVPG) reflects the portal pressure in cirrhotic portal hypertension regardless of the aetiology of liver disease. HVPG has been shown to correlate with variceal size and risk of haemorrhage. Maintenance of HVPG < 10 mmHg gives a 90% probability of not developing complications (including varices) at 4 years of follow-up.[23]

A recent review of the literature concluded that a reduction of HVPG to $\leq$ 12 mmHg or by $\geq$ 20% of baseline significantly reduced the risk of bleeding and mortality.[24]

Assessment of HVPG is invasive and seldom used outside of specialist centres. A potential surrogate marker for HVPG is variceal pressure measured during endoscopy. This has been attempted using a prototype pressure gauge developed by a Swiss group.[25] There appears to be some correlation between the two parameters but prospective studies are required to validate its clinical application. Interestingly, the same study demonstrated a significantly higher variceal pressure, but not HPVG, in patients with previous haemorrhage as compared to non-bleeders. In a patient group where coagulation is generally abnormal, the ability to gauge venous pressure without venous puncture is desirable.

HPVG measurement in the acute setting (*i.e.* variceal haemorrhage being treated pharmacologically and endoscopically) can also predict short-term prognosis. A prospective study showed that HVPG > 20 mmHg at the time of bleeding was associated with 5-day treatment failure (c statistic, 0.79).[26] Similar predictive power, however, was achieved using simple clinical parameters: systolic blood pressure < 100 mmHg, Childs–Pugh score and non-alcoholic aetiology (c statistic, 0.80) suggesting that, in this setting, there is little advantage in measuring HPVG.

CLINICAL SCORING SYSTEMS

The risk of bleeding may be predicted using simpler scoring systems. Tacke *et al.*[27] have devised a Bleeding Risk Score comprising serum cholinesterase < 2.25 kU/l, INR > 1.2, viral or alcoholic aetiology and presence of varices. This score was more sensitive and specific (AUROC 0.751) for risk of bleeding than either Childs–Pugh (AUROC 0.584) or MELD score (AUROC 0.577).[27] Interestingly, unlike the Childs–Pugh and MELD scores, the Bleeding Risk Score is not significantly predictive of the patient's overall survival (*i.e.* there do appear to be factors unrelated to the degree of liver disease which influence bleeding risk). The ability to predict excess mortality from re-bleeding allows those patients at high risk to be considered for early repeat endoscopy or continued high-dependency care.

The Rockall scoring system has been widely adopted in the UK to predict mortality and risk of re-bleeding for upper gastrointestinal bleeding of any source. It also has high predictive and discriminative value in the context of variceal bleeding: AUROC 0.798 for variceal re-bleeding and AUROC 0.834 for mortality.[28]

Unsurprisingly, the severity of underlying liver disease and evidence of multi-organ dysfunction (elevated creatinine) are associated with higher mortality. A retrospective analysis of predictors of mortality identified creatinine (> 133 μmol/l), bilirubin (> 51 μmol/l) and encephalopathy as variables associated with in-hospital death. In this study, re-bleeding within 24 h was associated with a 40% in-hospital mortality.[29]

Variceal haemorrhage is an important cause of death in cirrhotic patients with hepatocellular cancer. Subgroup analysis of these patients found that neither the presence nor size of tumour significantly affected bleeding risk. However, portal vein tumour thrombus was found to correlate significantly with the development of the endoscopic red sign in patients with hepatocellular cancer. Childs–Pugh score and low platelet count were also statistically significant risk factors for the red sign in both the presence and the absence of hepatocellular cancer.[30] In another retrospective study of 141

Table 2 Factors associated with early mortality in variceal haemorrhage

- Childs–Pugh C score
- Re-bleeding
- Elevated bilirubin
- Encephalopathy
- Elevated creatinine
- Shock
- Portal vein tumour

patients, active bleeding at endoscopy was not found to influence mortality at 1 year; however, Childs–Pugh C score and presence of hepatic or extrahepatic neoplasia did affect survival rates.[31] Predictors of early (*i.e.* 6-week) mortality were Childs–Pugh C score and shock on admission (Table 2). These findings highlight the need to pay attention to all systems when treating the patient with cirrhosis in the long term and when acute decompensation occurs.

ULTRASOUND

A further non-invasive method of assessing bleeding risk is sonographic measurement of flow volume in the portal trunk and splenic vein. In a controlled study of 158 patients with cirrhosis, flow volume in the splenic vein correlated with high-risk bleeders as assessed by endoscopy.[32] This investigation could be used to identify patients who would benefit from early diagnostic/interventional endoscopy when first diagnosed with cirrhosis but, in common with other ultrasound techniques, it is likely to be highly operator dependent.

PRIMARY PROPHYLAXIS OF FIRST VARICEAL HAEMORRHAGE

When considering the management of cirrhosis and portal hypertension, the ideal is to prevent the formation of varices at all. In practice, the first discovery of cirrhosis and portal hypertension frequently occurs when patients present with decompensated liver disease. In this situation, where there is no history of variceal haemorrhage, the traditional approach is non-selective β-blockers for small varices or endoscopic band ligation for larger varices. Risk of bleeding from small varices is relatively low (approximately 12% at 2 years); however, the natural history of small varices is progression to medium–large-sized varices at a rate of 12% at 1 year and 31% at 3 years.[33]

MONOTHERAPY

Meta-analysis has shown that variceal band ligation is superior to β-blockade in reducing the incidence of first bleeds but there is no difference in survival.[34] In subgroup analysis, variceal band ligation had a significant advantage in those trials which had < 30% patients with alcoholic cirrhosis, > 30% Childs–Pugh C score and > 50% patients with large varices. Importantly, there were significantly fewer severe adverse effects in the ligation groups.

An Italian group has also studied primary prophylaxis in Childs–Pugh B/C cirrhosis awaiting liver transplant. β-Blockers and variceal band ligation were similarly effective in preventing the primary end-point of variceal bleeding. Banding had the disadvantages of higher cost and bleeding from post-banding ulcers occurred in two out of 31 patients (one fatal). They recommend ligation only if patients are intolerant to β-blockers (16% in this study).[35]

COMBINATION THERAPY

In a randomised trial of patients with high-risk varices, addition of non-selective β-blockade to variceal band ligation did not give additional benefit in terms of decreasing risk of first bleed or preventing death, but did reduce the recurrence of varices.[36]

Randomised data of cirrhotic patients awaiting liver transplant, however, suggest that the combination of variceal band ligation and propranolol is superior to propranolol alone. Of patients in the combination treatment group, 6% bled compared to 31% in the monotherapy group.[37]

The data on the use of variceal band ligation in combination with β-blockade remain unclear and, at this point in time, the possible benefits would not seem to justify the likely increase in cost and potential adverse events.

COMPLICATIONS

The Baveno IV consensus[11] states that the long-term benefits of variceal band ligation are uncertain because of the short duration of follow-up. A Spanish study of 71 cirrhotic patients with no history of variceal bleeding assessed the long-term (up to 8 years) complication rates of portal hypertension whilst being treated. Those patients who demonstrated a significant HVPG reduction in response to propranolol ± nitrates) had a 90% probability of being free from variceal haemorrhage (compared to 45%). There were also lower rates of spontaneous bacterial peritonitis. There was no difference in development of ascites, encephalopathy or survival.[38] Meta-analysis of similar studies, however, has shown an increased survival in individuals with haemodynamic responses.

TREATMENT OF ACUTE VARICEAL HAEMORRHAGE

Acute variceal haemorrhage is a medical emergency and requires a multidisciplinary approach. Fluid resuscitation, attention to airway in addition to definitive endoscopic and pharmacological therapy are needed. Over-transfusion should be avoided. There is no data to suggest routine use of platelets, fresh frozen plasma or vitamin K, and these agents should be used on a case-by-case basis. A lower threshold for their use seems appropriate in cases of re-bleeding. On-going attention to the other features of decompensated liver disease should be delivered by physicians experienced in the field. Secondary prevention and consideration of referral for transplant assessment may be appropriate.

ENDOSCOPIC TREATMENT

Endoscopic therapy with sclerotherapy or variceal band ligation are effective in the treatment of active variceal bleeding. Meta-analysis has shown that

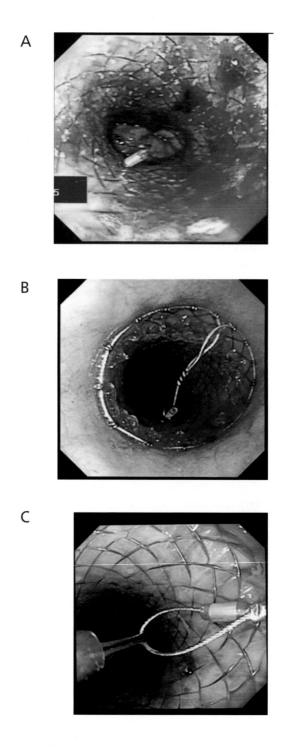

Fig. 2 The use of a self-expanding Danis stents for acute variceal bleeding.
(A) and (B): Self-expanding stents can be placed in the lower oesophagus during an acute variceal haemorrhage, with or without direct visualisation. (C): Stents can be removed endoscopically after several days using a specially designed loop system.
Courtesy of Dr David Patch, Royal Free Hospital, London UK.

endoscopic therapy alone is superior to vasoactive drugs alone in controlling active bleeding, preventing re-bleeding and improving mortality.[39]

Ligation is probably more effective than sclerotherapy both for acute bleeding and subsequent eradication. Randomised data have shown haemostasis is more frequently achieved with variceal band ligation (97%) than sclerotherapy (76%; $P = 0.009$).[40] In the setting of non-cirrhotic portal hypertension, variceal eradication was achieved with fewer sessions and fewer side effects using ligation when compared to sclerotherapy.[41] There are similar findings in varices of cirrhotic aetiology.

Most units routinely treating oesophageal varices have switched to band ligation as first-line therapy. Sclerotherapy remains a useful technique, however, when ligation is unavailable or technically difficult or in the treatment of gastric varices (discussed in more detail below).

BALLOON TAMPONADE

Sengstaken–Blakemore or Minnesota tubes are commonly used when variceal haemorrhage is uncontrollable, but can only be left *in situ* for 12–24 h. After this period, oesophageal necrosis may occur. A recent single-centre study found that overall effectiveness of balloon tamponade was 61%. This method was more effective in lower Childs–Pugh score and if endoscopic therapy had been attempted (75% versus 48% with no endoscopic therapy). Mortality associated with variceal bleeding requiring balloon tamponade was 33% in this centre.[42] Although effective at stopping bleeding, upon removal approximately 50% of patients will re-bleed. The rarity of the need to resort to balloon tamponade with the improvement of modern endoscopic interventional therapy is reflected in the scarcity of new literature; the only other published article in the last few years presented three cases of fatal complications including oesophageal rupture and mediastinitis.[43] Complications including aspiration, loss of traction and thoracic pain occur in about one-third of cases.

SELF-EXPANDING METAL STENTS

An exciting development in endoscopic treatment is the deployment of self-expanding metal stents for acute variceal bleeding (Fig. 2). Although not yet an established technique, there have been encouraging results in a pilot study of uncontrollable bleeding. Twenty patients who had failed standard combined endoscopic and vasoactive drug treatment were treated with stent insertion. Stents were left in place for 2–14 days. Bleeding ceased in all cases and extraction of the stents was uncomplicated.[44] Further studies are required to confirm these results.

PHARMACOTHERAPY

Vasoactive drugs
The aim of vasoactive drugs is acute reduction in portal pressure. Pharmacological treatment has the advantage of not requiring specialist teams and can be given rapidly while the patient is being resuscitated.

Meta-analysis has demonstrated that the use of terlipressin (a long-acting analogue of vasopressin) leads to a 34% relative risk reduction in mortality compared to placebo. However, it has not been demonstrated that terlipressin is superior to octreotide, somatostatin or endoscopic treatment alone.[45] There is experimental evidence that terlipressin has a more sustained haemodynamic effect than octreotide. In a randomised study of 42 cirrhotic patients with a history of variceal haemorrhage, both agents significantly decreased HVPG and portal venous flow; however, octreotide bolus followed by infusion had only a transient effect lasting 5 minutes whereas terlipressin exerted effects at all time points up to 25 minutes.[46] Terlipressin also achieved a reduction in HVPG of > 20% in 36% of cases versus 5% with high-dose somatostatin in a randomised, double-blind trial of 'non-responders' to a standard somatostatin dose.[47] Other potential benefits of terlipressin over somatostatin are increased renal sodium excretion.[48]

Meta-analysis of 939 patients demonstrated that the use of vasoactive drugs in combination with endoscopic therapy (either band ligation or sclerotherapy) is superior than endoscopic therapy alone in terms of initial control of bleeding and 5-day re-bleeding rates but there was no difference in overall mortality.[49]

A recent randomised trial comparing different doses of somatostatin (500 mg/h versus 250 mg/h) in combination with sclerotherapy demonstrated that higher doses were associated with significantly lower rates of re-bleeding for Childs–Pugh B/C patients (39% versus 13%).[50]

Terlipressin has the more robust evidence to advocate its use, and the above provide some further theoretical support. Side effects include cardiac and peripheral ischaemia and an ECG is mandatory before commencing treatment. Vasoactive treatment should ideally be continued for 5 days from the index bleed when the risk of re-bleeding is high.

Antibiotics

Bacterial infection may play a role in triggering variceal haemorrhage and is common in hospitalised cirrhotic patients. There is strong evidence that the use of prophylactic antibiotics reduces mortality in variceal bleeding.

Oral quinolones or intravenous cephalosporins have been the traditional antimicrobial of choice. Recent evidence from Fernandez et al.[51] suggests ceftriaxone is superior to norfloxacin. In 111 patients with advanced cirrhosis and gastrointestinal bleeding, use of oral norfloxacin was associated with proven infection in 26% of cases versus 11% with intravenous ceftriaxone ($P = 0.03$). There was no difference in mortality between the groups. Six out of seven patients in the norfloxacin group had Gram-negative bacilli which were quinolone resistant.[51] Other advantages of cephalosporins may be a decreased incidence of Clostridium difficile.

Recombinant factor VIIa

Activated factor VII transiently lowers the prothrombin time, the duration being dose-dependent. A randomised, double-blind trial showed no difference in mortality or adverse effects but found that factor VIIa increased haemostasis in Childs–Pugh B/C variceal bleeders.[52] In a single-centre, open-label study involving eight patients with variceal bleeding refractory to at least one standard treatment, haemostasis was achieved in all cases. However, re-bleeding occurred in 25% of cases and mortality was 50%.[53] At present its use appears safe and is justified for cases of uncontrollable haemorrhage; it should be considered on a case-by-case basis for early re-bleeders.

Transjugular intrahepatic portosystemic shunt

In the minority of cases where combined endoscopic and vasoactive drug therapy has not controlled bleeding, transjugular intrahepatic portosystemic shunts (TIPS) have been used to lower portal, and hence variceal pressure, acutely. In longitudinal studies, survival at 1 year is approximately 50%. The procedure is usually successful both technically and in reducing the portosystemic pressure gradient. A retrospective–prospective analysis found that patients receiving TIPS for variceal bleeding had a significantly longer survival than patients with refractory ascites, presumably reflecting the fact that refractory ascites often co-exists with severe end-stage liver disease.[54]

In cases of cirrhosis complicated by portal vein thrombosis, an American group has shown that TIPS placement is still technically feasible in 87% of cases with a 30-day mortality of 13%.[55] However, this was a small group of patients and results need to be confirmed with further studies – it is unlikely that such technically complex procedures will be undertaken in any but the most expert centres.

The main complication of TIPS placement is hepatic encephalopathy which can occur in up to one-third of patients, although it often improves after a number of weeks and can usually be managed medically. In a small number of refractory cases, shunt reduction (*i.e.* reducing the diameter of the shunt and thus the volume of blood bypassing the liver) may be required although the outcome is variable – 58% noted improvement and 42% remained unchanged or experienced worsening of hepatic encephalopathy in one study where the majority had TIPS insertion for variceal bleeding.[56]

One of the longer term complications of TIPS placement is shunt stenosis. Primary patency rates for TIPS are approximately 79–90% at 1 year,[57,58] and there remains no definitive answer to the question of whether, and how often, shunt patency should be assessed. Pseudo-intimal hyperplasia (*i.e.* granulation tissue forming along the tract between hepatic and portal veins) is thought to lead to TIPS stenosis. Brachytherapy has for some time been proposed to reduce pseudo-intimal hyperplasia in arterial stents and an interesting swine model[59] demonstrating improved TIPS patency following intraluminal irradiation has been repeated in a small human study. Seventeen patients randomised to receive a dose of 14 Gy from iridium-192 via intraluminal brachytherapy had a significantly lower incidence of shunt stenosis (29% versus 66.7%) at 1 year.[60] All patients had portal hypertension secondary to cirrhosis. Further studies on larger numbers of patients are required to determine if this translates to improved morbidity and mortality. In recent years, polytetrafluoroethylene-covered (PTFE) stents have been used more widely as they have been shown to increase long-term patency rates, and decrease the incidence of variceal bleeding and encephalopathy. However, in a single-centre, open study comparing 316 patients with uncovered stents and 157 patients with covered stents, no survival benefit was seen.[61] A smaller retrospective study by Barrio *et al.*[62] also showed improvements in various clinical and haemodynamic parameters with the use of covered stents but, again, no survival benefit.

Embolotherapy

A further approach to treating uncontrolled bleeding may be the combination of TIPS and adjunctive embolotherapy. In a single-centre study, patients treated with TIPS who continued to have a pressure gradient > 12 mmHg and varices which continued to fill were treated with sclerosing agents or coils to embolise vessels. The re-bleeding rate was significantly reduced at 2 years and 4 years (81% versus 53%, respectively).[63] Further studies are required to determine if these results are reproducible and to which patient groups this treatment is best applied.

Another radiological option is percutaneous transhepatic variceal embolisation where access to the portal system is gained percutaneously through the liver. This procedure has not been widely adopted due to high rates of variceal recurrence and re-bleeding. A recent randomised trial failed to show any survival advantage with embolisation as compared to ligation.[64] The group studied was heterogeneous including patients with acute or 'recent' variceal bleeding. Portocaval shunts can also be placed trans-hepatically in a method similar to TIPS and offers the theoretical advantage of improved patency rates (due to more direct control of shunt deployment). However, the two techniques have only been compared in a small head-to-head study of patients with portal hypertension in which only three had the procedure performed due to variceal bleeding.[65]

A similar technique pioneered in Leeds is percutaneous trans-splenic access with or without TIPS creation. This has been performed in patients with uncontrolled variceal haemorrhage secondary to portal vein thrombosis. Although performed in only three patients so far, it provides an additional route for endovascular treatment for refractory bleeding in patients for whom surgery is high risk and traditional TIPS placement is technically difficult or impossible.[66]

SURGICAL OPTIONS

Historically, surgery was one of the main-stays of treatment for uncontrolled variceal bleeding but it has been largely superseded by radiological techniques. As would be expected, surgical approaches are safer in patients with preserved liver function (Childs–Pugh A/B). In brief, the surgical methods are portosystemic shunting or oesophageal devascularisation.

Surgical shunts

Splenorenal shunts are the most often used although, in cases where previous surgery renders this impossible, mesogonadal shunts have been used with long-term success.[67] In a single-centre, retrospective, case review, distal splenorenal shunt (DSRS) performed in well-selected patients (*i.e.* Childs–Pugh A/B), 30-day mortality was 6.4%, recurrence of varices occurred in 5.4% and encephalopathy in 11.7%.[68]

Portosystemic shunting using a prosthetic H-graft mirrors the TIPS procedure in redirecting blood but introduces the risks of general anaesthesia and open surgery. Variceal re-bleeding rates are as low as 2% in some centres and long-term survival (> 10 years) was documented as 7% for Childs–Pugh C patients.[69]

DSRS was compared to TIPS in a multicentre, randomised, controlled trial. In terms of haemorrhage control, both interventions were similarly efficacious with no significant difference in 5-year survival or risk of encephalopathy. Interestingly, thrombosis, stenosis and re-intervention rates were significantly higher in the TIPS group (82% versus 11%), suggesting that, in skilled hands, DSRS may be a better alternative to TIPS.[70] This study did, however, exclude patients with Childs C cirrhosis in whom surgery is higher risk and in whom TIPS is likely to be a better option.

Surgical devascularisation

The Sugiura procedure (oesophageal devascularisation) has variable results and has undergone several modifications. The Japanese have reported low mortality (5%) and re-bleeding rates but these results have not been reproduced in the West.

In a long-term follow-up study in Saudi Arabia, transabdominal gastro-oesophageal devascularisation and oesophageal transection was performed on patients primarily with portal hypertension secondary to bilharzia. Complete variceal eradication was achieved in 70.6% of cases with an in-hospital mortality of 12.7%. The 15-year survival declined with Childs–Pugh grade (A, 44%; B, 22.5%; and C, 0%).[71] A recent retrospective analysis from India found that devascularisation without transection resulted in significantly fewer complications but a mortality of 31%.[72]

The choice between surgical and radiological treatment will depend to some extent on local resources and skills. In the West, radiological intervention has become standard; however, it is important not to loose the surgical expertise required to fashion portosystemic shunts for those patients where TIPS has failed or is not an option.

SECONDARY PROPHYLAXIS

Re-bleeding is highly likely to occur if there is no further treatment following the index bleed. Data from control groups indicate that around two-thirds of patients will re-bleed at 2 years leading to significant mortality (33%).[73]

Band ligation alone does not reduce bleeding risk completely; if portal pressure remains elevated, troublesome portal hypertensive gastropathy can occur as well as re-bleeding whilst the patient is enrolled in a banding programme. The methodology and timing of prophylactic band ligation is not well studied. It appears that the placement of large numbers of bands (> 6) in a single session has no advantage in terms of reducing the number of sessions required to achieve variceal eradication and may be associated with more complications.[74]

β-Blockers have been shown to decrease portal pressure and result in a lower incidence of re-bleeding by reducing cardiac output and producing splanchnic vasoconstriction. Meta-analysis has conclusively shown a reduction in re-bleeding and mortality but some patients have unacceptable side effects.

Other drugs considered for prophylaxis include angiotensin II receptor blockers. Olmesartan is a new angiotensin II (subtype I) receptor blocker. A third of patients with a history of variceal bleeding showed > 20% reduction in

HPVG after 14 days of treatment.[75] In contrast, candesartan is not effective in reducing portal pressure.[76]

The combination of band ligation and β-blockers has been shown to be more effective than either treatment modality alone. A randomised study of 80 patients with cirrhosis (Childs–Pugh grades A–C) showed that the re-bleeding rate was 38% in the ligation (monotherapy) group versus 14% in the nadolol and ligation group after a median follow-up period of 16 months with no difference in mortality.[77] Lowering portal pressure with drugs did not significantly affect the number of endoscopic treatments required to eradicate varices and there was no significant difference in recurrence rates of varices at 1 year.

EXTRA-OESOPHAGEAL VARICES AND TREATMENT

Gastric varices occur in approximately 15–20% of patients with portal hypertension and may occur in conjunction with oesophageal varices (primary) or following the eradication of oesophageal varices (secondary). The incidence of bleeding is approximately 20%.[78]

DIAGNOSIS

Endoscopic Doppler ultrasound has been piloted to aid differentiation of gastric varices from other gastric submucosal lesions.[79] Higher eradication rates and hence lower re-bleeding rates may be possible using endoscopic ultrasound to identify where perforating veins enter individual gastric varices. This is a time consuming and costly process and currently has only been used in a case series involving five patients and requires further validation.[80]

TREATMENT

The initial treatment is identical to that of oesophageal varices (*i.e.* fluid resuscitation and vasoactive drugs). Following endoscopic diagnosis of bleeding gastric varices, band ligation can control bleeding in the acute setting but is often followed by re-bleeding and is not recommended as routine treatment. Endoscopic techniques in common usage include sclerotherapy or the injection of cyanoacrylate tissue glue which achieves high rates of haemostasis. A Japanese group studied the effects of gastric variceal sclerotherapy with 5% ethanolamine oleate. Judging efficacy is difficult as patients were also treated with vasopressin and transdermal nitroglycerin patch. Complete haemostasis was achieved in 93.3%, with a 1-year re-bleeding rate of 13%, and a 1-year mortality of 31%.[81]

Recent evidence supports the earlier findings that re-bleeding rates are higher with ligation compared to glue/tissue adhesive injection, although efficacy for controlling acute bleeding is the same.[82] Interestingly, despite the much higher re-bleeding rates at 2 years and 3 years, there is no difference in survival. Another group found cyanoacrylate achieved haemostasis in all treated patients with re-bleeding occurring in 14% at 48 h.[78]

In a study assessing a combination of cyanoacrylate and band ligation, targeted ligation solely of the bleeding spot prior to cyanoacrylate injection

gave a haemostasis rate of 88.9% at 1 week. The final haemostasis rate was 81.5% although approximately a third had recurrent bleeding within the follow-up period of 5–53 months.[83]

A Taiwanese group has recently studied the effects of combining cyanoacrylate with hypertonic glucose injection. Patients with gastric variceal bleeding were treated with cyanoacrylate injection and subsequently randomised to receive adjuvant hypertonic glucose injection or not. Significantly more patients from the 'combined' group remained free of gastric varices at 2 years (92.8% versus 71.4%, respectively). Although no difference in survival was demonstrated, the use of adjuvant hypertonic glucose solution appears safe and relatively simple.[84]

A rare, but serious, side effect of tissue adhesive injection is cyanoacrylate embolism with anecdotal reports of both lung and brain emboli. Reduction in the risk of emboli might be made by refinement of injection techniques such as increasing the amount of glue used during a single injection – although there is, as yet, no evidence to support this.

TRANSJUGULAR INTRAHEPATIC PORTOSYSTEMIC SHUNT

TIPS has been shown to control bleeding from gastric varices by both reducing the portosystemic gradient and allowing access to the varices for coil embolisation. In a randomised comparison of TIPS and cyanoacrylate, after the initial control of bleeding, patients were randomised to cyanoacrylate (repeated until eradication) or TIPS. Variceal eradication was achieved in 51% of cyanoacrylate patients and 20% of TIPS patients but re-bleeding rates were lower in the TIPS group (38% versus 11%, respectively). Survival and frequency of complications were not significantly different.[85]

BALLOON-OCCLUDED RETROGRADE TRANSVENOUS OBLITERATION

This radiological technique developed in Japan has yet to find much support in the UK. Balloon-occluded retrograde transvenous obliteration (BORTO) involves cannulation of the gastric varix from the iliac vein via a naturally formed splenorenal shunt. Once in position, a balloon is inflated in the vessel lumen blocking blood flow and 5% ethanolamine oleate is injected retrogradely (Fig. 3). This technique can be used in the acute setting (after endoscopic treatment) or as an elective treatment for the eradication of gastric varices.

Clinical success rates are in the region of 75% with 2-year survival at 55%.[86] Although follow-up data suggest two-thirds of patients may experience worsening of oesophageal varices. Other complications included aggravation of ascites and portal hypertensive gastropathy. A further long-term follow-up study showed encouraging results with a 68% 5-year survival rate and haemostasis achieved in 94% of cases of bleeding gastric varices. Over 5 years, half of patients had worsening of oesophageal varices and 10% had oesophageal variceal haemorrhage. Re-bleeding from gastric varices was not observed after eradication.[87]

BORTO also appears to be effective as prophylaxis for gastric variceal bleeding. Non-randomised data demonstrated a lower bleeding rate at 1, 3 and

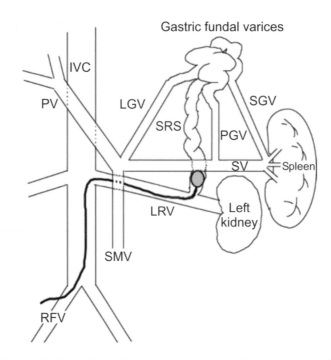

Fig. 3 Schematic illustrating balloon-occluded retrograde transvenous obliteration (BORTO) technique. Reproduced with permission from *J Gastroenterol Hepatol* 2003: **18**: 934–942 © 2003 Blackwell Publishing. IVC, inferior vena cava; LGV, left gastric vein; LRV, left renal vein; PGV, posterior gastric vein; PV, portal vein; RFV, right femoral vein; SGV, short gastric vein; SMV, superior mesenteric vein; SRS, splenorenal shunt; SV, splenic vein.

5 years with a significantly increased survival rate in patients treated with BORTO versus control.[88]

NON-CIRRHOTIC PORTAL HYPERTENSION

The majority of data pertain to portal hypertension secondary to cirrhosis. Rarely, conditions such as portal vein thrombosis, Budd–Chiari syndrome and congenital or acquired conditions can lead to portal hypertension in the absence of cirrhosis. The absence of clinical signs or clues in the history to chronic liver disease will diminish the clinician's suspicion that haematemesis may be of variceal origin. The absence of chronic liver disease means that patients are, in the main, better able to withstand the physiological stress of a major gastrointestinal bleed and, therefore, mortality is lower than in patients with established cirrhosis.

Endoscopic treatment and vasoactive drugs are still effective in this scenario; indeed, TIPS has been shown to be technically feasible even in the presence of portal vein thrombus although not in all cases with some centres advocating the use of both TIPS and local injection of thrombolytic agents in combination. As mentioned previously, trans-splenic access has recently been performed in patients with portal vein thrombosis with uncontrollable variceal bleeding. The consensus of current opinion is that patients with procoagulant tendencies and a history of variceal bleeding as a consequence of hepatic venous thrombosis should be anticoagulated (unless there are major contra-indications) in conjunction with standard prophylaxis of further variceal bleeding. There is a need for data on the risks and benefits in this difficult clinical scenario as there is no agreement on the duration of anticoagulation.[11]

SUMMARY

Variceal bleeding is a medical emergency with a high mortality. The majority occur on the background of cirrhosis, although non-cirrhotic portal hypertension should not be forgotten as a cause. The rising incidence of cirrhosis will present a challenge to health service planners in the future and effective treatment requires a multidisciplinary, multimodality approach. Attention to halting the progression of cirrhosis and lowering portal pressure are key in the long-term management.

During acute variceal haemorrhage, basic resuscitation should occur initially with the early use of vasoactive drugs and prophylactic antibiotics. Specialist endoscopy should be available within 12 h and should be performed by an endoscopist experienced in the management of portal hypertension and familiar with several techniques for haemostasis. Failure to control bleeding endoscopically should lead to consideration for radiological shunt insertion.

Advances in recent years have lead to many more therapeutic options in the management of portal hypertension; despite this, mortality remains high due to the underlying presence of liver disease. Attention to other aspects of liver support (nutrition, ascites management, control of sepsis) will improve outcome. The multidisciplinary nature of the control of complex variceal bleeding and degree of technical expertise required would suggest that patients will benefit from transfer to regional specialist centres, although not necessarily transplant centres.

There remains much work to be done to identify cost-effective non-invasive ways to detect varices and determine their potential to bleed, as well as refining methods to identify which interventional technique will best serve an individual patient.

Key points for clinical practice

- The incidence of cirrhosis and portal hypertension is increasing. With untreated portal hypertension the development and progression of varices is inevitable.

- The mortality associated with variceal bleeding is decreasing due to modern techniques.

- All patients with cirrhosis should be screened for varices at diagnosis until a reliable model has been developed.

- Patients with small varices should be treated with a β-blocker.

- Patients with medium or large varices should enter a band ligation programme if intolerant to β-blockers. High-risk patients may benefit from a combination of both treatments.

(continued)

Key points for clinical practice *(continued)*

- Acute treatment of variceal haemorrhage includes fluid resuscitation, vasoactive drugs, prophylactic antibiotics and early endoscopy with band ligation if possible. Balloon tamponade can be used as a bridge to other rescue treatments.

- Rescue therapy depends on local expertise. Transjugular intrahepatic portosystemic shunts and surgical shunts are effective in controlling bleeding and preventing re-bleeding. Liver transplant should be considered.

- Gastric varices should be treated with cyanoacrylate injection and subsequent radiological intervention.

- Novel techniques such as the use of self-expanding metal stents and balloon-occluded retrograde transvenous obliteration may become more widely adopted in the UK in the future.

References

1. Hearnshaw S, Travis S, Murphy M. The role of blood transfusion in the management of upper and lower intestinal tract bleeding. *Best Pract Res Clin Gastroenterol* 2008; **22**: 355–371.
2. Thabut D, Hammer M, Cai Y, Carbonell N. Cost of treatment of oesophageal variceal bleeding in patients with cirrhosis in France: results of a French survey. *Eur J Gastroenterol Hepatol* 2007; **19**: 679–686.
3. de Franchis R, Dell'Era A. Diagnosis and therapy of esophageal vascular disorders. *Curr Opin Gastroenterol* 2007; **23**: 422–427.
4. de Franchis R. (ed) *Portal Hypertension IV: Proceedings of the Fourth Baveno International Consensus Workshop.* Oxford: Blackwell, 2005.
5. Jalan R, Hayes PC. UK guidelines on the management of variceal haemorrhage in cirrhotic patients. British Society of Gastroenterology. *Gut* 2000; **46 (Suppl 3/4)**: III1–III15.
6. Garcia-Tsao G. Liver involvement in hereditary hemorrhagic telangiectasia (HHT). *J Hepatol* 2007; **46**: 499–507.
7. Goulis J, Patch D, Burroughs AK. Bacterial infection in the pathogenesis of variceal bleeding. *Lancet* 1999; **353**: 139–142.
8. Albillos A, Banares R, González M *et al.* The extent of the collateral circulation influences the postprandial increase in portal pressure in patients with cirrhosis. *Gut* 2007; **56**: 259–264.
9. Ferguson JW, Helmy A, Ludlam C, Webb DJ, Hayes PC, Newby DC. Hyperfibrinolysis in alcoholic cirrhosis: relative plasminogen activator inhibitor type 1 deficiency. *Thromb Res* 2008; **121**: 675–680.
10. Kovalak M, Lake J, Mattek N, Eisen G, Lieberman D, Zaman A. Endoscopic screening for varices in cirrhotic patients: data from a national endoscopic database. *Gastrointest Endosc* 2007; **65**: 82–88.
11. de Franchis R. Evolving consensus in portal hypertension. Report of the Baveno IV consensus workshop on methodology of diagnosis and therapy in portal hypertension. *J Hepatol* 2005; **43**: 167–176.
12. Kazemi F, Kettaneh A, N'kontchou *et al.* Liver stiffness measurement selects patients with cirrhosis at risk of bearing large oesophageal varices. *J Hepatol* 2006; **45**: 230–235.
13. Vanbiervliet G, Barjoan-Mariné E, Anty R *et al.* Serum fibrosis markers can detect large oesophageal varices with a high accuracy. *Eur J Gastroenterol Hepatol* 2005; **17**: 333–338.
14. Thabut D, Trabut JB, Massard J *et al.* Non-invasive diagnosis of large oesophageal varices with FibroTest in patients with cirrhosis: a preliminary retrospective study. *Liver*

Int 2006; **26**: 271–278.

15. Zardi EM, Uwechie V, Gentilucci UV *et al*. Portal diameter in the diagnosis of esophageal varices in 266 cirrhotic patients: which role? *Ultrasound Med Biol* 2007; **33**: 506–511.

16. Giannini EG, Zaman A, Kreil A *et al*. Platelet count/spleen diameter ratio for the noninvasive diagnosis of esophageal varices: results of a multicenter, prospective, validation study. *Am J Gastroenterol* 2006; **101**: 2511–2519.

17. Sanyal AJ, Fontana RJ, Di Bisceglie AM *et al*. for Halt-C Trial Group. The prevalence and risk factors associated with esophageal varices in subjects with hepatitis C and advanced fibrosis. *Gastrointest Endosc* 2006; **64**: 855–864.

18. Kim YJ, Raman SS, Yu NC, Too KJ, Jutabha R, Lu DSK. Esophageal varices in cirrhotic patients: evaluation with liver CT. *AJR Am J Roentgenol* 2007; **188**: 139–144.

19. Mifune H, Akaki S, Ida K, Sei T, Kanazawa S, Okada H. Evaluation of esophageal varices by multidetector-row CT: correlation with endoscopic 'red color sign'. *Acta Med Okayama* 2007; **61**: 247–254.

20. Pena LR, Cox T, Koch AG, Bosch A. Study comparing oesophageal capsule endoscopy versus EGD in the detection of varices. *Dig Liver Dis* 2008; **40**: 216–223.

21. Lapalus MG, Dumortier J, Fumex F *et al*. Esophageal capsule endoscopy versus esophagogastroduodenoscopy for evaluating portal hypertension: a prospective comparative study of performance and tolerance. *Endoscopy* 2006; **38**: 36–41.

22. Eisen GM, Eliakim R, Zaman A *et al*. The accuracy of PillCam ESO capsule endoscopy versus conventional upper endoscopy for the diagnosis of esophageal varices: a prospective three-center pilot study. *Endoscopy* 2006; **38**: 31–35.

23. Ripoll C, Groszmann R, Garcia-Tsao G *et al*. and Portal Hypertension Collaborative Group. Hepatic venous pressure gradient predicts clinical decompensation in patients with compensated cirrhosis. *Gastroenterology* 2007; **133**: 481–488.

24. D'Amico G, Garcia-Pagan JC, Luca A, Bosch J. Hepatic vein pressure gradient reduction and prevention of variceal bleeding in cirrhosis: a systematic review. *Gastroenterology* 2006; **131**: 1611–1624.

25. Spahr L, Giostra E, Morard I, Mentha G, Hadengue A. Perendoscopic variceal pressure measurement: a reliable estimation of portal pressure in patients with cirrhosis? *Gastroenterol Clin Biol* 2006; **30**: 1012–1018.

26. Abraldes JG, Villanueva C, Banares R *et al*. Hepatic venous pressure gradient and prognosis in patients with acute variceal bleeding treated with pharmacologic and endoscopic therapy. *J Hepatol* 2008; **48**: 229–236.

27. Tacke F, Fiedler K, Trautwein C. A simple clinical score predicts high risk for upper gastrointestinal hemorrhages from varices in patients with chronic liver disease. *Scand J Gastroenterol* 2007; **42**: 374–382.

28. Sarwar S, Dilshad A, Tariq S. Predictors of rebleed and mortality in patients with non-variceal upper gastrointestinal bleed. *J Coll Physicians Surg Pak* 2007; **17**: 384.

29. Ismail FW, Mumtaz K, Shah HA *et al*. Factors predicting in-hospital mortality in patients with cirrhosis hospitalized with gastro-esophageal variceal hemorrhage. *Indian J Gastroenterol* 2006; **25**: 240–243.

30. Kadouchi K, Higuchi K, Shiba M *et al*. What are the risk factors for aggravation of esophageal varices in patients with hepatocellular carcinoma? *J Gastroenterol Hepatol* 2007; **22**: 240–246.

31. Thomopoulos K, Theocharis G, Mimidis K, Lampropoulou-Karatza Ch, Alexandridis E, Nikolopoulou V. Improved survival of patients presenting with acute variceal bleeding. Prognostic indicators of short- and long-term mortality. *Dig Liver Dis* 2006; **38**: 899–904.

32. Tsubaki T, Sato S, Fujikawa H *et al*. Values of Doppler sonography predicts high risk variceal bleeding in patients with viral cirrhosis. *Hepatogastroenterology* 2007; **54**: 96–99.

33. Merli M, Nicolini G, Angeloni S *et al*. Incidence and natural history of small esophageal varices in cirrhotic patients. *J Hepatol* 2003; **38**: 266–272.

34. Khuroo MS, Khuroo NS, Farahat KL, Khuroo YS, Sofi AA, Dahab ST. Meta-analysis: endoscopic variceal ligation for primary prophylaxis of oesophageal variceal bleeding. *Aliment Pharmacol Ther* 2005; **21**: 347–361.

35. Norberto L, Polese L, Cillo U *et al*. A randomized study comparing ligation with propranolol for primary prophylaxis of variceal bleeding in candidates for liver transplantation. *Liver Transpl* 2007; **13**: 1272–1278.

36. Sarin SK, Wadhawan M, Agarwal SR, Tyagi P, Sharma BC. Endoscopic variceal ligation plus propranolol versus endoscopic variceal ligation alone in primary prophylaxis of variceal bleeding. *Am J Gastroenterol* 2005; **100**: 797-804.

37. Gheorghe C, Gheorghe L, Iacob S, Iacob R, Popescu I. Primary prophylaxis of variceal bleeding in cirrhotics awaiting liver transplantation. *Hepatogastroenterology* 2006; **53**: 552–557.

38. Turnes J, Garcia-Pagan JC, Abraldes JG, Hernandez-Guerra M, Dell'Era A, Bosch J. Pharmacological reduction of portal pressure and long-term risk of first variceal bleeding in patients with cirrhosis. *Am J Gastroenterol* 2006; **101**: 506–512.

39. Laine L, Cook D. Endoscopic ligation compared with sclerotherapy for treatment of esophageal variceal bleeding. A meta-analysis. *Ann Intern Med* 1995; **123**: 280–287.

40. Lo GH, Lai KH, Cheng JS *et al*. The additive effect of sclerotherapy to patients receiving repeated endoscopic variceal ligation: a prospective, randomized trial. *Hepatology* 1998; **28**: 391–395.

41. Zargar SA, Javid G, Khan BA *et al*. Endoscopic ligation vs. sclerotherapy in adults with extrahepatic portal venous obstruction: a prospective randomized study. *Gastrointest Endosc* 2005; **61**: 58–66.

42. Pinto-Marques P, Romaozinho JM, Ferreira M, Amaro P, Freitas D. Esophageal perforation – associated risk with balloon tamponade after endoscopic therapy. Myth or reality? *Hepatogastroenterology* 2006; **53**: 536–539.

43. Chong CF. Esophageal rupture due to Sengstaken–Blakemore tube misplacement. *World J Gastroenterol* 2005; **11**: 6563–6565.

44. Hubmann R, Bodlaj G, Czompo M *et al*. The use of self-expanding metal stents to treat acute esophageal variceal bleeding. *Endoscopy* 2006; **38**: 896–901.

45. Ioannou G, Doust J, Rockey DC. Terlipressin for acute esophageal variceal hemorrhage. *Cochrane Database of Systematic Reviews* 2002, Issue 4. Art. No.: CD002147. DOI: 10.1002/14651858.CD002147.

46. Baik SK, Jeong PH, Ji S *et al*. Acute hemodynamic effects of octreotide and terlipressin in patients with cirrhosis: a randomized comparison. *Am J Gastroenterol* 2005; **100**: 631–635.

47. Villanueva C, Planella M, Aracil C *et al*. Hemodynamic effects of terlipressin and high somatostatin dose during acute variceal bleeding in nonresponders to the usual somatostatin dose. *Am J Gastroenterol* 2005; **100**: 624–630.

48. Kalambokis G, Economou M, Paraskevi K *et al*. Effects of somatostatin, terlipressin and somatostatin plus terlipressin on portal and systemic hemodynamics and renal sodium excretion in patients with cirrhosis. *J Gastroenterol Hepatol* 2005; **20**: 1075–1081.

49. Banares R, Albillos A, Rincon D *et al*. Endoscopic treatment versus endoscopic plus pharmacologic treatment for acute variceal bleeding: a meta-analysis. *Hepatology* 2002; **35**: 609–615.

50. Palazon JM, Such J, Sánchez-Payá J *et al*. A comparison of two different dosages of somatostatin combined with sclerotherapy for the treatment of acute esophageal variceal bleeding: a prospective randomized trial. *Rev Esp Enferm Dig* 2006; **98**: 249–254.

51. Fernández J, Ruiz del Arbol L, Gomez C *et al*. Norfloxacin vs ceftriaxone in the prophylaxis of infections in patients with advanced cirrhosis and hemorrhage. *Gastroenterology* 2006; **131**: 1049–1056.

52. Bosch J, Thabut D, Albillos A *et al*. for International Study Group on rFVIIa in UGI Hemorrhage. Recombinant factor VIIa for variceal bleeding in patients with advanced cirrhosis: a randomized, controlled trial. *Hepatology* 2008; **47**: 1604–1614.

53. Romero-Castro R, Jimenez-Saenz M, Pellicer-Bautista F *et al*. Recombinant-activated factor VII as hemostatic therapy in eight cases of severe hemorrhage from esophageal varices. *Clin Gastroenterol Hepatol* 2004; **2**: 78–84.

54. Membreno F, Baez AL, Pandula R, Walser E, Lau DT. Differences in long-term survival after transjugular intrahepatic portosystemic shunt for refractory ascites and variceal bleed. *J Gastroenterol Hepatol* 2005; **20**: 474–481.

55. Van Ha TG, Hodge J, Funaki B *et al*. Transjugular intrahepatic portosystemic shunt placement in patients with cirrhosis and concomitant portal vein thrombosis. *Cardiovasc Intervent Radiol* 2006; **29**: 785–790.

56. Kochar N, Tripathi D, Ireland H, Redhead DN, Hayes PC. Transjugular intrahepatic portosystemic stent shunt (TIPSS) modification in the management of post-TIPSS

refractory hepatic encephalopathy. *Gut* 2006; **55**: 1617–1623.

57. Vignali C, Bargellini I, Grosso M *et al.* TIPS with expanded polytetrafluoroethylene-covered stent: results of an Italian multicenter study. *AJR Am J Roentgenol* 2005; **185**: 472–480.

58. Rössle M, Siegerstetter V, Euringer W *et al.* The use of a polytetrafluoroethylene-covered stent graft for transjugular intrahepatic portosystemic shunt (TIPS): Long-term follow-up of 100 patients. *Acta Radiol* 2006; **47**: 660–666.

59. Park JS, Oh JH, Kim DY *et al.* Effects of intraluminal irradiation with holmium-166 for TIPS stenosis: experimental study in a swine model, *Korean J Radiol* 2007; **8**: 127–135.

60. Hidajat N, Stupavsky A, Gellermann J. Intraluminal brachytherapy of *de novo* TIPS: a prospective randomized double-blind study. *AJR Am J Roentgenol* 2006; **186**: 1133–1137.

61. Tripathi D, Ferguson J, Barkell H *et al.* Improved clinical outcome with transjugular intrahepatic portosystemic stent-shunt utilizing polytetrafluoroethylene-covered stents. *Eur J Gastroenterol Hepatol* 2006; **18**: 225–232.

62. Barrio J, Ripoll C, Banares R *et al.* Comparison of transjugular intrahepatic portosystemic shunt dysfunction in PTFE-covered stent-grafts versus bare stents. *Eur J Radiol* 2005; **55**: 120–124.

63. Tesdal IK, Filser T, Weiss C, Holm E, Dueber C, Jaschke W. Transjugular intrahepatic portosystemic shunts: adjunctive embolotherapy of gastroesophageal collateral vessels in the prevention of variceal rebleeding. *Radiology* 2005; **236**: 360–367.

64. Zhang CQ, Liu FL, Liang B *et al.* A modified percutaneous transhepatic variceal embolization with 2-octyl cyanoacrylate versus endoscopic ligation in esophageal variceal bleeding management: randomized controlled trial. *Dig Dis Sci* 2008; **53**: 2258–2267.

65. Hoppe H, Wang SL, Petersen BD. Intravascular US-guided direct intrahepatic portocaval shunt with an expanded polytetrafluoroethylene-covered stent-graft. *Radiology* 2008; **246**: 306–314.

66. Tuite DJ, Rehman J, Davies MH, Patel JV, Nicholson AA, Kessel DO. Percutaneous transsplenic access in the management of bleeding varices from chronic portal vein thrombosis. *J Vasc Interv Radiol* 2007; **18**: 1571–1575.

67. Kim HB, Pomposelli JJ, Lillehei CW *et al.* Mesogonadal shunts for extrahepatic portal vein thrombosis and variceal hemorrhage. *Liver Transpl* 2005; **11**: 1389–1394.

68. Elwood DR, Pomposelli JJ, Pomfret EA, Lewis WD, Jenkins RL. Distal splenorenal shunt: preferred treatment for recurrent variceal hemorrhage in the patient with well-compensated cirrhosis. *Arch Surg* 2006; **141**: 385–388.

69. Rosemurgy A, Thometz D, Clark W *et al.* Survival and variceal rehemorrhage after shunting support small-diameter prosthetic H-graft portacaval shunt. *J Gastrointest Surg* 2007; **11**: 325–332.

70. Henderson JM. Surgery versus transjugular intrahepatic portal systemic shunt in the treatment of severe variceal bleeding. *Clin Liver Dis* 2006; **10**: 599–612.

71. Qazi SA, Khalid K, Hameed AM *et al.* Transabdominal gastro-esophageal devascularization and esophageal transection for bleeding esophageal varices after failed injection sclerotherapy: long-term follow-up report. *World J Surg* 2006; **30**: 1329–1337.

72. Johnson M, Rajendran S, Kannan TG *et al.* Transabdominal modified devascularization procedure with or without esophageal stapler transection – an operation adequate for effective control of a variceal bleed. Is esophageal stapler transection necessary? *World J Surg* 2006; **30**: 1507–1518.

73. Lebrec D. Review: pharmacotherapeutic agents in the treatment of portal hypertension. *J Gastroenterol Hepatol* 1997; **12**: 159–166.

74. Ramirez FC, Colon VJ, Landan D, Grade AJ, Evanich E. The effects of the number of rubber bands placed at each endoscopic session upon variceal outcomes: a prospective, randomized study. *Am J Gastroenterol* 2007; **102**: 1372–1376.

75. Hidaka H, Kokubu S, Nakazawa T *et al.* New angiotensin II type 1 receptor blocker olmesartan improves portal hypertension in patients with cirrhosis. *Hepatol Res* 2007; **37**: 1011–1017.

76. Heim MH, Jacob L, Beglinger C. The angiotensin II receptor antagonist candesartan is not effective in reducing portal hypertension in patients with cirrhosis. *Digestion* 2007;

75: 122–123.

77. de la Pena J, Brullet E, Sanchez-Hernandez E *et al.* EVL Study Group. Variceal ligation plus nadolol compared with ligation for prophylaxis of variceal rebleeding: a multicenter trial. *Hepatology* 2005; **41**: 572–578.

78. Mumtaz K, Majid S, Shah HA *et al.* Prevalence of gastric varices and results of sclerotherapy with N-butyl-2-cyanoacrylate for controlling acute gastric variceal bleeding. *World J Gastroenterol* 2007; **13**: 1247–1251.

79. Wong RC, Farooq FT, Chak A. Endoscopic Doppler US probe for the diagnosis of gastric varices (with videos). *Gastrointest Endosc* 2007; **65**: 491–496.

80. Romero-Castro R, Pellicer-Bautista FJ, Jimenez-Saenz M *et al.* EUS-guided injection of cyanoacrylate in perforating feeding veins in gastric varices: results in 5 cases. *Gastrointest Endosc* 2007; **66**: 402–407.

81. Kojima K, Imazu H, Matsumura M *et al.* Sclerotherapy for gastric fundal variceal bleeding: is complete obliteration possible without cyanoacrylate? *J Gastroenterol Hepatol* 2005; **20**: 1701–1706.

82. Tan PC, Hou MC, Lin HC *et al.* A randomized trial of endoscopic treatment of acute gastric variceal hemorrhage: N-butyl-2-cyanoacrylate injection versus band ligation. *Hepatology* 2006; **43**: 690–697.

83. Sugimoto N, Watanabe K, Watanabe K *et al.* Endoscopic hemostasis for bleeding gastric varices treated by combination of variceal ligation and sclerotherapy with N-butyl-2-cyanoacrylate. *J Gastroenterol* 2007; **42**: 528–532.

84. Kuo MJ, Yeh HZ, Chen GH *et al.* Improvement of tissue-adhesive obliteration of bleeding gastric varices using adjuvant hypertonic glucose injection: a prospective randomized trial. *Endoscopy* 2007; **39**: 487–491.

85. Lo GH, Liang HL, Chen WC *et al.* A prospective, randomized controlled trial of transjugular intrahepatic portosystemic shunt versus cyanoacrylate injection in the prevention of gastric variceal rebleeding. *Endoscopy* 2007; **39**: 679–685.

86. Cho SK, Shin SW, Lee IH. Balloon-occluded retrograde transvenous obliteration of gastric varices: outcomes and complications in 49 patients. *AJR Am J Roentgenol* 2007; **189**: 1523.

87. Hiraga N, Aikata H, Takaki S *et al.* The long-term outcome of patients with bleeding gastric varices after balloon-occluded retrograde transvenous obliteration. *J Gastroenterol* 2007; **42**: 663–672.

88. Takuma Y, Nouso K, Makino Y, Saito S, Shiratori Y. Prophylactic balloon-occluded retrograde transvenous obliteration for gastric varices in compensated cirrhosis. *Clin Gastroenterol Hepatol* 2005; **3**: 1245–1252.

Simon J.W. Monkhouse
Justin D.T. Morgan Sally A. Norton

Obesity surgery

Obesity is a world-wide epidemic and a leading public health priority.[1] According to the US National Center for Health Statistics, the prevalence of obesity (defined as a body mass index (BMI) > 30 kg/m^2) has risen exponentially from 12.8% in 1962 to 27% in 2002.[2] The data from the US are mirrored in many countries including the UK (22% prevalence) and Australia (20% prevalence).[3] This has massive health and economic implications.

Obesity is associated with many significant co-morbidities: these include hypertension, coronary heart disease, type 2 diabetes, dyslipidaemias, non-alcoholic hepatic steatosis, obstructive sleep apnoea, osteoarthritis, reduced fertility and a greater susceptibility to a range of cancers.[4] No less important are the psychological co-morbidities of depression, social stigmatisation and isolation.[5] In addition, obesity is associated with a reduced life expectancy. A large prospective study demonstrated that an elevated BMI (> 30 kg/m^2) is associated with an increased risk of death, irrespective of sex, age or ethnic background.[6]

Obesity is complex and causes include genetics, the environment and learned behaviour. Research using animal models suggest that mutations in genes controlling the hormones and receptors in the appetite signalling pathway, can cause dramatic changes in eating behaviour and subsequent weight change. A mutation in the melanocortin-4-receptor, for example, disrupts satiety signalling and accounts for about 5% of morbidly obese

Simon J.W. Monkhouse MA MBBChir(Hons) MRCS (for correspondence)
Specialist Registrar in General Surgery, Southmead Hospital, Bristol BS10 5NB, UK
E-mail: sjwmonkhouse@hotmail.com

Justin D.T. Morgan MB BCh MD PGCME FRCS
Consultant General, Endocrine and Transplant Surgeon, Southmead Hospital, Bristol BS10 5NB, UK

Sally A. Norton MB ChB MD FRCS(Ed)
Consultant General, Laparoscopic and Upper GI Surgeon, Southmead Hospital, Bristol BS10 5NB, UK

patients (BMI > 40 kg/m^2). Other genes have been identified; currently, over 430 genes or chromosomal regions have been implicated in the aetiology of obesity. Obesity tends to run in families and this is perhaps a reflection of a shared genetic susceptibility together with exposure to similar environmental and cultural influences. A large UK twin study looking at the effect of genetic influence on childhood obesity in over 5000 twins, concluded that genetic factors were responsible for 40% of the abdominal adiposity. The remainder was attributed to the force of the obesogenic environment.[6] The environment and composition of the diet seem to influence weight at a more rapid rate in those genetically pre-disposed individuals than in those with a normal genotype. An increased tendency towards a sedentary life-style exacerbates the problem further.

Another major cause is previous emotional trauma and psychological illness. This can manifest as obesity as these individuals derive comfort from eating to excess.

Management of the obesity epidemic must focus on prevention. However, for established cases, a combination of diet, exercise, counselling and pharmacological treatments are often encouraged. Although these measures may have impressive initial results, the weight loss is rarely maintained.[8] The clinical and psychological associated problems generally return with weight re-gain. Obesity surgery has been shown to be the only long-term effective method to control weight. Some studies report an excess weight loss of up to 61.2%[9] sustained for up to 16 years after surgery.[10]

An increased awareness of the implications of obesity, together with advances in laparoscopic technology has meant that obesity surgery has become much more prevalent and continues to grow in popularity.

This chapter explores the subject of obesity surgery. It highlights the complex problems associated with this unique group of patients and demonstrates the advantages and disadvantages of surgical intervention.

DEFINITION OF OBESITY

The degree of obesity in adults should be defined in accordance with the 2006 guidelines of the National Institute for Health and Clinical Excellence (NICE) as summarised in Table 1.

BMI does not always provide an accurate measure of adiposity in adults. In highly muscular individuals, for example, the BMI may be misleadingly high.

Table 1 Definition of obesity

Classification	BMI (kg/m^2)	Other terms in use
Healthy weight	18.5–24.9	
Overweight	25–29.9	
Obesity I	30–34.9	
Obesity II	35–39.9	Morbid obesity (if associated with co-morbidity)
Obesity III	40–50	Morbid obesity
	50 or more	Super obesity

Source: NICE guidelines 2006.

There is no one accurate tool for measuring the degree of obesity but waist circumference has proved useful in those with a BMI < 35 kg/m^2. Waist circumference is not recommended as a measure of obesity in those with a BMI > 35 kg/m^2 but is a useful predictor for developing long-term health problems such as the metabolic syndrome and its consequences. This syndrome describes the clustering of risk factors including dyslipidaemia, glucose intolerance and hypertension with central obesity. Those with metabolic syndrome are at risk of developing cardiovascular problems and type 2 diabetes. Early identification of those at risk and weight loss are paramount in preventing the onset of these complications.

NON-SURGICAL TREATMENTS

NICE produced extensive guidelines on obesity management in 2002, which were revised in 2006. A combination of diet, graded exercise and education/behavioural changes were recommended as first-line measures to tackle obesity. Pharmacological treatments should only be used when first-line treatment has failed or reached a plateau. They are absolutely contra-indicated in children under 12 years of age.

Orlistat and sibutramine are the most frequently prescribed anti-obesity drugs. Orlistat prevents the absorption of fat by inhibiting the key enzymes required to convert dietary fat into its absorbable form. Sibutramine, in contrast, acts centrally to inhibit serotonin and noradrenaline re-uptake and this creates a feeling of satiety. Sibutramine is also thermogenic and thus increases energy expenditure through heat production.

A 2005 meta-analysis of drug treatments for obesity showed that the mean weight loss at 1 year for orlistat was 2.9 kg and for sibutramine was 4.5 kg.[3] A new drug, rimonabant (a cannabinoid-1 receptor antagonist), undergoing clinical trials, produced 6.6 kg weight loss at 1 year. Although promising, this degree of weight loss is clearly insufficient for most obese patients. Long-term compliance with medication is poor due to unsatisfactory side effect profiles; when stopped, weight is almost invariably regained.

A randomised, controlled trial compared a group of patients undergoing pharmacological treatment to a matched group of patients undergoing voluntary obesity surgery. At 8-year follow-up, the surgically treated arm had lost on average 20 kg but the medically treated arm had not lost any weight compared with baseline.[11]

Drug therapy may, however, have a role in weight loss reduction prior to surgery or in those individuals not suitable for surgery.

INDICATIONS FOR SURGERY

The 2006 UK NICE guidelines recommend obesity surgery as a treatment option if the following criteria are met:

1. The patient must have a BMI > 40 kg/m^2 or BMI > 35 kg/m^2 associated with serious obesity related co-morbidity (type 2 diabetes, hypertension, *etc.*).
2. All reasonable non-surgical methods have been tried and failed to produce clinically significant weight loss over a 6-month period.

3. The patient will receive intensive follow-up in a specialist obesity service.

4. The patient is considered fit for anaesthesia.

5. The patient commits to the need for long-term follow-up.

These revised guidelines also recognise that, in patients with a BMI > 50 kg/m^2, drugs are unlikely to be effective and surgery can be offered without a trial of medication.

OBESITY SURGERY

Obesity is not just a disease of the modern age. There are many references to obesity throughout history. Hippocrates (460–377 BC), the father of modern medicine, recognised the serious problems associated with obesity, commenting that 'sudden death is more common in those who are naturally fat than in the lean'.[2]

There are anecdotal reports of surgical attempts to cure obesity in the late 19th century but obesity surgery, as we know it, was introduced in 1950s. The surgery can be divided into three broad categories: (i) purely malabsorptive procedures; (ii) purely restrictive procedures; and (iii) a combination of both types.

Victor Henrikson in the 1950s performed an extensive small bowel resection in an attempt to cure obesity by reducing the absorptive capacity of the gut.[12] This was followed by various small bowel bypasses, such as the jejuno-ileal bypass, but the complication rate was unacceptably high. Problems included blind loop syndrome due to bacterial overgrowth, electrolyte imbalances, liver failure, migratory arthralgias, bloating and intractable diarrhoea.[13]

This problem was partially overcome by the introduction of a 'Roux' loop which meant that all segments of bowel received some flow of luminal contents. Continual refinement and revision of the surgery, over a decade, by various surgical pioneers such as Mason, Ito and Griffen, led to the Roux-en-Y

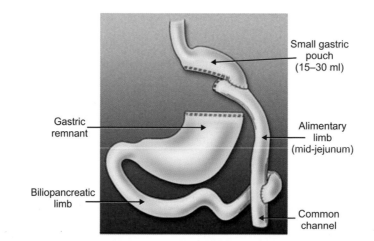

Fig. 1 The Roux-en-Y gastric bypass (RYGB), a restrictive and malabsorptive procedure. **Alimentary limb** – Roux limb that extends from the gastrojejunostomy to the jejuno-jejunostomy (purely undigested food and stomach secretions). **Biliopancreatic limb** – jejunum from the duodenojejunal junction to the jejunojejunostomy (purely biliary and pancreatic secretions). **Common channel** – from the jejunojejunostomy to the ileocaecal valve (length of small bowel where absorption takes place).

A

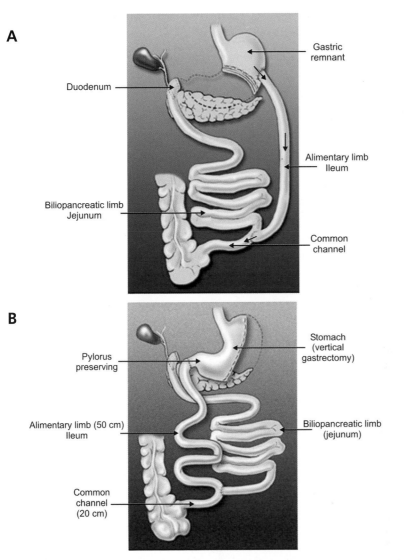

Gastric
remnant

Duodenum

Alimentary limb
Ileum

Biliopancreatic limb
Jejunum

Common
channel

B

Stomach
(vertical
gastrectomy)

Pylorus
preserving

Alimentary limb (50 cm)
Ileum

Biliopancreatic limb
(jejunum)

Common
channel
(20 cm)

Fig. 2 (A) The biliopancreatic diversion (BPD), mainly malabsorptive but with a degree of restriction. (B) The biliopancreatic diversion with duodenal switch (BPD/DS), mainly malabsorptive but with a degree of restriction. Reprinted with permission of American Society for Metabolic and Batiatric Surgery, © 2008, all rights reserved.

gastric bypass (RYGB; Fig. 1). There are many variations of this technique; by varying the length of the common channel, the degree of malabsorption can be modified. The size of the gastric pouch can also be altered. These variations have an impact on the rate and extent of weight loss.

In the 1970s, Scopinaro developed a modification of the RYGB called bilio-pancreatic diversion (BPD).[14] This operation produced dramatic, sustainable weight loss (Fig. 2A).

In 1998, Hess and Marceau modified the Scopinaro BPD, to create a BPD with duodenal switch (BPD/DS; Fig. 2B).[2] This created similar malabsorption to the Scopinaro BPD but the preservation of the pylorus controlled flow down

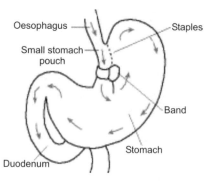

Oesophagus

Staples

Small stomach pouch

Band

Duodenum

Stomach

Fig. 3 Vertical banded gastroplasty, purely restrictive. Courtesy of National Institute of Diabetes and Digestive and Kidney Diseases, National Institutes of Health.

the enteric limb and ameliorated problems with diarrhoea and dumping syndrome. The transection of the stomach in this case is along the greater curvature and is known as a sleeve gastrectomy. This can be performed alone as a definitive surgical procedure or can be performed as the first of a two-part procedure to reduce weight before the bypass element is introduced. Sleeve gastrectomy can result in excess weight loss of up to 50% in the first year but may suffer from a long-term failure rate as the pouch enlarges.[15]

Both the BPD and BPD/DS procedures are in use today. They have initial gastric restriction in the first 12–18 months but, as the pouch slowly enlarges, this becomes less effective. The weight loss is maintained in the long-term by the malabsorptive element; however, there is a requirement for long-term vitamin and mineral supplements and a risk of protein malnutrition.

Mason described the first purely gastric restrictive procedure in 1971 which involved partially transecting the stomach. This technique evolved over several years and, in 1982, vertical banded gastroplasty[2] was developed (Fig. 3). A few surgeons still perform this technique but it has largely been abandoned (due to its long-term failure rate) in favour of gastric banding.

Molina developed the first fixed gastric band, which was placed in 1992. In contemporary practice, the band is made from silicone and has an adjustable saline reservoir. The saline can be instilled or removed via a subcutaneous port depending on the degree of restriction required (Fig. 4A). The banding procedure is mainly performed laparoscopically and has the benefit of total reversibility (Fig. 4B).

Before the advent of minimally invasive surgery, open obesity procedures were associated with a high rate of complications, due in large part to the morbidity of the incision itself. Laparoscopic surgery brought with it a new range of possibilities and had many inherent advantages. These included reduced postoperative pain, decreased respiratory complications, faster recovery, reduced stress response and a reduction in wound infection and incisional hernia rates.[16] As a result, the vast majority of surgeons choose the laparoscopic approach for all the current techniques described.

The choice of which operation is most suited for an individual is determined by a number of factors. Surgeon preference and patient requirements are taken into account.

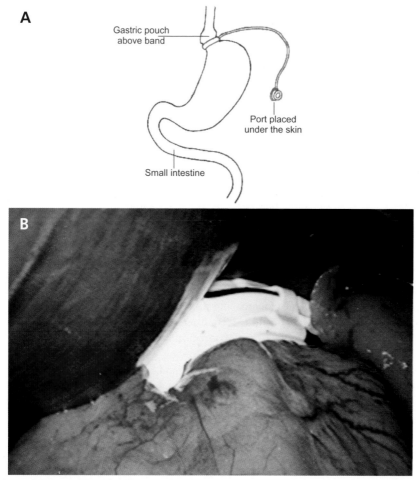

Fig. 4 (A) Laparoscopic adjustable gastric banding (LAGB), purely restrictive. Reprinted with permission of the author, Michael France (www.laparoscopicsurgeon.com). (B) An adjustable gastric band *in situ*.

There are demographic trends of note with a predominance of laparoscopic adjustable gastric banding in Europe and Australasia over North America with the reverse trend for gastric bypass.[17]

PAEDIATRIC OBESITY SURGERY

Obesity is also a major problem in the adolescent population. A rapid increase in the obesity-related co-morbidities among adolescents indicates that adolescent obesity is a major health problem. As with adults, medical treatments for obesity often fail. Recently, obesity surgery has been introduced for this group and early results are encouraging. The surgery appears to be safe and is associated with reduction in co-morbidity and improvement in self-image. The need for a specialist multidisciplinary team and life-long follow-up was stressed in the 2006 NICE guidelines which endorses surgery for this group only after conservative measures have failed. There are, as yet, no good long-term results for paediatric obesity surgery as it remains restricted to a highly selected group of patients.

MECHANISMS OF WEIGHT LOSS

Restrictive procedures promote early satiety by gastric and oesophageal distension. This distension activates afferent nerves via mechanoreceptors and neuropeptides, such as Substance P, which in turn causes brain activity in areas associated with appetite signalling. This may help to control food intake.[18] Dixon *et al.*[19] showed that the degree of restriction afforded by the band had a direct impact on appetite and satiety that was independent of food intake. The mechanism of this is uncertain although parasympathetic vagal stimulation via mechanoreceptors seems likely.

Gastric bypass causes massive changes in gut hormone levels. Ghrelin, a hormone derived from the stomach, stimulates food intake and its plasma levels are reduced following bypass. Leptin, another satiety hormone, interacts with ghrelin and acts on the mesolimbic reward pathway in the ventral tegmental area of the midbrain. A reduction in both these hormones, following gastric bypass, seems to reduce the reward of hedonic eating.[18]

There is a simultaneous increase in peptide YY and glucagon-like peptide 1 (GLP-1). These hormones are released from the distal gut in response to the increased stimulation of this part of the gut following bypass, and may contribute to weight loss by decreasing food intake. Bypass procedures tend to exclude foregut-derived hormones, such as cholecystokinin[18] and the altered hormone milieu contributes to malabsorption and subsequent weight loss.

There is a degree of learned behaviour following surgery which has an impact on weight loss. Over-eating or eating the wrong food types may lead to unpleasant consequences such as nausea, excessive diarrhoea, vomiting or pain. This sets up a negative feedback loop which encourages the patient to avoid that stimulus in the future.[20]

This is an area that is not fully understood and attracts keen research interest. Over time, it may become possible to mimic the changes induced by surgery through synthetic hormone or endocrine analogues.

IMPACT OF SURGERY ON WEIGHT LOSS

The success of surgery is often measured in terms of weight loss, not least by the patient. Percentage excess weight loss (EWL), defined as the percentage of weight lost above the ideal body weight, is a more useful marker of success.

A recent meta-analysis showed mean percentage excess weight loss 2 years following surgery was 61.2% for all obesity procedures. This ranged from 47.5% for gastric banding, 61.6% for gastric bypass to 70.1% for biliopancreatic diversion with duodenal switch.[20] The superior results from BPD/DS are at the expense of increased complications.

Figure 5 shows a weight loss comparison between adjustable gastric banding and gastric bypass. Weight loss is more rapid and extensive with gastric bypass in the first 2 years after the procedure but the difference in excess weight loss is not significant at 3 years and 4 years.[3] Indeed, the EWL at 5 years for laparoscopic adjustable gastric banding (LAGB) and RYGB are similar and appear to be independent of starting BMI. In a series of 1000 LAGB patients from Birmingham, 174 had a starting BMI > 50 kg/m^2. At 18 months, the EWL for this subgroup was 39 ± 8.2% which was not significantly different to the rest of the patients in the series.[21]

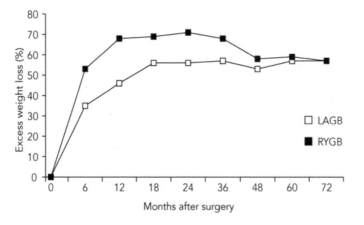

Fig. 5 Weight loss comparison between RYGB and LAGB over time. From O'Brien P *et al*.[3] Copyright © 2005, *The Medical Journal of Australia*; reproduced with permission.

The long-term success of these procedures is difficult to establish accurately, not least because long-term follow-up is poor in many studies. In some cases, 50% or more of subjects were lost to follow-up. Despite this, various studies have reported a 40% failure rate in the long-term.[20] A study of patients who underwent biliopancreatic diversion showed that the failure rate doubled every 5 years.[22] A Swiss study looking specifically at laparoscopic adjustable gastric banding, reported a 40% 5-year failure rate (defined as EWL < 25%) and only a 43% 7-year success rate (defined as EWL > 50%).[23] Without careful postoperative management and psychological counselling, poor eating habits can return and the rate of weight loss can decline. With restrictive procedures, in particular, there is the possibility that the pouch can slowly enlarge to accommodate a greater food intake. A long follow-up period is needed to support patients, monitor progress, identify signs of failure early and intervene as necessary. With good postoperative support, however, gastric banding can produce excellent results with up to 79% EWL sustained at 3 years (personal communication).

It is important to define markers of success. The aim of surgery is to reduce the BMI to the point where the impact from co-morbidities is reduced. It is not to achieve a normal BMI; after all, obesity surgery is not designed as cosmetic surgery.

IMPACT OF SURGERY ON CO-MORBIDITIES

The impact of obesity surgery on type 2 diabetes and impaired glucose tolerance is dramatic. The surgically-induced weight loss appears to improve both insulin resistance and β-cell function with resulting improvement in glycaemic control. This leads not only to resolution of diabetes in established cases but also to non-progression of impaired glucose tolerance to fulminant diabetes.[24] Most studies have shown that the benefit of surgery is greatest in those patients with early diabetes, before the β-cell mass has been irreversibly impaired.[24] Interestingly, in LAGB patients the improvement seems to be directly attributable to weight loss, but in the RYGB group, subtle metabolic

Table 2 Percentage of patients with resolution or improvement of major co-morbidities according to obesity operation

Major co-morbidity	Operation			
	Adjustable gastric banding	Vertical banded gastroplasty	Gastric bypass	Biliopancreatic bypass
Diabetes	48 (9; 29–67)	72 (11; 55–88)	84 (26; 77–90)	99 (9; 87–100)
Dyslipidaemia	59 (6; 82–89)	74 (7; 61–86)	97 (6; 94–100)	99 (3; 98–100)
Hypertension	43 (12; 30–56)	69 (20; 57–79)	68 (20; 58–77)	83 (7; 73–94)
Sleep apnoea	95 (5; 89–100)	78 (10; 54–100)	80 (13; 68–92)	92 (6; 82–100)

The table shows the mean percentage of patients (with number of studies; and 95% CI).
Reprinted from Kral and Naslund[18] with permission from Macmillan Publishers Ltd, ©2007.

improvements occur before weight loss becomes apparent. This is likely to be mediated by hormonal changes, particularly with glucagon like peptide-1. This is an area of intense research interest.

The prospective Swedish Obese Subjects Study produced 10-year follow-up data on the impact of surgery on co-morbidities. It compared a surgically treated obese population (24% LAGB, 5% RYGB and 70% vertical banded gastroplasty) to a matched control group. The surgical group had a statistically significant odds ratio for recovery from diabetes (3.45), hypertension (1.68), hypertriglyceridaemia (2.57) and low HDL cholesterol (2.35). Recovery from hypercholesterolaemia did not reach statistical significance, however.[24] The Swedish Obese Subjects Study, although the largest study of its kind, was not randomised and is purely an observational study.

Other co-morbidities can also be improved. A study involving 33 asthma sufferers showed that at 1-year postoperatively, a third of those had no symptoms and no need for medication. Another study showed an 89% reduction in the symptoms of reflux oesophagitis in the 12 months following LAGB.[3]

The impact of surgery on the associated conditions is not uniform; the type of operation influences the degree of improvement. This is illustrated in Table 2 which shows long-term results of various operations on co-morbidity resolution. The data were complied from multiple studies with different end-points. As with all decisions in surgery, a risk–benefit analysis must be undertaken. Although, the BPD option appears to be the best in terms of resolution of co-morbidities, it does have the highest complication rate and highest associated mortality.

Psychological well-being is also promoted by surgery. The quality of life of nearly 500 obese subjects was assessed prior to surgery using the SF-36 questionnaire. Abnormally low scores were seen in all eight sub-sections of the questionnaire before surgery, indicating a great deal of psychological morbidity. At 1-year post surgery, all scores had returned to normal and this change in mood appeared to be maintained at 4 years following surgery.[25]

IMPACT ON MORTALITY

One of the main goals of surgery is to reduce the mortality associated with obesity. The Swedish Obese Subjects Study reported its 10-year follow-up data in 2006. In the surgically treated group, there was significantly lower mortality over 10 years than in the group who were treated without surgical intervention.[18] The main cause of death in each group was myocardial infarction. This landmark observational study suggests the effectiveness of obesity surgery. It is somewhat limited, however. There was no randomisation, patients under 37 years of age were excluded and there was limited statistical power.[26] Also, the type of surgery was not controlled – some subjects underwent RYGB, whereas others under went either VBG or LAGB.

Another important study, from Washington, looked at mortality from gastric bypass 15 years after surgery. They reported a mortality of 11.3% compared to 16.3% in non-treated obese controls.[27] Both these studies suggest that obesity surgery has a positive effect on survival.

COMPLICATIONS OF SURGERY

All surgery carries some degree of risk and the decision to operate is made after a careful balance of the risks versus the benefits. This particular group of patients often have limited physiological reserves and this, together with their size, may make the surgery high-risk. Early detection and appropriate management of complications is crucial to prevent long-term morbidity and mortality.

PERI-OPERATIVE COMPLICATIONS

Pulmonary embolism (all procedures)
Postoperative pulmonary embolism is the major cause of death in this group. The incidence is 1–2% in this population. Measures taken to reduce this risk include pre-operative low molecular weight heparin, intra-operative pneumatic calf compression and early mobilisation postoperatively.

Anastomotic leak (RYGB/BPD/BPD/DS)
An anastomotic leak is a serious, life-threatening problem and can be difficult to diagnose due to the patient's size. Radiological investigations are difficult as the patient may not fit into a conventional scanner and also the scans do not have a high sensitivity for leaks. Most present with non-specific signs of sepsis (tachycardia, leukocytosis, fever) within the first 10 postoperative days. A large case series of 63 patients with 68 leaks following RYGB showed that 44% were not detectable by CT scanning, 63% required surgery and 10% died.[28,29] Any patient with tachycardia and sepsis within 10 days of bypass surgery should be considered for re-laparoscopy. It is sometimes possible to stent leaks endoscopically with small expandable metal stents; in another case series, 16 out of 17 leaks were successfully managed in this way.[30]

Wound dehiscence (open procedures)
Wound dehiscence incidence is 1%.[29] This may result from technical failure (early dehiscence) or from sepsis/nutritional deficiencies (delayed dehiscence).

Gastrointestinal bleeding (bypass procedures)
Bleeding within 72 h of operation is usually due to an intra-operative complication or ischaemia at the anastomosis.[29] At this stage, endoscopy

should be avoided and early re-operation is indicated if conservative, supportive measures fail.

Peri-operative mortality rate

This is of major importance to both patients and clinicians. According to Buchwald et al.[17], in a 2007 meta-analysis on the subject, operative mortality depends on a number of factors including:

1. The technical skill of the surgeon and the stage of the 'learning curve' that the surgeon and the institution are on.

2. The availability of pre- and postoperative care including anaesthetic support.

3. The type of operation (restrictive, malabsorptive or a mixture of both).

4. Laparoscopic versus open surgery.

5. Patient selection with respect to age, sex, ethnic background and body habitus.

6. The presence of significant co-morbidities (for example, type 2 diabetes or hypertension).

Mortality analysis from the literature is often difficult because of the tendency only to report positive outcomes and some centres do not publish data at all. There is frequent selection bias. However, the overwhelming finding is that obesity surgery has a relatively low mortality. The 30-day mortality for obesity surgery as a whole is 0.28%. This rises to 1% or more with the more complex procedures such as laparoscopic BPD/DS and open revisional surgery.[17] The 30-day mortality after LAGB is less than 0.2% with many large series reporting no 30-day mortality.[21] This makes LAGB a very attractive option to the patient.

The 30-day to 2-year mortality for obesity surgery is < 1%. Restrictive operations have the lowest mortality followed by the restrictive/malabsorptive gastric bypass (RYGB) followed by the purely malabsorptive BPD/DS. Also, there is a higher mortality for open procedures than laparoscopic procedures, with the exception of BPD/DS.

The other interesting finding from the literature is that mortality rates are improving and this is almost certainly due to increasing expertise, wide-spread adoption of the laparoscopic approach18 and better peri-operative care for these patients.

LATE COMPLICATIONS

Gallstones (all operations)

Cholelithiasis is common following obesity surgery (incidence of up to 30%)[29] and may be precipitated by rapid weight loss.[31] As a result, gallstones are more common following gastric bypass surgery compared to banding. Prophylactic cholecystectomy during bariatric surgery remains controversial.

Incisional hernia (all operations)

Incisional hernia has a reported incidence of 10–20%. Hernias mainly follow open surgery but smaller laparoscopic port site hernias are possible. These are more likely to be symptomatic and require operative intervention.

Rapid weight regain (all operations)

This raises the possibility of staple line dehiscence and creation of a gastro-gastric fistula where the excluded portion of stomach suddenly starts filling again.[32] Early oral contrast X-ray studies should demonstrate this and highlight the need to return to theatre. In the case of gastric banding, early weight gain may be attributed to pouch enlargement or band slippage as discussed below.

Mineral and vitamin deficiencies (RYGB/BPD/BPD/DS)

The stomach, duodenum and proximal jejunum contribute to the absorption of vitamin B_{12}, calcium and iron[20] and, as such, it is possible to have deficiencies in these nutrients after bypass procedures.

Vitamin B_{12} deficiency tends not to present clinically due to the presence of a normal functioning terminal ileum, maintenance of intrinsic factor production by the residual stomach and routine exogenous vitamin B_{12} intake post surgery.

Changes in calcium malabsorption have been demonstrated post-operatively[33] but this has not equated to clinically significant osteoporosis in the short term. Elder and Wolfe[20] postulate this is due to the relatively young age of the patient group, routine oral intake of calcium after surgery, the increased bone mass due to obesity and excess oestrogen production by adipocytes. Circulating parathormone levels have been noted to be high following BPD/DS34 but, again, no serious bone pathology resulted.

Iron deficiency is often due to exclusion of stomach and duodenum and may be exacerbated by intra-operative blood loss. Routine iron administration after surgery is advised with regular serum monitoring.[20]

Electrolyte disturbances are common if there is excessive diarrhoea postoperatively.

Anastomotic stricture (RYGB/BPD/BPD/DS)

Strictures can follow any gastrointestinal anastomosis. Causes include technical error, ischaemia, subclinical leak, tension or delayed fibrosis secondary to ulceration.[20] Diagnosis is made on endoscopy and, in general terms, an anastomosis of less than 10 mm in diameter requires endoscopic balloon dilation. Perforation remains a real risk, particularly within 4 weeks of operation. Late strictures may require serial dilatation due to fibrosis.

Dumping syndrome (RYGB/BPD/BPD/DS)

This syndrome is characterised by facial flushing, light-headedness, fatigue and post-prandial diarrhoea after the consumption of sugars and starches.[29] It is caused by inappropriately high insulin secretion and reactive hypo-glycaemia. Most gastric bypass patients experience this for up to 18 months following surgery but the incidence of chronic dumping is only 5–10%.[29] The inclusion of the pylorus in the BPD/DS prevents this condition by slowing down transit time. Dietary modifications, such as consuming carbohydrates mid-meal and eating slowly, can dramatically improve dumping syndrome.

Gastrointestinal bleeding (mainly bypass procedures)

From 72 h to 1 week, erosions and ulceration can occur at anastomoses. Aetiology for such ulceration includes, *Helicobacter pylori* infection, use of a non-absorbable suture, postoperative stress response, increased acid production and ischaemia.[20] Endoscopy can be attempted at this stage. A standard endoscope can be used to examine the gastrojejunostomy, pouch and Roux limb but a paediatric colonoscopy is required to look at the jejuno-jejunostomy and retrogradely at the biliopancreatic limb.[29]

Band slippage (LAGB)

Band slippage is an acute, serious complication. It is defined as a cephalic prolapse of the stomach's inferior portion with consequent caudal slippage of the band. The angle of the band is reduced on X-ray images with evidence of pouch enlargement. Symptoms include dysphagia and vomiting.[35]

Band slippage is an acute emergency and band deflation, followed by immediate surgery if symptoms do not rapidly resolve, is essential to avoid the risk of gastric ischaemia. In a case series, Vertruyen[36] concluded that laparoscopic band removal, reduction of the prolapsed stomach and replacement by a new band is the safest and best long-term method for treating these cases; however, the risk of recurrent slippage has prompted other centres to convert to bypass at this stage.[37] Band slippage is now less common due to improved surgical technique. Some centres advocate gastro-gastric fixation sutures around the band to prevent slippage although others believe they may contribute to erosion (see below).[38]

Band erosion (LAGB)

This is rare but can be a cause of bleeding though more commonly presents with weight gain. Erosion of the band through the stomach wall is a slow process such that it rarely results in perforation and subsequent peritonitis and requires band removal, usually by laparoscopic surgery.

HEALTH ECONOMICS

Obesity places a great financial burden on society. National Audit Office figures suggest that the economic burden of obesity in the UK amounts to approximately £2 billion. This not only includes the direct healthcare costs related to obesity and its treatment (amounting to £479.4 million) but also the impact of loss of productivity in the workforce.

The actual cost effectiveness of surgery is very difficult to work out. It relies on complex economic modelling often using artificial hypothetical scenarios. A Swedish study attempted to model the cost effectiveness of obesity surgery compared to conventional management. They used the data from the Swedish Obese Subjects Study to estimate the prevalence of hypertension and diabetes in a surgically treated group and a control group over 10 years. They concluded that the cost is £199/patient/year greater in the control group than the surgical group.[39]

Another observational study, in which severely obese patients undergoing surgery were matched to controls, looked at the implications of surgery on healthcare costs. It found that the surgical cohort had a statistically significant reduced cost over the 5-year study period (US$8813 compared to US$11,854 for the controls).[10] Interestingly, when the costs were broken down into their component parts, the costs of drugs were similar between the two cohorts. The decrease in the use of drugs to treat diabetes and hypertension were offset by an increase in the use of drugs to manage gastrointestinal tract disorders.[24]

THE FUTURE

Progress is being made in endoscopic techniques to complement or replace existing surgical techniques. The intragastric balloons, introduced in the 1980s as a means of gastric capacity restriction, have been shown to be ineffective in randomised clinical trials.[3] A new intragastric balloon (BioEnterics) has been introduced into clinical practice in Australia but long-term results are still awaited.

Gastric electrical stimulation, first introduced in 1999 by Cigaina, is showing some promise. Here, electrodes placed in the wall of the stomach connected to a subcutaneous pacer create gastric paresis. Animal models showed encouraging results but the results from human clinical trials are still awaited.[2]

Robotically assisted surgery (using the da Vinci robot) is currently being used in America to perform obesity surgery in a few specialised centres.[16] Reported advantages include less wound infection, greater mechanical advantage with the super-obese population (BMI > 60 kg/m^2), superior quality anastomoses and reduced hospital stays. This technique is still under investigation and has not been subject to randomised control trials.[40] It is likely to take on an increasingly important role in the future.

Key points for clinical practice

- Obesity surgery is not suitable for every patient. Specific criteria must be met and the patient must be motivated and fully informed. Obesity surgery may be considered for adolescent obese patients.

- Management of obese patients is complex requiring physicians, psychiatrists, dieticians, counsellors and surgeons. Patients require long-term follow-up to ensure success and appropriate support. This requires specialist facilities and teams with experience in obesity surgery.

- The type of surgery offered will depend on the patient, the associated morbidities and the experience of the surgeon.

- The operations offered include purely malabsorptive, purely restrictive and a combination of the two. Laparoscopic adjustable gastric banding and gastric bypass (laparoscopic or open) are the two most common operative procedures performed world-wide.

- Surgery conveys advantages in terms of co-morbidity reduction, particularly with type 2 diabetes and hypertension. There is also a notable survival advantage.

- After obesity surgery, most patients do not reach 'normal' weight. However, the excess weight loss is usually sufficient to ameliorate co-morbidities and to improve long-term survival.

- Obesity surgery can have complications. The type of operation, whether it is done laparoscopically or not and the patient's characteristics will influence the nature and frequency of complications. Signs of complications may be subtle and insidious in this special group of patients due to their unique physiology and physical size.

- Obesity surgery is cost-effective with life-long savings to be made. This is due to reduced healthcare utilisation post-surgery and increased productivity.

References

1. Prentice AM. The emerging epidemic of obesity in developing countries. *Int J Epidemiol* 2006; **35**: 93–99.
2. Gillison W, Buchwald H. *Pioneers in Surgical Gastroenterology*. London: tfm Publishing, 2007.
3. O'Brien PE, Brown WA, Dixon JB. Obesity, weight loss and bariatric surgery. *Med J Aust* 2005; **183**: 310–314.
4. Bray GA. Medical consequences of obesity. *J Clin Endocrinol Metab* 2004; **89**: 2583–2589.
5. Puhl R, Brownell KD. Bias, discrimination and obesity. *Obes Res* 2001; **9**: 788–805.
6. Adams KF, Schatzkin A, Harris TB *et al*. Overweight, obesity and mortality in a large prospective cohort of persons 50–71 years old. *N Engl J Med* 2006; **355**: 763–778.
7. Wardle J, Haworth CM, Plonin R, Carnell S. Evidence for strong genetic influence on childhood adiposity despite the force of the obesogenic environment. *Ann J Clin Nutr* 2008; **87**: 398–404.
8. North American Association for the Study of Obesity and the National Heart, Lung, and Blood Institute. *The Practical Guide: Identification, Evaluation, and Treatment of Overweight and Obesity in Adults*. Bethesda, MD: National Institutes of Health; 2000.
9. Buchwald H, Avidor Y, Braunwald E *et al*. Bariatric surgery: a systematic review and meta-analysis. *JAMA* 2004; **292**: 1724–1737.
10. Christou NV, Sampalis JS, Liberman M *et al*. Surgery decreases long-term mortality, morbidity and health care use in morbidly obese patients. *Ann Surg* 2004; **240**: 416–424.
11. Maggard MA, Shugarman LR, Suttorp M *et al*. Meta-analysis: surgical treatment of obesity. *Ann Intern Med* 2005; **142**: 547–559.
12. Henrikson V. Can small bowel resection be defended as therapy for obesity? *Obes Surg* 1994; **4**: 54.
13. Dietel M. A synopsis of the development of bariatric operations. *Obes Surg* 2007; **17**: 707–710.
14. Scopinaro N, Gianetta E, Civalleri D, Bonalumi U, Bachi V. Bilio-pancreatic bypass for obesity: II. Initial experience in man. *Br J Surg* 1979; **66**: 618–620.
15. Mognol P, Chosidow D, Marmuse JP. Laparoscopic sleeve gastrectomy as an initial bariatric operation for high risk patients; initial results in 10 patients. *Obes Surg* 2005; **15**: 1030–1033.
16. Nguyen NT, Goldman C, Rosenquist J *et al*. Laparoscopic versus open gastric bypass: a randomised study of outcomes, quality of life and costs. *Ann Surg* 2001; **234**: 279–291.
17. Buchwald H, Estok R, Fahrbach K, Banel D, Sledge I. Trends in mortality in bariatric surgery: a systematic review and meta-analysis. *Surgery* 2007; **142**: 621–635.
18. Kral JG, Naslund E. Surgical treatment of obesity. *Nat Clin Pract Endocrinol Metab* 2007; **3**: 574–583.
19. Dixon AFR, Dixon JB, O'Brien PE. Laparoscopic adjustable gastric banding induces prolonged satiety: a randomised blind cross-over study. *J Clin Endocrinol Metab* 2005; **90**: 813–819.
20. Elder KA, Wolfe BM. Bariatric surgery: a review of procedures and outcomes. *Gastroenterology* 2007; **132**: 2253–2271.
21. Bennett JMH, Mehta S, Rhodes M. Surgery for morbid obesity. *Postgrad Med J* 2007; **83**: 8–15.
22. Biron S, Hould FS, Lebel S *et al*. Twenty years of biliopancreatic diversion: what is the goal of surgery? *Obes Surg* 2004; **14**: 160–164.
23. Suter M, Calmes JM, Paroz A, Giusti V. A 10-year experience with laparoscopic gastric banding for morbid obesity: high long-term complication and failure rates. *Obes Surg* 2006; **16**: 829–835.
24. Meneghini LF. Impact of bariatric surgery on type 2 diabetes. *Cell Biochem Biophys* 2007; **48**: 97–102.
25. Dixon JB, Dixon ME, O'Brien PE. Quality of life after lap-band placement: influence of time, weight loss and co-morbidities. *Obes Res* 2001; **9**: 713–721.
26. Barclay L. Bariatric surgery improves survival in obese patients. *N Engl J Med* 2007; **357**: 741–752, 818–820.
27. Flum DR, Dellinger EP. Impact of gastric bypass operation on survival: a population-based analysis. *J Am Coll Surg* 2004; **199**: 543–551.

28. Gonzalez R, Sarr MG, Smith CD *et al.* Diagnosis and contemporary management of anastomotic leaks after gastric bypass for obesity. *J Am Coll Surg* 2007; **204**: 47–55.

29. Lee C, Kelly J, Wassef W. Complications of bariatric surgery. *Curr Opin Gastroenterol* 2007; **23**: 636–643.

30. Salinas A, Baptista A, Santiago E *et al.* Self-expandable metal stents to treat gastric leaks. *Surg Obes Relat Dis* 2006; **2**: 570–572.

31. Fakhry SM, Herbst CA, Buckwalter JA. Cholecystectomy in morbidly obese patients. *Am Surg* 1987; **53**: 26–28.

32. Stanczyk M, Deveney CW, Traxler SA *et al.* Gastro-gastric fistula in the era of the divided Roux-en-Y gastric bypass: strategies for prevention diagnosis and management. *Obes Surg* 2006; **16**: 359–364.

33. Riedt CS, Brolin RE, Sherrell RM, Field MP, Shapses SA. True fractional calcium absorption is decreased after Roux-en-Y gastric bypass surgery. *Obes Surg* 2006; **14**: 1940–1948.

34. Slater GH, Ren CJ, Siegel N *et al.* Serum fat-soluble vitamin deficiency and abnormal calcium metabolism after malabsorptive bariatric surgery. *J Gastrointest Surg* 2004; **8**: 48–55.

35. Moser F, Gorodner MV, Galvani CA, Baptista M, Chretien C, Horgan S. Pouch enlargement and band slippage: two different entities. *Surg Endosc* 2006; **20**: 1021–1029.

36. Vertruyen M. Repositioning the lap-band for proximal pouch dilatation. *Obes Surg* 2003; **13**: 285–288.

37. Gumbs AA, Pomp A, Gagner M. Revisional bariatric surgery for inadequate weight loss. *Obes Surg* 2007; **17**: 1137–1145.

38. Singhal R, Kitchen M, Ndirika S, Hunt K, Bridgwater S, Super P. The 'Birmingham stitch' – avoiding slippage in laparoscopic gastric banding. *Obes Surg* 2008; **18**: 359–363.

39. Sjostrom L, Narbro K, Sjostrom D. Costs and benefits when treating obesity. *Int J Obes Relat Metab Disord* 1995; **19 (Suppl 6)**: S9–S12.

40. Jacobsen G, Berger R, Horgan S. The role of robotic surgery in morbid obesity. *J Laparoendosc Adv Surg Tech* 2003; **13**: 279–283.

Richard Parker C. Anne McCune

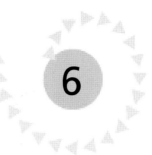

6

Non-alcoholic fatty liver disease – management of a burgeoning epidemic

Non-alcoholic fatty liver disease (NAFLD) is now the commonest chronic liver disorder in Western populations, being strongly associated with visceral obesity, insulin resistance, hypertension and hyperlipidaemia. Around 30% of adults in the US are thought to be affected and the number is projected to rise. NAFLD is widely regarded as the hepatic manifestation of the metabolic syndrome. The majority of individuals will not develop serious liver disease but a significant minority, mostly those with non-alcoholic steatohepatitis (NASH), will progress to cirrhosis. Non-liver related morbidity and mortality, mainly due to cardiovascular disease, is also higher in NAFLD subjects.

NAFLD is an umbrella term describing a spectrum of disease associated with excessive fat accumulation in the liver (steatosis), in the absence of excessive alcohol consumption (defined as no more than one standard drink a day for women and two standard drinks per day for men). The spectrum of pathology ranges from simple bland steatosis, to steatohepatitis (NASH), through to advanced fibrosis/cirrhosis and even hepatocellular carcinoma, but the histological changes seen are indistinguishable from those seen in alcohol-related liver disease. This chapter focuses on recent advances in epidemiological and clinical data as a guide to investigation and management of primary NAFLD, where the commonest risk factors are obesity, diabetes and hypertriglyceridaemia but secondary causes of NAFLD require careful exclusion (Table 1). Future potential therapies are also included. The management of NAFLD in children and adolescents will not be addressed,

Richard Parker MB ChB
Clinical Fellow, Department of Hepatology, Bristol Royal Infirmary, Marlborough Street, Bristol BS2 8HW, UK

C. Anne McCune BSc MBBS MRCP MD (for correspondence)
Consultant Gastroenterologist and Hepatologist, Clinical Effectiveness Lead, Medicine, Department of Hepatology, Bristol Royal Infirmary, Marlborough Street, Bristol BS2 8HW, UK
E-Mail: Anne.McCune@ubht.nhs.uk

Table 1 Secondary causes of fatty liver

Drugs	Tamoxifen, corticosteroids, diltiazem, methotrexate, amiodarone, nifedipine, valproate, synthetic oestrogens, antiretroviral therapy (HAART)
Toxins	Alcohol, hydrocarbons, industrial solvents, pesticides
Surgery	Jejuno-ileal bypass and biliopancreatic diversion, extensive small bowel loss
Nutritional	Total parenteral nutrition, rapid weight loss or starvation, severe small bowel bacterial overgrowth
Viral	Hepatitis C
Genetic	Wilson's disease
Metabolic	Polycystic ovary syndrome, hypothyroidism, lipodystrophy syndromes, abetalipoproteinaemia, mitochondrial disorders, Prader–Willi syndrome

although this has clearly become a major child health issue and likely to impact significantly on adult healthcare resources in the future.

EPIDEMIOLOGY

NAFLD can lead to end-stage liver disease and hepatocellular carcinoma, so there is an urgent need to define its natural history and prevalence. Obesity, type 2 diabetes, hypertension and dyslipidaemia are common features of the metabolic syndrome (Table 2). NAFLD, hepatic component of this syndrome, is very prevalent in diabetic (~70%), hypertensive (~30%), obese (~75%), and morbidly obese (~90%) patients. The World Health Organization (WHO) now recognises a global obesity epidemic. In England, over a fifth of adults are clinically obese with a further half of men and third of women being overweight (Office for National Statistics, UK).

Table 2 Adult Treatment Panel III report (ATP III) criteria for the metabolic syndrome

Risk factor	Defining level
Waist circumference	
Men	> 102 cm (> 40 inches)
Women	> 88 cm (> 35 inches)
Triglycerides*	≥ 150 mg/dl
HDL cholesterol*	
Men	< 40 mg/dl
Women	< 50 mg/dl
Blood pressure	≥ 130/85 mmHg
Fasting glucose*	≥ 110 mg/dl

Adapted from Executive Summary of 3rd report of the National Cholesterol Education Program expert panel on detection, evaluation, and treatment of high cholesterol in adults (Adult Treatment Panel III), 2001.
*Patients are considered to meet defining level if already established on cholesterol- or glucose-lowering medication.

In the US, the incidence of type 2 diabetes mellitus has doubled in the last 30 years. Given the association of NAFLD with obesity and diabetes, this rising tide of metabolic disease preludes a similar epidemic of chronic liver disease. NASH was first described in the 1970s in obese female patients denying alcohol consumption[1] but generated little interest until the end of the 1980s. Since then, attempts have been made to describe its prevalence but an accurate measure is lacking for a number of reasons. First, simple tests such as liver transaminases are normal in many subjects with NAFLD and so population studies relying on liver function tests alone will under-estimate disease prevalence. Second, radiological modalities are only sensitive once a significant amount of steatosis (usually greater than a third) has developed[2] and are operator subjective. Third, only histology can reliably distinguish NASH from simple steatosis. Liver biopsy is limited by sampling error and is invasive; it is thus unsuitable for large population studies. Additionally, many histological series have been undertaken in tertiary referral centres and/or within high-risk patient populations such as diabetics making it impossible to generalise the findings.

Despite these limitations, the prevalence of NAFLD has been estimated at between 3–23% on the basis of unexplained raised aminotransferase levels, 14–23% using liver ultrasonography and 31% using sensitive magnetic resonance (MR) spectroscopy.[3–5] Two large population studies – the Dallas Heart Study and the Third National Health and Nutrition Examination Survey (NHANES III) – have provided the most accurate prevalence data and have been reviewed elsewhere.[3,4,6] In the former study, 2200 adults in the US were screened using MR-spectroscopy: a third were found to have steatosis. This means that > 70 million US citizens potentially have NAFLD and are at higher risk of more serious liver disease.[3] A higher prevalence of steatosis was found amongst Hispanics (45%) than whites (33%) or blacks (24%). In the NHANES III study, over 15,000 adults were identified by detecting abnormal transaminases and excluding other liver diseases: up to 22% of the study population were thought to have NAFLD, if recently advocated 'healthy ranges' for transaminases are applied.[7] A recent study of biopsy-proven NAFLD from two tertiary centres in the US found an equal number of men and women to be affected but women were at higher risk of more advanced disease.[8] Finally, the Dionysus study in Italy, confirmed a similar high prevalence of NAFLD in an unselected population screened with liver ultrasonography.[9]

The true prevalence of the more serious entity NASH is unknown because liver biopsy is not feasible in large population studies. NASH could be present in a third of all NAFLD cases,[5] with current estimates suggesting the prevalence of NASH is around 2–7% in Western populations.[5]

NATURAL HISTORY AND PROGNOSIS

The natural history of NAFLD has yet to be fully determined and large, prospective studies which include histological data are still lacking. Generally, steatosis without inflammation (bland steatosis) does not progress,[3–5,10–12] whilst histological series suggest that up to a third of NASH fibrosis cases will slowly progress.[5] Predictors of progression are obesity, type 2 diabetes mellitus and fibrosis at index biopsy.[5,13] Of patients with NASH, 10–15% will develop cirrhosis, most commonly after the fifth decade.[5,12,13]

These projections are based largely on histological series of limited size but two recent studies merit further discussion. The Olmsted County study is one of the largest and best natural history studies in NAFLD.[12] A total of 420 patients with NAFLD from within a well-defined community-based population in the US were studied. Individuals with radiologically and/or histologically confirmed NAFLD were rigorously identified and overall survival compared to the age- and sex-matched controls. Although cardiovascular events remained the commonest cause of death, those with NAFLD had a higher liver-related mortality (1.7% over 7 years) than controls. These data imply that the liver-related mortality is significantly raised in NAFLD although the absolute liver-related mortality is still relatively low. However, considering the number of individuals affected globally, this represents a significant mortality-burden world-wide.

Swedish researchers following a NAFLD cohort for a mean of 14 years were able to show mortality was not increased in patients with simple steatosis but liver fibrosis progressed in 47% of NASH cases.[13] Again, mortality was higher in the NAFLD cohort than in controls and the third most common cause of death was complications of liver disease, with cardiovascular disease being the primary cause of death. Strikingly, the vast majority (78%) developed either type 2 diabetes mellitus or glucose intolerance during follow-up.[13] Further evidence that NAFLD is not a benign disease is provided by 'cryptogenic' cirrhosis data showing a higher than expected prevalence of obesity, diabetes mellitus and hypertension,[14] and by the finding that type 2 diabetes mellitus is a risk factor for hepatocellular carcinoma. Thus there is compelling circumstantial evidence that many cases of 'cryptogenic' cirrhosis are in fact attributable to 'burned-out' NASH.[14] Whether the risk of hepatocellular carcinoma in NASH cirrhosis is as high as in cirrhosis of other aetiologies remains controversial and requires further study.

PATHOGENESIS

The pathogenesis of NAFLD is subject to intense scrutiny and a complete account is beyond the scope of this chapter. Figure 1 demonstrates the various pathways from initial insult through to mechanisms for inflammation, and the potential targets for treatment. A 'two-hit' hypothesis currently serves best to explain the progression of steatosis through to steatohepatitis. It should be noted that this is probably an oversimplification of several overlapping processes.

The initial insult is the development of steatosis due to dysregulation of lipid metabolism, largely from the combined effects of obesity and insulin resistance. Increased delivery of fatty acids to the liver coupled with the metabolic effects of hyperinsulinaemia increases hepatocyte fat and 'primes' the liver for inflammation. This represents the first 'hit'. These fat-laden hepatocytes become overwhelmed and vulnerable to a 'second hit' from a variety of insults including oxidative stress (and ultimately lipid peroxification), gut-derived endotoxin, pro-inflammatory cytokines and adipose-derived adipocytokines (Fig. 1). The resultant cell injury and necro-inflammatory

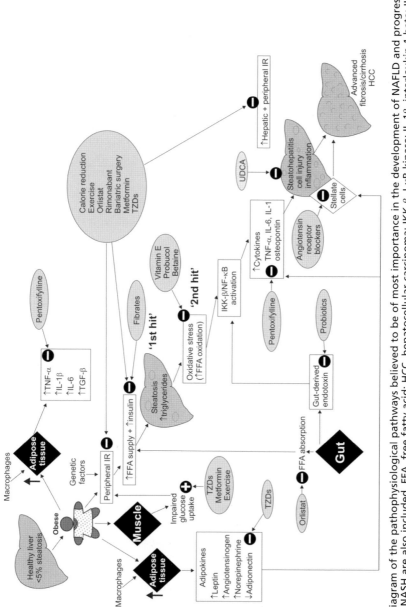

Fig. 1 Simplified schematic diagram of the pathophysiological pathways believed to be of most importance in the development of NAFLD and progression to NASH. Tested therapies in NASH are also included. FFA, free fatty acid; HCC, hepatocellular carcinoma; IKK-β, I-κB kinase; IL-1β, interleukin 1 beta; IL-6, interleukin 6; IR, insulin resistance; NF-κB, nuclear factor κB; TNF-α, tumour necrosis factor alpha; TGF-β, transforming growth factor beta; TZDs, thiazolidinediones.

reaction can lead to fibrosis and, ultimately, cirrhosis. Fibrosis, part of an attempted healing response, is mediated by various agents via hepatic stellate cells. Leptin and sympathetic nervous system tone, via angiotensin-II and norepinephrine, have been implicated (Fig. 1).

DIAGNOSIS AND INVESTIGATION

Patients with NAFLD commonly present when abnormal liver function tests are discovered incidentally or routine abdominal imaging suggests hepatic steatosis. Although patients may complain of malaise or a vague ache in the right upper quadrant (ascribed to capsular distension), most are asymptomatic. A pro-active approach is required in individuals with conditions associated with NAFLD and/or insulin resistance, such as polycystic ovarian syndrome, obstructive sleep apnoea and older diabetic patients, because the majority of NAFLD patients have normal liver function. A small but increasing proportion of patients will present with complications of end-stage liver disease.

Physical examination commonly reveals hepatomegaly. Mildly elevated AST and ALT are characteristic with the ALT:AST ratio > 1. A ratio < 1 supports alcohol-related damage, but in advanced disease the ratio can reverse. Less commonly, patients may have isolated, mildly-elevated alkaline phosphatase, but infiltrative liver disease should be excluded. Hyperferritinaemia (with normal transferrin saturation) is present in up to 60% of patients and low titre autoantibodies are also common. As NAFLD is largely a diagnosis of exclusion, other chronic liver disorders should be sought. Liver function tests cannot reliably distinguish between steatosis and advanced fibrosis/cirrhosis but failing synthetic liver function (low albumin, prolonged insulin resistance) may signify cirrhosis and thrombocytopenia may herald the development of portal hypertension.

Exclusion of patients with a history of excessive alcohol consumption is imperative but there is no clear consensus on the definition of 'excessive'. In an attempt to standardise clinical research trials, the National Institute of Health Clinical Network Research group defined that men should consume no more than 140 g/week and women no more than 70 g/week, equivalent to a maximum of 2 standard drinks/day for men and less for women.[15] The importance of life-time alcohol consumption, rather than recent consumption, levels requires further study.

Routine assessment should include appropriate investigations for other components of the metabolic syndrome (Table 2). NAFLD patients have a very high risk of developing diabetes or glucose intolerance over a 10–15-year period[13] and should, therefore, be monitored closely. Measures of insulin resistance (*e.g.* homeostasis model assessment) are costly and remain research tools. Body mass index (BMI) and waist circumference are an integral part of routine assessment with the understanding that cut-offs for such anthropometric criteria vary according to ethnicity.[15,16] Interestingly, whilst abdominal obesity (*i.e.* waist circumference) predicts the severity of metabolic risk in NAFLD, dorsocervical lipohypertrophy correlates more closely with the presence of steatohepatitis and fibrosis.[17] It remains to be seen whether the finding is clinically useful.

Imaging

Ultrasound can detect hepatic steatosis with reasonable accuracy but truncal obesity can make the examination technically difficult. Characteristically, NAFLD patients have a 'bright' diffusely echogenic liver. Ultrasonography does not have sufficient sensitivity or specificity for wide-spread screening; however, when more than a third of the liver is fatty, sensitivity improves.[2] Currently, no imaging modality can accurately distinguish simple steatosis from steatohepatitis or fibrosis; however, imaging can be useful to define complications of advanced disease (e.g. portal hypertension, ascites) and ultrasonography is the modality of choice for hepatocellular carcinoma surveillance in those with cirrhosis. MR-spectroscopy remains a research/epidemiological tool and newer imaging techniques such as contrast bubble ultrasonography remain largely untested.

DISTINGUISHING NASH FROM NAFLD AND STAGING FIBROSIS

Who should have a liver biopsy?

The decision regarding liver biopsy remains contentious. There is a need to distinguish NASH with fibrosis from bland steatosis, and to exclude other pathology. Patients with NASH have the highest cirrhosis risk and pre-existing fibrosis is a strong predictor of fibrosis progression.[12,13] Without a reliable indicator, treatment decisions are relatively uninformed and surveillance of disease progression difficult. Liver biopsy remains the gold standard test to stage hepatic fibrosis and offer prognostic advice to patients.

Biopsy, however, is invasive, carries a small but definite risk, and is costly and impractical due to the large number of patients affected. Biopsy is associated with both sampling error and interobserver variability. A recent study found the negative predictive value of a single liver biopsy in the diagnosis of NAFLD was just 0.74.[18] Those who argue against biopsy often do so because there is no definitive pharmacological therapy for NASH. However, biopsy can identify other aetiologies not previously considered and in one study biopsy led to a change in patient management in 18%.[19] Liver biopsy should be considered for those with atypical clinical features (e.g. lean patients), hyperferritinaemia associated with HFE (haemochromatosis) mutations or in those found to have positive autoantibodies.

The characteristic histological features include macrovesicular steatosis, lobular inflammation, ballooning of hepatocytes and Mallory bodies. Fibrosis in NAFLD is characteristically perisinusoidal or perivenular in the early stages; with progression, bridging fibrosis and cirrhosis is seen. A structured histology scoring system for NAFLD was developed by Brunt and colleagues in 1999. More recently, in an attempt to reach wider consensus on classification, a NAFLD activity scoring system has been promoted to ensure uniformity in clinical research.[20]

Clinical scoring systems

There are no universally accepted algorithms to aid decisions regarding either the necessity or timing of biopsy, and there remains a pressing need to detect disease and fibrosis non-invasively. Many surrogate markers of inflammation or fibrosis have been proposed with the aim of distinguishing NASH from

NAFLD and identifying bridging fibrosis/cirrhosis. The surrogate markers of advanced disease include older age, raised BMI, presence of diabetes or glucose intolerance, raised ALT, AST:ALT ratio > 1, thrombocytopenia, hyaluronic acid and serum ferritin. Scoring systems using one or more clinical or laboratory measurements have been enthusiastically promoted by research groups in an attempt to identify patients with advanced fibrosis. Such systems not only identify patients in whom biopsy is indicated, but also have the potential to monitor disease progression especially during treatment, avoiding the impracticalities of serial biopsy.[6,8,21–23] Scoring systems perform best when used to identify advanced fibrosis in NASH and are less accurate in predicting mild-to-moderate fibrosis.

The NAFLD fibrosis score[6] has been developed based on 733 patients all of whom had biopsy-proven NAFLD; 480 in an estimation group and a further 253 in a validation group. Six readily available biochemical and clinical variables found to be most significant were included in the score: BMI, age, AST/ALT, presence or absence of diabetes or fasting hyperglycaemia, platelet count and albumin. Using these variables, a risk score is calculated with high (0.676) and low (–1.455) cut off values.[6] The area under the curve (AUC) in receiver operator characteristic (ROC) analysis of the scoring system was 0.88 and 0.82 in the estimation and validation groups, respectively. The negative predictive value for exclusion of advanced fibrosis at the lower end of the score was 93% and 88% in the estimation and validation groups, respectively. Conversely, a high cut-off score gave a positive predictive value of 90% and 82% in the estimation and validation groups. Less than a third of patients fell into an indeterminate group but, more importantly, the authors concluded that biopsy could be avoided in just over 70% of patients.[6]

Others have promoted differing scoring methods. Patients with a negative BARD score (BARD – BMI, AST:ALT ratio and diabetes) appear at low risk for advanced fibrosis and could also potentially avoid biopsy.[8] The BARD and NAFLD fibrosis scores were compared in 92 patients and found to be at least equivalent in excluding patients with stage 3/4 fibrosis.[8] BARD score appears to be more accurate in predicting advanced fibrosis in non-diabetics.[8]

Non-invasive markers of fibrosis

There has also been wide-spread interest in the use of 'panel testing' to aid fibrosis detection as in other liver diseases such as hepatitis C. They are more accurate in their ability to exclude fibrosis and perform less well in those with mild-to-moderate fibrosis. One such panel, FibroTest-FibroSURE (Biopredictive),[24] has been extensively validated in hepatitis C patients. In ROC analysis, the AUC is comparable to the NAFLD fibrosis score for presence of advanced fibrosis with a negative predictive value of 90% and positive predictive value of 70%. The Original European Liver Fibrosis (OELF) panel[25] uses a different approach by employing a number of serum fibrosis-specific markers. In common with the NAFLD fibrosis score, OELF also includes age in the algorithm[25] and an AUC of 0.87 (95% CI, 0.66–1.0) suggests OELF has good diagnostic accuracy. It should be noted, however, that of the large number of patients (> 1000) studied, relatively few had NAFLD. In a recent validation study, the original panel algorithm was simplified (ELF – Enhanced Liver Fibrosis panel).[26] The utility of combining the ELF markers with the NAFLD activity score was also examined in 196 biopsy-proven NAFLD patients enrolled from two UK centres. The clinical utility of both ELF and NAFLD fibrosis score in predicting fibrosis was similar and combining the two improved accuracy further, avoiding liver biopsy in up to 88%.

Other biomarkers

Hepatocyte apoptosis, as a marker of liver cell inflammation, has been the subject of recent interest and research. Caspase cleaved cytokeratin 18 (CK-18) appears to be a useful biomarker of NASH but remains an experimental tool. It is currently being evaluated in wider 'panels' to differentiate steatosis from NASH.[27,28] Several other biomarkers including reactive oxygen species and the adipocytokines leptin and adiponectin are under investigation.

Transient elastography

A recent development in ultrasound technique is transient elastography, marketed as FibroScan®. The technique measures the velocity of low-frequency ultrasound through liver tissue and, as wave velocity is proportional to elasticity, the harder and stiffer the liver tissue the faster the wave travels. Although early studies (mainly in patients with hepatitis C) showed good correlation between stiffness measurements and fibrosis stage, it has reduced reproducibility in those with a high BMI: in a recent, large, prospective study of those with a BMI of greater than 28 kg/m^2, it was also associated with technical failure.[29] This is an obvious drawback in the context of NAFLD staging because the majority of patients will be overweight or obese. At present, FibroScan® technology cannot be recommended for NAFLD outside clinical trials.

In the absence of any universally accepted algorithms, the authors employ a pragmatic approach and do not biopsy all patients with suspected NAFLD. We use risk stratification (presently the NAFLD fibrosis score) and offer liver biopsy to those in intermediate- or high-risk groups. Local validation of any employed scoring algorithm is, however, recommended.

MANAGEMENT

Unfortunately, a paucity of randomised, controlled studies means there is currently no proven therapy for NAFLD. Relatively few patients have been studied and clinical end-points are heterogeneous, limiting the conclusions that can be drawn. In broad terms, management strategies, both current and experimental, can be generally divided into four main components:

1. Treatment strategies targeting the metabolic syndrome.

2. Treatments targeting the liver injury itself (steatohepatitis).

3. Treatments focusing on hepatocyte cytoprotection.

4. Management of complications of cirrhosis (e.g. hepatocellular carcinoma and variceal surveillance).

General management

The vast majority of patients have one or more features of the metabolic syndrome so the cornerstone of overall management should be tackling obesity, hypertension, dyslipidaemia and diabetes. As the cardiovascular event rate and mortality in NAFLD exceeds liver-related death, especially in those with early fibrosis, aggressive management of the metabolic syndrome can reduce mortality. It is reasonable to assume that such a strategy will also eventually reduce liver-related morbidity. Indeed, a multifactorial intervention which focused on aggressive management of individual components of the metabolic syndrome in non-diabetic NAFLD patients was beneficial.[30] HMG-CoA reductase inhibitors (statins) can be recommended as safe and should be initiated as indicated by the patient's cardiovascular/diabetic risk profile. Primary care physicians can be re-assured there is no excess risk of a statin-induced hepatitis[31] even if serum transaminases are raised, and little evidence exists to support the wide-spread costly monitoring currently undertaken in primary care. There is no consensus guidance on even minimal/modest alcohol consumption once a diagnosis of NAFLD is made and studies are required to address this, especially in those patients with marked necro-inflammatory activity on biopsy. The safest course, for a concerned patient, is complete abstinence.

Life-style intervention: weight loss and exercise

NAFLD patients are commonly overweight or obese and, almost without exception, have insulin resistance. Weight reduction as a management strategy in NAFLD is biologically plausible because weight loss reduces adipose tissue, lowers insulin levels and improves insulin sensitivity (Fig. 1). In diabetes prevention programmes, life-style intervention significantly reduces development of the metabolic syndrome[32] and has potential to reduce NAFLD development and/or progression as well. However, there are few studies substantiating this hypothesis, most of which are uncontrolled and largely investigate calorie reduction and/or exercise rather than dietary manipulation *per se*. The benefits of life-style modification in NAFLD have recently been reviewed[33] but there remains no consensus on how this should be achieved. A carbohydrate, rather than fat, restricted diet lowers transaminases more in insulin resistant adults[34] but more controlled studies in this area are merited. Surprisingly, there has been only one controlled study of calorie-restricted diet and exercise in NAFLD which included an evaluation of histological response.[35] Twenty-five obese Japanese patients were enrolled, 15 of whom followed a restricted diet combined with an exercise programme for 3 months and compared to 10 patients with no life-style changes. Biochemical tests including transaminases and histological steatosis improved significantly in the group who had life-style intervention.

Patients with NAFLD should enrol on a weight-reduction programme to achieve a 10% weight reduction over a 6-month period, or no more than 1.5 kg/week, because rapid or excessive weight loss can result in deterioration of the underlying liver disease. A calorie-restricted diet should be combined with 30 min of daily aerobic exercise. The ideal diet composition for NAFLD patients has not been established and further, larger, controlled studies are required.

Pharmacological treatment of obesity

Pharmacological therapy should be considered for those who fail to respond adequately to the life-style changes described above.

Orlistat

Orlistat is a non-absorbed inhibitor of gastric and pancreatic lipases, reducing the absorption of dietary triglycerides by a third. It is a licensed and proven anti-obesity agent and, although generally well-tolerated, unpleasant gastrointestinal side effects (*e.g.* loose fatty stools) can lead to compliance problems. Early pilot data suggested a beneficial effect in two small series of obese individuals with biopsy-proven NASH when combined with appropriate dietary advice. Improved aminotransferases, histological steatosis, necro-inflammation and, in some cases, fibrosis were described.[36,37] However, the period of follow-up was short and both studies were uncontrolled. Subsequently, there have been two randomised controlled trials (RCTs) examining orlistat in NASH but only one full publication.[38] Fifty-two patients with confirmed NAFLD were randomised to treatment with orlistat or placebo for 6 months.[38] Patients were also given additional dietary and exercise advice. Just over half of the patients in whom an index biopsy was performed underwent a second biopsy at end-of-study period. Orlistat was found to improve both aminotransferases and radiological steatosis, as measured by ultrasonography, and this effect appeared independent of weight reduction.

Rimonabant

Rimonabant is a selective antagonist of cannabinoid type-1 receptors and indicated in obese adults as an adjunct to diet and exercise. Cannabinoid type-1 receptors, both central and peripheral, are up-regulated in obesity. Rimonabant is undergoing clinical investigation in NASH following a positive animal study which indicated a role beyond that of simple weight loss.[39,40] Rimonabant is contra-indicated in patients with major depression or those taking antidepressants as depressive reactions occur in up to 10% of those treated.

Sibutramine

Sibutramine is a serotonin and norepinephrine re-uptake inhibitor that mainly acts to increase satiety. In type II diabetics, sibutramine was efficacious in achieving weight loss and has beneficial effects on insulin resistance and dyslipidaemia amongst other metabolic effects. There has been a small, uncontrolled, pilot study showing some benefit in NAFLD.[41]

Bariatric surgery

Bariatric surgery is widely accepted as the treatment modality of choice in the severely obese because it is associated with durable long-term weight control and improves insulin resistance, obstructive sleep apnoea, hypertension and hyperlipidaemia when compared to controls.[42] Recent data have also confirmed an overall reduction in mortality following bariatric surgery.[43] It is gaining further support in the subgroup with NAFLD because of emerging evidence that the liver insult also appears to benefit.

'Restrictive' bariatric surgery includes the current 'gold standard' of laparoscopic adjustable gastric banding (LAGB) and older operations such as vertical gastric banding, horizontal gastroplasty and open adjustable banding. 'Malabsorptive' bariatric surgery, such as jejuno-ileal bypass and biliopancreatic diversions, is less frequently performed now in large part because of high number of operative complications but also because the dramatic weight loss associated with this type of surgery was associated with worsening liver disease. Bariatric surgery is approved by the National Institute for Health and Clinical Excellence (<www.nice.org.uk>) for morbidly obese patients (BMI ≥ 40 kg/m^2) or patients with a lower BMI (BMI ≥ 35 kg/m^2) and a co-morbidity which may improve with weight loss (type 2 diabetes mellitus, hypertension). The average weight loss achieved with bariatric surgery is approximately 50–60% from baseline.

Bariatric surgery of differing types is associated with improvement in liver function tests and, to varying degree, histological improvement.[44–52] LAGB has gained in popularity, particularly in Europe and the UK, due to the minimally-invasive approach and reduced complication rate. In Australian patients undergoing bariatric surgery, LAGB was found to be a highly efficacious method of achieving and maintaining weight loss.[44,45] There were also major improvements identified on repeat biopsy, with resolution of NASH observed in 80%. Those with the metabolic syndrome benefited the most from surgery.[44,45] In a novel study, weight loss was associated with significantly reduced hepatic expression of factors regulating fibrogenesis and inflammation in NAFLD as well as a predicted reduction insulin resistance, although numbers studied were small.[49] Whether bariatric surgery will lead to the predicted long-term reductions in liver-related morbidity and mortality still remains to be established. The length of histological follow-up in bariatric series has been inconsistent and, in general, relatively short. In a recent study,[18] consecutive patients with NAFLD (two-thirds of whom had NASH) undergoing Roux-en-Y gastric bypass surgery were evaluated 2 years' post-surgery.[53] Wedge liver biopsies were performed at time of surgery and patients underwent a further percutaneous biopsy 2 years later. The mean weight loss was approximately 60% at follow-up and associated with improved steatosis, steatohepatitis and fibrosis. More importantly, this massive weight loss was not associated with histological progression of disease but again the number studied was small. Finally, a recent systematic review published in abstract form concluded steatosis and necro-inflammatory changes improve or completely resolve in the majority of patients following bariatric surgery with a low risk of fibrosis progression or worsening of steatohepatitis.[54]

Patients considering bariatric surgery should be assessed and counselled by a multidisciplinary team including an obesity surgeon and clinician with expertise in obesity management. The vast majority of patients (around 90%) offered bariatric surgery will have NAFLD and additional advice/input from a hepatologists is important; some experts advocate routine liver biopsy to aid management.[55] Well-compensated liver disease should not automatically preclude surgery as those with NASH cirrhosis can benefit from bariatric surgery.[56] Incidental cirrhosis is present in a small, but significant, number of patients undergoing surgery[57] but patients should be managed on an individual basis and there are no large series to guide practice.

In summary, bariatric surgery has the potential to induce marked, durable weight loss with associated improvement in necro-inflammation (normalisation of LFTs) and fibrosis. It is the treatment modality of choice for the morbidly obese patient with NAFLD, especially with co-morbidity.

Management of insulin resistance

Insulin resistance plays a central role in pathogenesis of NAFLD (Fig. 1) and NAFLD itself may also play a key role in the development and progression of other components of the metabolic syndrome.[58] Treatment of insulin resistance has focused on metformin and thiazolidinediones.

Thiazolidinediones 'glitazones'

Thiazolidinediones (TZDs) agonise nuclear transcription factor peroxisome proliferation-activated receptor γ (PPAR-γ) and improve insulin sensitivity. The receptor is up-regulated in animal models of fatty liver[59] and a number of animal studies have shown beneficial effects of PPAR-γ agonists on liver steatosis, inflammation and fibrosis. Unfortunately, an early TZD (troglitazone) was associated with severe hepatotoxicity and withdrawn, but rosiglitazone and pioglitazone are now widely used in the management of type II diabetes.

Rosiglitazone (4 mg twice daily) for 48 weeks was found beneficial in a small (n = 22) non-placebo controlled study of biopsy-proven NASH improving insulin sensitivity, histological scores and mean transaminase levels.[60] Similarly, 18 normoglycaemic NASH subjects were given 30 mg pioglitazone daily for 48 weeks with demonstrable improvement in all liver enzymes, radiological steatosis/liver volume and improved fibrosis scores in some patients.[61] The first RCT involving TZDs,[62] studied 55 biopsy-proven NASH patients with either type 2 diabetes mellitus or impaired glucose tolerance. Patients were randomised to receive pioglitazone 45 mg daily and low calorie diet or treated with diet alone. Although there was significant improvement in steatosis, inflammation and hepatocyte ballooning with pioglitazone compared to placebo, the improvement in fibrosis did not reach statistical significance. In a larger RCT (published in abstract form only), rosiglitazone was also beneficial.[63] Finally, Aithal et al.[64] recently presented an abstract of findings of a small double-blind RCT (n = 74). Non-diabetic patients with NASH were either treated with pioglitazone together with diet and exercise, or prescribed diet and exercise alone for 12 months. Pioglitazone was superior to placebo in reducing insulin resistance, liver function tests, serum ferritin and tissue inhibitor of metalloproteinase (TIMP)-1 but was associated with significant weight gain (see below). The histological findings were rather inconsistent; in comparison to placebo there were no significant changes in steatosis or lobular inflammation, although hepatocellullar injury was significantly reduced ($P = 0.005$) and an improvement in fibrosis was also significant ($P = 0.05$). Further studies with extended follow-up are required to validate these findings and assess pioglitazone's long-term efficacy.

TZDs are generally well tolerated by patients with fatigue and peripheral oedema being the main adverse events reported. Pioglitazone was found to increase weight in patients with NASH due to an increase in adipose tissue mass rather than water retention,[65] a particularly undesirable effect in NAFLD although the fat increase tends to be peripheral rather than visceral. Unfortunately, the long-term safety of TZDs has been questioned after an increase in cardiovascular events in male diabetics treated with rosiglitazone was reported. Larger RCTs are required to assess their efficacy and safety because the treatment effect in NAFLD is likely to require long-term therapy.[66]

Metformin
Metformin, a biguanide, is widely used in the management of hyperglycaemia in overweight patients with type 2 diabetes mellitus. It is an insulin-sensitising agent and was associated with a reduction in liver fat/size and transaminases in studies with obese ob/ob mice.[67] Its precise action is unknown but it appears to decrease hepatic glucose production, improve insulin resistance and free fatty acid uptake by hepatocytes, most likely through inhibited expression of tumour necrosis factor-α (TNF-α) and TNF-α inducible factors.[67] Initial pilot studies[68–72] reported biochemical improvement but histological evaluation was incomplete. In a randomised open-label comparison study of metformin or vitamin E with diet alone, metformin was superior to vitamin E or diet in reducing transaminase levels ($P < 0.0001$).[73] Treatment was associated with improvement in histological inflammation and fibrosis but few patients in the metformin group underwent repeat liver biopsy limiting the conclusions that can be drawn. In another non-blinded RCT. 6-months' treatment with metformin (850 mg b.d.), in combination with a lipid and calorie reduction diet, led to significantly lower mean aminotransferase levels and improved insulin resistance in comparison to controls treated with diet alone.[74] Disappointingly, there was no significant improvement in necro-inflammatory activity nor fibrosis on liver histology but the treatment duration was relatively short and histological follow-up incomplete. Metformin was generally well-tolerated and not associated with symptomatic hypoglycaemia or significant lactic acidosis. Further, larger, well-powered, double-blind RCTs are warranted including larger number of patients with advanced fibrosis before metformin can be recommended for non-diabetic patients with NAFLD.

Other modifiers of insulin resistance
Nateglinide, an insulin secretagogue, has been studied in five patients with both diabetes and NASH with favourable results.[75] In a short-term, pilot study, oligofructose, an inulin-type fructan, improved liver biochemistry in patients with NASH.[76] Exenatide, an incretin analogue, is a newer diabetic agent and improves insulin resistance. Early animal data have recently been published but human data are limited.

Lipid-lowering agents
Dyslipidaemia is common in patients with NAFLD, especially hyper-triglyceridaemia. In NASH patients with hypercholesterolaemia, statins reduce serum cholesterol, serum transaminases,[77–80] ultrasonographic steatosis[77,78] and, in a small study of five patients treated with pravastatin, also steatohepatitis.[80] The studies are too small to make wide-spread recommendations. Their therapeutic efficacy in NASH is likely to be limited because, although effective at reducing cholesterol, they have lesser impact on serum

triglyceride levels. However, statins in NAFLD patients are well-tolerated and safe (see above).

The use of fibrates (PPAR-α agonists) is more rational and, indeed, beneficial effects have been confirmed in murine models of NASH. However, there is limited human data and only one RCT (46 patients were randomised to receive 600 mg gemfibrozil daily or placebo). Although biochemical improvement occurred, histological data were lacking and the treatment duration was short.[81] Conversely, clofibrate proved non-beneficial when examined in a 1-year pilot study.[82]

Probucol is a lipid-lowering medication which also has additional antioxidant properties. A small RCT showed promising results[83,84] but there is insufficient data to recommend wide-spread use in NAFLD.

Angiotensin-receptor blockers

Increased sympathetic nervous system (SNS) tone has been demonstrated in obese mice with NASH. In similar animal models, angiotensin II has been shown to be profibrotic via the activation of hepatic stellate cells. The SNS could be an exciting potential therapeutic target to switch off both necro-inflammation and fibrosis in NASH. Angiotensin receptor blockers also decrease insulin resistance and, in a recent small pilot study in hypertensive NASH patients, losartan was beneficial, meriting further study.[85,86]

Antioxidants

Vitamin E

Oxidative stress is known to play a central key role in the pathogenesis of NASH so research has focused on agents with the potential to reduce this. There have been a number of small studies involving vitamin E with conflicting results. Vitamin E acts as radical scavenger, preventing lipid peroxification. In a RCT comparing both vitamin E (1000 IU) and vitamin C (1000 mg) daily for 6 months to placebo, necro-inflammation was not reduced but there was significant improvement in fibrosis.[87] In addition to its antioxidant properties, vitamin E may also reduce insulin resistance and PPAR-α expression in NASH.[88]

Betaine

Betaine is a choline metabolite with antioxidant properties. One small, uncontrolled study has suggested potential benefit in NASH but more data are required.

Iron

Insulin and iron pathways are interlinked with iron status, influencing hepatic insulin signalling and glucose uptake. This is supported by the evidence that venesection therapy can improve insulin resistance in healthy volunteers and type 2 diabetes mellitus patients with hyperferritinaemia. A few, small, uncontrolled studies have also shown a beneficial effect of venesection in those identified with NAFLD. Recently, in an observational study, Valenti et al.[89] studied the effects of 4 months' venesection therapy in 64 Italian subjects with NAFLD who had failed to respond to a 4-month period of initial life-style modification compared to controls matched for age, sex, BMI, ferritin and ALT level. Phlebotomy reduced insulin resistance but had no effect on transaminases. Those with a higher baseline ferritin seemed to benefit most. A major limitation of this study was a lack of histological data. Although early studies suggested hepatic iron was a significant source of oxidative stress in NAFLD, more recent data suggest haemosiderosis and HFE mutations do not contribute significantly to fibrosis development in NAFLD and iron burden is largely below a fibrogenic level previously described in hereditary haemochromatosis.[90] Increased ferritin levels in NAFLD are a surrogate marker for the presence of severe fibrosis rather than iron overload *per se*.

Cytoprotective agents

Pentoxifylline
TNF-α is an important anti-inflammatory cytokine in the pathogenesis of NASH and remains a future potential target. Pentoxifylline, an oral TNF-α antagonist, has not been evaluated in a RCT, although pilot data reported significant biochemical improvement in NASH.

Ursodeoxycholic acid
Ursodeoxycholic acid (UDCA), a bile acid, is used in a wide spectrum of chronic liver diseases and is associated with an excellent safety profile. Its action is not precisely understood but it is postulated to be of benefit in NASH through a direct cytoprotective and anti-apoptotic effect. A large, randomised, double-blinded, placebo-controlled study of 166 NASH patients showed no benefit above placebo for the group given UDCA for 1 year at a dose equivalent to 13–15 mcg/kg/day,[91] although a later pilot, randomised, smaller study found improved LFTs and steatosis in those treated for 2 years with UDCA and vitamin E in comparison to placebo after 2 years of therapy.[92]

Probiotics
There has been recent interest, as in other liver diseases, in a potential imbalance in normal gut flora and gut bacterial toxins in the pathogenesis of NASH making manipulation of small bowel bacterial flora a novel, attractive and potentially safe therapeutic target.[93] Probiotics (such as VSL#3) may be of use but further study is required.[94]

Other agents
The IKK2–NF-κB signalling pathway (Fig. 1) is believed to play a key role in NASH progression. Pharmacological blockade of IKK2 improved dietary-induced NASH in mice[95] and IKK2 appears a promising target for future therapy.

CONCLUSIONS

Non-alcoholic fatty liver disease has now become the commonest cause of chronic liver disease world-wide. Strong evidence that NAFLD is part of the metabolic syndrome indicates that NAFLD will become more prevalent in the future. Although many patients have silent disease and will ultimately die of non-hepatic causes, NAFLD should not be considered a benign condition as a significant proportion of patients will progress to cirrhosis and liver failure.

The burden on all health services, especially gastroenterology/hepatology services, is thus likely to increase.

The investigation of patients with possible NAFLD should exclude other liver pathology and secondary causes of fatty liver. The balance between biopsy and surrogate markers of fibrosis must be judged, and clinical scoring systems exist to aid decision making but require further validation in different patient populations. Attention should be paid to surveillance of associated conditions, particularly the development of type 2 diabetes mellitus and hypertension.

The treatment of NAFLD is currently being intensely investigated, but at present there is no established treatment for those with the more severe NASH. Despite this, weight loss with life-style measures should be pursued and bariatric surgery has a proven role in the treatment of the morbidly obese patient with NASH. The evidence for therapeutic agents in non-diabetic patients, such as thiazdioneliodiones and metformin, remains weak. There is, therefore, a pressing need for further novel treatment therapies, targeting one or more of the multiple interactive pathways now elucidated in NAFLD development, if the burgeoning epidemic of fatty liver disease is to be contained in a cost effective manner.

Key points for clinical practice

- Non-alcoholic fatty liver disease (NAFLD) is a common clinical problem with evidence of an increasing burden of liver-related mortality globally, especially in Western 'developed' nations where up to a third of adults are thought to be affected.

- NAFLD is a spectrum of disorders ranging from simple bland steatosis to non-alcoholic steatohepatitis (NASH), cirrhosis and hepatocellular carcinoma.

- NAFLD is the hepatic manifestation of the metabolic syndrome. The global obesity epidemic predicts an increase in advanced disease.

- Steatosis alone has a benign prognosis and rarely progresses to cirrhosis. Conversely, individuals with NASH are at risk of developing cirrhosis with current estimates suggesting 10–15% will develop end-stage liver disease.

- Liver biopsy is the only reliable way to diagnose and stage NASH but is not without limitations. It should be reserved for those at risk of more serious liver disease.

- Although non-invasive tests of fibrosis lack sensitivity and specificity in screening for mild-to-moderate fibrosis, clinical scoring systems such as the NAFLD fibrosis score are practical and may help the busy clinician target biopsy, especially in practices where resources and biopsy availability are limited.

- Management of NAFLD/NASH should primarily focus on the underlying MS; life-style changes, namely dietary calorie restriction and regular aerobic exercise, remain the cornerstone of therapy.

(continued next page)

Key points for clinical practice *(continued)*

- There is insufficient data to recommend wide-scale pharmacological intervention in NAFLD. Further research is required to study the risk–benefit and cost-effectiveness of experimental therapies. Statins are safe in patients with NAFLD. Individuals with NASH (with or without more advanced liver disease) are no more likely to develop a drug-induced liver injury than those without fatty liver disease.

- Bariatric surgery can be recommended in the morbidly obese patient with NAFLD and is most successful when the patient is managed by an expert centre with a multidisciplinary team approach.

- Patients diagnosed with NAFLD should be screened annually for diabetes and hypertension.

References

1. Ludwig J, Viggiano TR, McGill DB, Oh BJ. Nonalcoholic steatohepatitis: Mayo Clinic experiences with a hitherto unnamed disease. *Mayo Clin Proc* 1980; **55**: 434–438.
2. Saadeh S, Younossi ZM, Remer EM *et al*. The utility of radiological imaging in nonalcoholic fatty liver disease. *Gastroenterology* 2002; **123**: 745–750.
3. Angulo P. GI epidemiology: nonalcoholic fatty liver disease. *Aliment Pharmacol Ther* 2007; **25**: 883–889.
4. McCullough AJ. The epidemiology and risk factors of NASH. In: Farrell GC, George J, de la M.Hall P, McCullough AJ. (eds) *Fatty liver disease. NASH and related disorders.* Oxford: Blackwell, 2005; 23–37.
5. Farrell GC, Larter CZ. Nonalcoholic fatty liver disease: from steatosis to cirrhosis. *Hepatology* 2006; **43 (Suppl 1)**: S99–S112.
6. Angulo P, Hui JM, Marchesini G *et al*. The NAFLD fibrosis score: a noninvasive system that identifies liver fibrosis in patients with NAFLD. *Hepatology* 2007; **45**: 846–854.
7. Clark JM, Brancati FL, Diehl AM. The prevalence and etiology of elevated aminotransferase levels in the United States. *Am J Gastroenterol* 2003; **98**: 960–967.
8. Harrison S, Oliver D, Arnold HL, Gogia S, Neuschwander-Tetri BA. Development and validation of a simple NAFLD clinical scoring system for identifying patients without advanced disease. *Gut* 2008; doi: 10.11136/gut.2007.146019.
9. Bedogni G, Miglioli L, Masutti F, Tiribelli C, Marchesini G, Bellentani S. Prevalence of and risk factors for nonalcoholic fatty liver disease: the Dionysos nutrition and liver study. *Hepatology* 2005; **42**: 44–52.
10. Dam-Larsen S, Franzmann M, Andersen IB *et al*. Long term prognosis of fatty liver: risk of chronic liver disease and death. *Gut* 2004; **53**: 750–755.
11. Teli MR, James OF, Burt AD, Bennett MK, Day CP. The natural history of nonalcoholic fatty liver: a follow-up study. *Hepatology* 1995; **22**: 1714–1719.
12. Adams LA, Lymp JF, St Sauver J *et al*. The natural history of nonalcoholic fatty liver disease: a population-based cohort study. *Gastroenterology* 2005; **129**: 113–121.
13. Ekstedt M, Franzen LE, Mathiesen UL *et al*. Long-term follow-up of patients with NAFLD and elevated liver enzymes. *Hepatology* 2006; **44**: 865–873.
14. Maheshwari A, Thuluvath PJ. Cryptogenic cirrhosis and NAFLD: are they related? *Am J Gastroenterol* 2006; **101**: 664–668.
15. Chitturi S, Farrell GC, Hashimoto E, Saibara T, Lau GK, Sollano JD. Non-alcoholic fatty liver disease in the Asia-Pacific region: definitions and overview of proposed guidelines. *J Gastroenterol Hepatol* 2007; **22**: 778–787.
16. Chan HL, de Silva HJ, Leung NW, Lim SG, Farrell GC. How should we manage patients with non-alcoholic fatty liver disease in 2007? *J Gastroenterol Hepatol* 2007; **22**: 801–808.

17. Cheung O, Kapoor A, Puri P *et al.* The impact of fat distribution on the severity of nonalcoholic fatty liver disease and metabolic syndrome. *Hepatology* 2007; **46**: 1091–1100.

18. Ratziu V, Charlotte F, Heurtier A *et al.* Sampling variability of liver biopsy in nonalcoholic fatty liver disease. *Gastroenterology* 2005; **128**: 1898–1906.

19. Skelly MM, James PD, Ryder SD. Findings on liver biopsy to investigate abnormal liver function tests in the absence of diagnostic serology. *J Hepatol* 2001; **35**: 195–199.

20. Kleiner DE, Brunt EM, Van NM *et al.* Design and validation of a histological scoring system for nonalcoholic fatty liver disease. *Hepatology* 2005; **41**: 1313–1321.

21. Dixon JB, Bhathal PS, O'Brien PE. Nonalcoholic fatty liver disease: predictors of nonalcoholic steatohepatitis and liver fibrosis in the severely obese. *Gastroenterology* 2001; **121**: 91–100.

22. Angulo P, Keach JC, Batts KP, Lindor KD. Independent predictors of liver fibrosis in patients with nonalcoholic steatohepatitis. *Hepatology* 1999; **30**: 1356–1362.

23. Ratziu V, Giral P, Charlotte F *et al.* Liver fibrosis in overweight patients. *Gastroenterology* 2000; **118**: 1117–1123.

24. Ratziu V, Massard J, Charlotte F *et al.* Diagnostic value of biochemical markers (FibroTest-FibroSURE) for the prediction of liver fibrosis in patients with non-alcoholic fatty liver disease. *BMC Gastroenterol* 2006; **6**: 6.

25. Rosenberg WM, Voelker M, Thiel R *et al.* Serum markers detect the presence of liver fibrosis: a cohort study. *Gastroenterology* 2004; **127**: 1704–1713.

26. Guha IN, Parkes J, Roderick P *et al.* Noninvasive markers of fibrosis in nonalcoholic fatty liver disease: Validating the European Liver Fibrosis Panel and exploring simple markers. *Hepatology* 2008; **47**: 455–460.

27. Wieckowska A, McCullough AJ, Feldstein AE. Noninvasive diagnosis and monitoring of nonalcoholic steatohepatitis: present and future. *Hepatology* 2007; **46**: 582–589.

28. Wieckowska A, Zein NN, Yerian LM, Lopez AR, McCullough AJ, Feldstein AE. *In vivo* assessment of liver cell apoptosis as a novel biomarker of disease severity in nonalcoholic fatty liver disease. *Hepatology* 2006; **44**: 27–33.

29. Foucher J, Chanteloup E, Vergniol J *et al.* Diagnosis of cirrhosis by transient elastography (FibroScan): a prospective study. *Gut* 2006; **55**: 403–408.

30. Athyros VG, Mikhailidis DP, Didangelos TP *et al.* Effect of multifactorial treatment on non-alcoholic fatty liver disease in metabolic syndrome: a randomised study. *Curr Med Res Opin* 2006; **22**: 873–883.

31. Lewis JH, Mortensen ME, Zweig S, Fusco MJ, Medoff JR, Belder R. Efficacy and safety of high-dose pravastatin in hypercholesterolemic patients with well-compensated chronic liver disease: results of a prospective, randomized, double-blind, placebo-controlled, multicenter trial. *Hepatology* 2007; **46**: 1453–1463.

32. Orchard TJ, Temprosa M, Goldberg R *et al.* The effect of metformin and intensive lifestyle intervention on the metabolic syndrome: the Diabetes Prevention Program randomized trial. *Ann Intern Med* 2005; **142**: 611–619.

33. Harrison SA, Day CP. Benefits of lifestyle modification in NAFLD. *Gut* 2007; **56**: 1760–1769.

34. Ryan MC, Abbasi F, Lamendola C, Carter S, McLaughlin TL. Serum alanine aminotransferase levels decrease further with carbohydrate than fat restriction in insulin-resistant adults. *Diabetes Care* 2007; **30**: 1075–1080.

35. Ueno T, Sugawara H, Sujaku K *et al.* Therapeutic effects of restricted diet and exercise in obese patients with fatty liver. *J Hepatol* 1997; **27**: 103–107.

36. Harrison SA, Fincke C, Helinski D, Torgerson S, Hayashi P. A pilot study of orlistat treatment in obese, non-alcoholic steatohepatitis patients. *Aliment Pharmacol Ther* 2004; **20**: 623–628.

37. Hussein O, Grosovski M, Schlesinger S, Szvalb S, Assy N. Orlistat reverse fatty infiltration and improves hepatic fibrosis in obese patients with nonalcoholic steatohepatitis (NASH). *Dig Dis Sci* 2007; **52**: 2512–2519.

38. Zelber-Sagi S, Kessler A, Brazowsky E *et al.* A double-blind randomized placebo-controlled trial of orlistat for the treatment of nonalcoholic fatty liver disease. *Clin Gastroenterol Hepatol* 2006; **4**: 639–644.

39. Banasch M, Goetze O, Schmidt WE, Meier JJ. Rimonabant as a novel therapeutic option for nonalcoholic steatohepatitis. *Liver Int* 2007; **27**: 1152–1155.

40. Gary-Bobo M, Elachouri G, Gallas JF *et al.* Rimonabant reduces obesity-associated hepatic steatosis and features of metabolic syndrome in obese Zucker fa/fa rats. *Hepatology* 2007; **46**: 122–129.

41. Sabuncu T, Nazligul Y, Karaoglanoglu M, Ucar E, Kilic FB. The effects of sibutramine and orlistat on the ultrasonographic findings, insulin resistance and liver enzyme levels in obese patients with non-alcoholic steatohepatitis. *Rom J Gastroenterol* 2003; **12**: 189–192.

42. Scheen AJ, Letiexhe M, Rorive M, De FJ, Luyckx FH, Desaive C. Bariatric surgery: 10-year results of the Swedish Obese Subjects Study. *Rev Med Liege* 2005; **60**: 121–125.

43. Sjostrom L, Narbro K, Sjostrom CD *et al.* Effects of bariatric surgery on mortality in Swedish obese subjects. *N Engl J Med* 2007; **357**: 741–752.

44. Dixon JB, Bhathal PS, O'Brien PE. Weight loss and non-alcoholic fatty liver disease: falls in gamma-glutamyl transferase concentrations are associated with histologic improvement. *Obes Surg* 2006; **16**: 1278–1286.

45. Dixon JB, Bhathal PS, Hughes NR, O'Brien PE. Nonalcoholic fatty liver disease: Improvement in liver histological analysis with weight loss. *Hepatology* 2004; **39**: 1647–1654.

46. Shaffer EA. Bariatric surgery: a promising solution for nonalcoholic steatohepatitis in the very obese. *J Clin Gastroenterol* 2006; **40 (Suppl 1)**: S44–S50.

47. Stratopoulos C, Papakonstantinou A, Terzis I *et al.* Changes in liver histology accompanying massive weight loss after gastroplasty for morbid obesity. *Obes Surg* 2005; **15**: 1154–1160.

48. Jaskiewicz K, Raczynska S, Rzepko R, Sledzinski Z. Nonalcoholic fatty liver disease treated by gastroplasty. *Dig Dis Sci* 2006; **51**: 21–26.

49. Klein S, Mittendorfer B, Eagon JC *et al.* Gastric bypass surgery improves metabolic and hepatic abnormalities associated with nonalcoholic fatty liver disease. *Gastroenterology* 2006; **130**: 1564–1572.

50. Mathurin P, Gonzalez F, Kerdraon O *et al.* The evolution of severe steatosis after bariatric surgery is related to insulin resistance. *Gastroenterology* 2006; **130**: 1617–1624.

51. Barker KB, Palekar NA, Bowers SP, Goldberg JE, Pulcini JP, Harrison SA. Non-alcoholic steatohepatitis: effect of Roux-en-Y gastric bypass surgery. *Am J Gastroenterol* 2006; **101**: 368–373.

52. Kral JG, Thung SN, Biron S *et al.* Effects of surgical treatment of the metabolic syndrome on liver fibrosis and cirrhosis. *Surgery* 2004; **135**: 48–58.

53. Furuya Jr CK, de Oliveira CP, de Mello ES *et al.* Effects of bariatric surgery on nonalcoholic fatty liver disease: preliminary findings after 2 years. *J Gastroenterol Hepatol* 2007; **22**: 510–514.

54. Mummadi R, Kasturi K, Sood G. Effect of bariatric surgery on non-alcoholic fatty liver disease (NAFLD): a meta-analysis. *Hepatology* 2007; **46 (Suppl 1)**: 294A.

55. Shalhub S, Parsee A, Gallagher SF *et al.* The importance of routine liver biopsy in diagnosing nonalcoholic steatohepatitis in bariatric patients. *Obes Surg* 2004; **14**: 54–59.

56. Dallal RM, Mattar SG, Lord JL *et al.* Results of laparoscopic gastric bypass in patients with cirrhosis. *Obes Surg* 2004; **14**: 47–53.

57. Machado M, Marques-Vidal P, Cortez-Pinto H. Hepatic histology in obese patients undergoing bariatric surgery. *J Hepatol* 2006; **45**: 600–606.

58. Targher G, Bertolini L, Padovani R *et al.* Prevalence of nonalcoholic fatty liver disease and its association with cardiovascular disease among type 2 diabetic patients. *Diabetes Care* 2007; **30**: 1212–1218.

59. Yamaguchi K, Yang L, McCall S *et al.* Inhibiting triglyceride synthesis improves hepatic steatosis but exacerbates liver damage and fibrosis in obese mice with nonalcoholic steatohepatitis. *Hepatology* 2007; **45**: 1366–1374.

60. Neuschwander-Tetri BA, Brunt EM, Wehmeier KR, Oliver D, Bacon BR. Improved nonalcoholic steatohepatitis after 48 weeks of treatment with the PPAR-gamma ligand rosiglitazone. *Hepatology* 2003; **38**: 1008–1017.

61. Promrat K, Lutchman G, Uwaifo GI *et al.* A pilot study of pioglitazone treatment for nonalcoholic steatohepatitis. *Hepatology* 2004; **39**: 188–196.

62. Belfort R, Harrison SA, Brown K *et al.* A placebo-controlled trial of pioglitazone in subjects with nonalcoholic steatohepatitis. *N Engl J Med* 2006; **355**: 2297–2307.

63. Ratziu V, Charlotte F, Jacqueminent S *et al.* A one year randomized, placebo-controlled,

double-blind trial of rosiglitazone in non-alcoholic steatohepatitis: results of the FLIRT pilot trial. *J Hepatol* 2006; **44 (Suppl 2)**: S272.

64. Aithal GP, Thomas JA, Kaye P *et al*. A randomized, double blind, placebo controlled trial of one year of pioglitazone in non-diabetic subjects with nonalcoholic steatohepatitis. *Hepatology* 2007; **46 (Suppl 1)**: 295A.

65. Balas B, Belfort R, Harrison SA *et al*. Pioglitazone treatment increases whole body fat but not total body water in patients with non-alcoholic steatohepatitis. *J Hepatol* 2007; **47**: 565–570.

66. Lutchman G, Modi A, Kleiner DE *et al*. The effects of discontinuing pioglitazone in patients with nonalcoholic steatohepatitis. *Hepatology* 2007; **46**: 424–429.

67. Lin HZ, Yang SQ, Chuckaree C, Kuhajda F, Ronnet G, Diehl AM. Metformin reverses fatty liver disease in obese, leptin-deficient mice. *Nat Med* 2000; **6**: 998–1003.

68. Magalotti D, Marchesini G, Ramilli S, Berzigotti A, Bianchi G, Zoli M. Splanchnic haemodynamics in non-alcoholic fatty liver disease: effect of a dietary/pharmacological treatment. A pilot study. *Dig Liver Dis* 2004; **36**: 406–411.

69. Marchesini G, Brizi M, Bianchi G, Tomassetti S, Zoli M, Melchionda N. Metformin in non-alcoholic steatohepatitis. *Lancet* 2001; **358**: 893–894.

70. Nair S, Diehl AM, Wiseman M, Farr Jr GH, Perrillo RP. Metformin in the treatment of non-alcoholic steatohepatitis: a pilot open label trial. *Aliment Pharmacol Ther* 2004; **20**: 23–28.

71. Schwimmer JB, Middleton MS, Deutsch R, Lavine JE. A phase 2 clinical trial of metformin as a treatment for non-diabetic paediatric non-alcoholic steatohepatitis. *Aliment Pharmacol Ther* 2005; **21**: 871–879.

72. Tiikkainen M, Hakkinen AM, Korsheninnikova E, Nyman T, Makimattila S, Yki-Jarvinen H. Effects of rosiglitazone and metformin on liver fat content, hepatic insulin resistance, insulin clearance, and gene expression in adipose tissue in patients with type 2 diabetes. *Diabetes* 2004; **53**: 2169–2176.

73. Bugianesi E, Gentilcore E, Manini R *et al*. A randomized controlled trial of metformin versus vitamin E or prescriptive diet in nonalcoholic fatty liver disease. *Am J Gastroenterol* 2005; **100**: 1082–1090.

74. Uygun A, Kadayifci A, Isik AT *et al*. Metformin in the treatment of patients with non-alcoholic steatohepatitis. *Aliment Pharmacol Ther* 2004; **19**: 537–544.

75. Morita Y, Ueno T, Sasaki N *et al*. Nateglinide is useful for nonalcoholic steatohepatitis (NASH) patients with type 2 diabetes. *Hepatogastroenterology* 2005; **52**: 1338–1343.

76. Daubioul CA, Horsmans Y, Lambert P, Danse E, Delzenne NM. Effects of oligofructose on glucose and lipid metabolism in patients with nonalcoholic steatohepatitis: results of a pilot study. *Eur J Clin Nutr* 2005; **59**: 723–726.

77. Kiyici M, Gulten M, Gurel S *et al*. Ursodeoxycholic acid and atorvastatin in the treatment of nonalcoholic steatohepatitis. *Can J Gastroenterol* 2003; **17**: 713–718.

78. Hatzitolios A, Savopoulos C, Lazaraki G *et al*. Efficacy of omega-3 fatty acids, atorvastatin and orlistat in non-alcoholic fatty liver disease with dyslipidemia. *Indian J Gastroenterol* 2004; **23**: 131–134.

79. Gomez-Dominguez E, Gisbert JP, Moreno-Monteagudo JA, Garcia-Buey L, Moreno-Otero R. A pilot study of atorvastatin treatment in dyslipemic, non-alcoholic fatty liver patients. *Aliment Pharmacol Ther* 2006; **23**: 1643–1647.

80. Rallidis LS, Drakoulis CK, Parasi AS. Pravastatin in patients with nonalcoholic steatohepatitis: results of a pilot study. *Atherosclerosis* 2004; **174**: 193–196.

81. Basaranoglu M, Acbay O, Sonsuz A. A controlled trial of gemfibrozil in the treatment of patients with nonalcoholic steatohepatitis. *J Hepatol* 1999; **31**: 384.

82. Laurin J, Lindor KD, Crippin JS *et al*. Ursodeoxycholic acid or clofibrate in the treatment of non-alcohol-induced steatohepatitis: a pilot study. *Hepatology* 1996; **23**: 1464–1467.

83. Merat S, Malekzadeh R, Sohrabi MR *et al*. Probucol in the treatment of non-alcoholic steatohepatitis: a double-blind randomized controlled study. *J Hepatol* 2003; **38**: 414–418.

84. Merat S, Aduli M, Kazemi R *et al*. Liver histology changes in nonalcoholic steatohepatitis after one year of treatment with probucol. *Dig Dis Sci* 2008; **53**: 2246–2250.

85. Yokohama S, Tokusashi Y, Nakamura K *et al*. Inhibitory effect of angiotensin II receptor antagonist on hepatic stellate cell activation in non-alcoholic steatohepatitis. *World J Gastroenterol* 2006; **12**: 322–326.

86. Yokohama S, Yoneda M, Haneda M *et al.* Therapeutic efficacy of an angiotensin II receptor antagonist in patients with nonalcoholic steatohepatitis. *Hepatology* 2004; **40**: 1222–1225.

87. Harrison SA, Torgerson S, Hayashi P, Ward J, Schenker S. Vitamin E and vitamin C treatment improves fibrosis in patients with nonalcoholic steatohepatitis. *Am J Gastroenterol* 2003; **98**: 2485–2490.

88. Yakaryilmaz F, Guliter S, Savas B *et al.* Effects of vitamin E treatment on peroxisome proliferator-activated receptor-alpha expression and insulin resistance in patients with non-alcoholic steatohepatitis: results of a pilot study. *Intern Med J* 2007; **37**: 229–235.

89. Valenti L, Fracanzani AL, Dongiovanni P *et al.* Iron depletion by phlebotomy improves insulin resistance in patients with nonalcoholic fatty liver disease and hyperferritinemia: evidence from a case-control study. *Am J Gastroenterol* 2007; **102**: 1251–1258.

90. Bugianesi E, Manzini P, D'Antico S *et al.* Relative contribution of iron burden, HFE mutations, and insulin resistance to fibrosis in nonalcoholic fatty liver. *Hepatology* 2004; **39**: 179–187.

91. Lindor KD, Kowdley KV, Heathcote EJ *et al.* Ursodeoxycholic acid for treatment of nonalcoholic steatohepatitis: results of a randomized trial. *Hepatology* 2004; **39**: 770–778.

92. Dufour JF, Oneta CM, Gonvers JJ *et al.* Randomized placebo-controlled trial of ursodeoxycholic acid with vitamin e in nonalcoholic steatohepatitis. *Clin Gastroenterol Hepatol* 2006; **4**: 1537–1543.

93. Li Z, Yang S, Lin H *et al.* Probiotics and antibodies to TNF inhibit inflammatory activity and improve nonalcoholic fatty liver disease. *Hepatology* 2003; **37**: 343–350.

94. Loguercio C, Federico A, Tuccillo C *et al.* Beneficial effects of a probiotic VSL#3 on parameters of liver dysfunction in chronic liver diseases. *J Clin Gastroenterol* 2005; **39**: 540–543.

95. Beraza N, Malato Y, Vander BS *et al.* Pharmacological IKK2 inhibition blocks liver steatosis and initiation of non-alcoholic steatohepatitis. *Gut* 2008; **57**: 655–663.

Mark P. Callaway

7

Imaging the liver

The incidence of liver disease is increasing whether this is diffuse inflammation due to fatty infiltration or hepatocellular carcinoma. Precise non-invasive diagnosis of liver disease at an early stage of these disease processes is important.

MAGNETIC RESONANCE

Magnetic resonance (MR) technology has improved greatly over the last 5 years with enhanced magnetic gradients allowing rapid image acquisition, coupled with liver cell-specific contrast. Increased magnetic gradients allow the acquisition of a large volume of tissue within a single breath hold. These produce an assessment of the whole liver in each of the arterial, portal and parenchymal phases of enhancement. The versatility of unenhanced MR has increased; multiple different sequences can be used, each of which can provide unique information about diffuse disease processes within the liver. Extracellular intravenous contrast agents are routinely used; these can demonstrate different patterns of enhancement within a focal abnormality. Tissue-specific contrast media can be used; this contrast can be used to identify the presence of either hepatocytes or reticulo-endothelial cells within a lesion further classifying a specific lesion. MR is emerging as a problem solving modality when the results from multislice computed tomography (CT) or ultrasonography is inconclusive or incomplete. MR of the liver is also effective for the presurgical assessment of patients who are candidates for transplantation, surgical resection or ablative treatment.

By combining all the information available from both the unenhanced and contrast enhanced imaging, an accurate, non-invasive diagnosis of most liver lesions is possible.

Mark P. Callaway MRCP FRCR
Consultant GI Radiologist, Bristol Royal Infirmary, Marlborough Street, Bristol BS2 8HW, UK
E-mail: mark.callaway@UHBristol.nhs.uk

LIMITATIONS OF MR IMAGING

There are several contra-indications to MR imaging (MRI); these include cardiac pacemakers, implantable defibrillators, certain metallic neurosurgical aneurysm clips, metallic orbital foreign bodies, cochlear implants and epicardial pacing leads. MRI should be avoided in the first trimester of pregnancy and the use of MR contrast agents is not licensed in the UK for the duration of pregnancy.

Even with faster sequencing and single-breath hold acquisition, a standard liver MR takes much longer than the equivalent CT. Thus, this type of imaging is not suited to the very ill or unco-operative patient. This can be relevant if the patient has a large amount of ascites present or is encephalopathic. A small proportion of patients are claustrophobic and will refuse to undergo an examination.

NON-CONTRAST SEQUENCING

The appearance of liver lesions is extremely variable on MRI but the majority of centres use breath hold in and out-of-phase T1-weighting, and a fat-saturated breath hold T2-weighted as baseline imaging. This simple combination of sequences can indicate the likely nature of a lesion or if there is extensive fatty infiltration in the liver, and can be achieved in less than 15 min. The appearance of a malignant lesion is extremely variable, but most often these lesions will have a low signal on T1-weighted imaging and an intermediate high signal on T2-weighted imaging. This differentiates these lesions from both cysts and haemangiomas. Both these benign lesions have a much higher signal on T2-weighted imaging and, although cysts should not require MRI for diagnosis, haemangiomas can be a great mimic, occasionally iso-echoic or hypo-echoic on ultrasound and hypodense post-contrast on CT.

CONTRAST-ENHANCED MRI

The most common MR contrast agent used in imaging the liver is based on the gadolinium chelates. These are non-specific paramagnetic substances, which can be used to enhance the extracellular fluid spaces. These agents work in a very similar way to iodinated contrast in CT imaging. This is the largest group of products and includes the first MR contrast media Gd-DTPA Magnevist (Schering Germany). It also includes Dotaram (Guerbet, France), Omniscan (Nycomed, USA) and ProHance (Bracco, Italy). When using gadolinium to assess a lesion enhancement, most centres use triple-phase acquisition. This is performed using a gradient echo volume acquisition allowing rapid accumulation of a 3-D data set in any orthogonal plane. The application of fat saturation banding maximises the contrast-to-liver signal. The three phases of acquisition are: arterial 20–25 s, portal venous 60–90 s and parenchymal 120–150 s post injection. A small timing bolus of gadolinium can be used to determine the optimum time to acquisition.

Hepatocyte-targeted contrast agents

Hepatocyte-selective contrast agents undergo uptake by hepatocytes and are eliminated, at least in part, through the biliary system. Until recently, the only primary hepatocyte contrast medium was mangafodipir trisodium. As a paramagnetic contrast agent, mangafodipir trisodium primarily affects T1 relaxation. This contrast medium is taken up by normally functioning hepatocytes and so lesions that do not contain hepatocytes do not take up contrast. The increased signal intensity generated in functioning hepatocytes improves the contrast in non-enhancing tissues on T1-weighted images. The use of fat saturation improves contrast.

Agents with combined extracellular and hepatocyte specific distribution

Gadobenate dimeglumine (Gd-BOPTA, Multihance. Bracco Imaging) was released for use in Europe in 1998 for use in the liver. More recently, gadoxetic acid disodium (Primovist, Schering) has become available. Both of these compounds differ from the purely extracellular gadolinium agents by combining the properties of a conventional non-specific gadolinium agent with those of an agent targeted specifically to hepatocytes. This has a major advantage over the pure hepatocyte-directed contrast media as both the enhancement of a lesion and tissue specific assessment can be achieved using the same contrast bolus. A triple-phase acquisition exploiting the gadolinium component can be acquired immediately after injection, and then delayed imaging at 10 min and 20 min post injection can be performed to assess a lesions hepatocellular uptake. One area where this is very useful is in identifying small metastases, which do not contain hepatocytes. These lesions remain low signal on the delayed contrast. This, in combination with the volume acquisition, allows identification of small lesions.

Reticulo-endothelial specific contrast agents (SPIO-MRI)

Iron oxide particulate agents (SPIO) are selectively taken up by Kupffer cells in the reticulo-endothelial system (RES) primarily in the liver. There are two formulations available in the UK – Endorem (Guerbet, Paris) and Resovist (Schering); however, Resovist is not licensed in the UK. Endorem is given as an infusion, with the contrast added to 100 ml of 5% dextrose. This infusion is administered over 30 min with imaging at 60 min post infusion. Endorem has a particulate size of between 50–180 nm. Resovist is administered as an intravenous slow bolus preparation; the particulate size is 45–60 nm. Moderate-to-severe backache has been reported in between 3–8% of patients receiving SPIO; the backache is usually self-limiting in the majority.

The principal effect of the particles is on T2 relaxation, and thus the post contrast imaging is performed using T2-weighted sequences. Gradient echo sequencing is used to exploit the susceptibility artefact between normal liver containing Kupffer cells, and lesions that do not contain Kupffer cells. A recent study has shown that a gradient echo sequence with an echo time of 15 ms is the most sensitive post SPIO sequence; this allowed detection of 70% of subcentimetre lesions. Some authors use fat saturation in addition and there is a move to reduce slice thickness to 6 mm to facilitate even better rates of detection.

INDICATIONS FOR HEPATIC MRI

The demand for complex MR examination continues to exceed the availability of MRI in the UK, so MRI of the liver is often reserved for specific indications.

As with all other areas of imaging, a clear clinical history is vital to ensure the correct examination is performed. There are four major areas where MRI has an expanding role.

DIFFUSE LIVER DISEASE – FAT WITHIN THE LIVER

The incidence of fat within the liver continues to increase, with hepatic steatosis becoming a common occurrence. Hepatic steatosis is caused by the accumulation of triglycerides within the cytoplasm of hepatocytes. Steatosis is most commonly diffuse, which can be easily detected by transabdominal ultrasound. Diffuse steatosis is often combined with areas of focal fatty sparing. Occasionally, however, focal or lobar areas of steatosis can be seen. This appearance can mimic focal liver lesion. Typical geographical regions include anterior to the right portal vein, the gallbladder fossa, adjacent to the fissure of the ligament terres or in the subcapsular region.[1] With areas of focal steatosis or sparing, there should be no mass effect on the adjacent parenchyma or displacement of the vascular structures. If the areas of focal sparing is wedge-shaped, the presence of an underlying tumour near the apex of the focal sparing needs to be excluded.[2]

Gradient echo in- and opposed-phase T1-weighted MRI allows reliable detection and characterisation of these pseudo-lesions, often sparing the patient from additional imaging or even a percutaneous biopsy. This non-contrast sequence will detect and characterise focal, as well as diffuse, steatosis of the liver by using the chemical shift cancellation artefact, also known as the black line artefact or the Indian ink artefact. The two separate phases of imaging are acquired in the same examination – a normal T1-weighted sequence and an opposed-phase T1-weighted sequence. Opposed-phase, or out-of-phase, imaging can be identified by the presence of a strong, sharply-defined, black line surrounding the organ interface. These sequences are designed to exploit the similar properties of fat and water within the cellular structure. On the in-phase imaging, fat has a high signal, water a low signal.

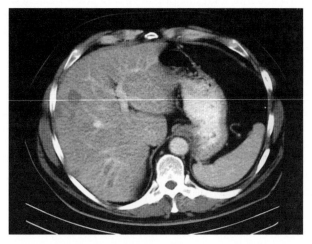

Fig. 1 Fat in the liver. This patient presented with multiple low attenuation lesions in the liver on this axial CT scan. These were thought to be multiple metastasis of an unknown primary.

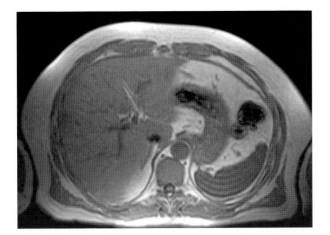

Fig. 2 Fat in the liver. T1-weighted in-phase MR of the liver. The liver has a uniform signal characteristic, with no evidence of a focal abnormality.

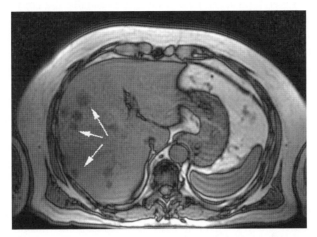

Fig. 3 Fat in the liver. T1-weighted out-of-phase MR of the liver. This sequence is performed to identify fat in the liver. When fat and water are imaged and are out of phase, the area containing fat becomes dark. The areas of concern demonstrated on the CT have now become dark indicating fatty focal deposition. The out-of-phase sequence can be identified by the presence of a dark line at the organ interface.

Opposed-phase imaging is performed at the phase when the signal from water is 180° to that of fat and the subsequent summation results in no signal being produced. Hence, if a lesion contains only water the signal will change little on the opposed phase; however, if there is a high fat content in addition to the background water content, the lesion will become darker on the opposed-phase imaging. This is specific for fat and means a pseudo-lesion can be differentiated easily without the need for contrast media (Figs 1–3).

ATYPICAL LESION IN A NON-CIRRHOTIC LIVER

One of the areas where the use of MRI continues to expand is in the diagnosis of lesions that are often identified by other imaging modalities within the liver.

The availability of transabdominal ultrasound continues to increase and, with the higher resolution of modern machines, more asymptomatic lesions are being detected. MRI provides the opportunity to provide an accurate, non-invasive diagnosis without the need for percutaneous biopsy.

Haemangioma

The liver haemangioma is the most common benign lesion identified. The haemangioma occurs with a frequency in post-mortem series of between 6–30%, with a 5:1 frequency in females.[3] Haemangiomas occur with most frequency in postmenopausal women. While the vast majority of lesions are asymptomatic, large haemangiomas cause symptoms by compression of adjacent structures. Rupture and thrombosis with associated pain have both been reported.

Haemangiomas are multiple in over 50% of cases and can range in size up to 20 cm, although anything over 10 cm is defined as a giant haemangioma.

On ultrasonographic examination, the typical appearance of a haemangioma is of a well-defined hyperechoic lesion, usually 1–2 cm in maximum diameter. However, haemangioma is a great mimic and can have an atypical appearance in up to 30% of cases, with the lesion either hypo-echoic or iso-echoic to the background liver on a transabdominal examination.[4] This can lead to diagnostic uncertainty and MRI can be used to confirm the diagnosis.

The hypo-echoic region can often correspond to regions of cystic degeneration. In some cases, there is evidence of faint acoustic enhancement. Rarely, these lesions calcify. On colour Doppler examination, large peripheral feeding vessels can be demonstrated.

MR has a major role in the diagnosis of haemangioma; this can be achieved without the necessity for intravenous contrast media. Haemangiomas characteristically demonstrate marked hyperintensity on T2-weighted imaging. In some cases, small areas of lower intensity can be identified, corresponding to areas of fibrosis within the lesion. The T2-relaxation time of haemangiomas is much longer than the surrounding soft tissue and longer than metastasis, because of the high water content. The optimum T2-weighting of a lesion occurs when the echo time (TE) is equivalent to the T2-relaxation time heavily weighted T2-imaging can aid in the diagnosis. If T2-weighted imaging is performed at 80 ms and 160ms, haemangiomas with high water content will increase in signal. One study has identified the optimum T2 relaxation for malignant tumours as 76 ms at 1.5 Tesla, as compared to 142 ms for haemangioma.[5] Consequently, these lesions will have a high signal on the initial sequence but the signal will reduce on the heavily T2 sequence.

Haemangiomas have a very similar pattern of enhancement following the injection of gadolinium as occurs on post contrast-enhanced CT. This is a peripheral globular enhancement which gradually fills the lesion over time. This appearance is unique to haemangioma and, if present, is diagnostic. However, three patterns of enhancement, depending on the size of the lesion have been described the classic pattern described.[6] Small lesions, less than 1.5 cm, have a uniform, bright rapid enhancement. In larger lesions, an area of hypo-intensity within the centre of the lesion remains following gadolinium. This is due to the presence of a central fibrotic scar; these appearances should not be confused with the scar found in an area of focal nodular hyperplasia.

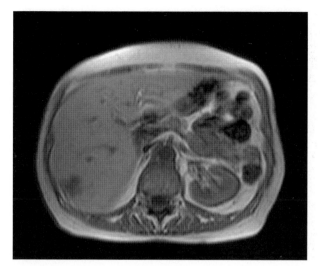

Fig. 4 Haemangioma. T1-weighted in-phase MR of the liver. There is a well-demarcated lesion in segment 6 of the liver. This is low signal on T1 weighting. The background liver has a normal appearance.

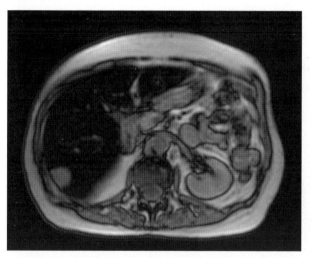

Fig. 5 Haemangioma. T1-weighted out-of-phase MR of the liver. On the out-of-phase imaging the background liver becomes very dark, this is because the signal from fat and water have cancelled out in the out-of-phase imaging. This suggests extensive fatty infiltration. The haemangioma does not contain fat so appears to be high signal on this phase. The signal is maintained appearing high on this phase.

Haemangiomas have a lack of Kupffer cells and, theoretically, should have no uptake of SPIO particles. However, because these small particles remain in the blood pool for a period of time and the blood can pool within a haemangioma, this can mimic uptake of SPIO by the lesion. Following the administration of SPIO, haemangioma may enhance at T1-weighting, with a decreased signal on T2-weighting as a result of blood pooling of contrast.[7] These appearances can lead to confusion with what appears to be uptake of iron oxide within the lesion; this is particularly important if the initial

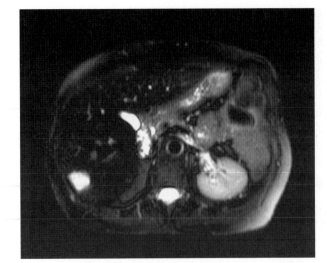

Fig. 6 Haemangioma. T2-weighted MR of the liver. There is a well-demarcated, low-signal lesion in segment 6 of the liver on T1-weighting. This lesion is bright on T2-weighting and is higher signal than usually noted with metastatic disease.

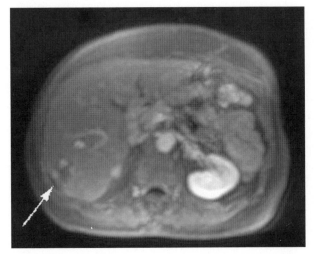

Fig. 7 Haemangioma. Post gadolinium T1-weighted MR in the arterial phase of enhancement. The lesion demonstrates peripheral globular centripetal enhancement (arrowed) which is characteristic of a haemangioma.

ultrasound was iso-echoic as these appearances mimic an area of focal nodular hyperplasia.

Hepatocyte-specific contrast media demonstrate haemangioma well. There is the initial gadolinium effect with peripheral globular centripetal infilling of the lesion which becomes iso-intense in the parenchyma phase; however, in the delay, because of the absence of hepatocytes within a haemangioma, the lesion washes out completely.

Overall, the MR diagnosis of haemangioma can often be made without the need for MR contrast with high T2-weighted image on the unenhanced images. If uncertainty remains, either gadolinium or a hepatocyte-specific contrast should

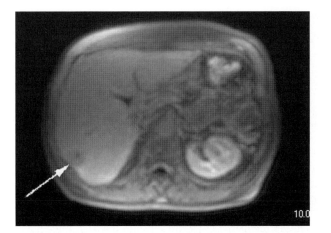

Fig. 8 Haemangioma. Post gadolinium T1-weighted MR in the delayed phase of enhancement. The lesion has 'filled in' with contrast becoming almost isodense against the background liver.

be used as this will demonstrate the classic peripheral centripetal enhancement pattern and wash out on the delayed phase. The use of SPIO should be avoided as this can add confusion as there can be pooling of iron-rich blood within the lesion which can mimic the presence of Kupffer cells (Figs 4–8).

Focal nodular hyperplasia

Focal nodular hyperplasia (FNH) is the second most common benign focal lesion within the liver, accounting for 8% of all primary hepatic tumours.[8] The tumour is thought to arise as a localised hepatocyte reaction to a congenital vascular malformation.[9] There is a link with oral contraceptives although, unlike adenoma, the role of oral contraceptives is to promote rather than induce growth within the lesion. Over 90% of FNH occur in women in the 3rd to 5th decade. Most FNHs are small, well-circumscribed, subcapsular lesions occurring in the right lobe of the liver. Over 90% of FNHs are less than 5 cm in diameter.

Currently, FNHs are divided into two sub types – classic and non-classic. The non-classic variety is then further subdivided into telangiectatic FNH, FNH with cytological atypia and mixed hyperplastic and adenomatous FNH. Classic FNH accounts for approximately 80% of cases. It contains the following histological features: abnormal nodular architecture, malformed vessels and bile duct proliferation. Non-classic FNH lacks one of the first two features of classic FNH but always contains bile duct proliferation. Both classic and non-classic FNHs have been shown to contain a variable number of Kupffer cells. Unlike adenoma, it is extremely unusual for FNH to necrose or for a haemorrhage to occur, because the tumour's rate of development is proportional to its blood supply. Once the diagnosis of an area of focal nodular hyperplasia has been made, there is little need to follow-up the patient, and the patient can be re-assured.

The classic ultrasound appearance of FNH is a well-demarcated, homogeneous mass often as an incidental finding. This mass is usually hyperechoic or iso-echoic to normal liver. In only 20% of cases can a central scar be identified on ultrasound;

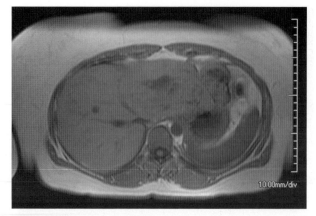

Fig. 9 Focal nodular hyperplasia. T1-weighted MR of the liver. There is a large isodense lesion arising from the left lobe of the liver. A large low signal central scar can be seen (arrowed).

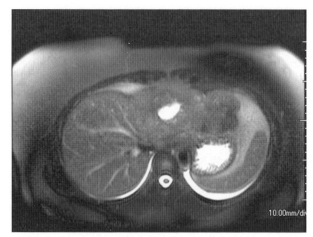

Fig. 10 Focal nodular hyperplasia. T2-weighted MR of the liver. The large lesion remains isodense with the background liver with no increase in signal, the central scar becomes high signal.

colour Doppler can be used to demonstrate flow in the vessels of the central scar.[10] It can be difficult to be certain of the diagnosis of an FNH on ultrasound particularly if the central feeding vessel is not clearly visualised.

MRI can produce certain diagnostic characteristics that are diagnostic of FNH. Focal nodular hyperplasias are predominantly composed of normal hepatocytes with a disorganised internal architecture; on standard T1-imaging, it is often either iso- or hypodense to normal surrounding liver. On T2-weighting, the lesion can be either iso- or hyperdense to surrounding tissue. The central scar, a classic feature of FNH, can be a helpful diagnostic feature with low signal on T1 and high signal on T2. Intravenous contrast has an important role in the diagnosis of FNH. Overall, the lesion is often difficult to visualise on unenhanced MRI as the signal produced is very similar to the background liver. The absence of an increased signal on T2-weighted examination is useful and supports the presence of a benign lesion.

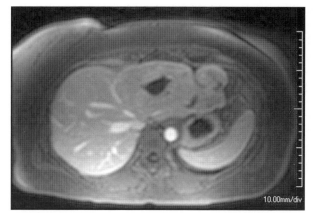

Fig. 11 Focal nodular hyperplasia. Post gadolinium T1-weighted MR of the liver in the arterial phase. There is uniform enhancement of the lesion which is usually supplied via the hepatic artery.

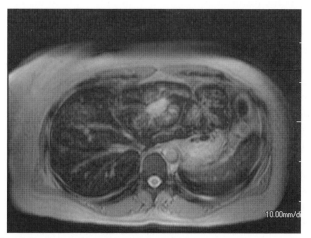

Fig. 12 Focal nodular hyperplasia. Post iron oxide T2-weighted MR of the liver. The liver appears black because of the uniform uptake of iron oxide. The large lesion has also taken up contrast. This confirms that Kuppfer cells are contained within the lesion and differentiates focal nodular hyperplasia from adenoma.

Contrast-enhanced MR is vital to confirm the diagnosis of a FNH. Focal nodular hyperplasia derives the majority of its arterial supply from the hepatic artery; therefore, on initially following intravenous gadolinium, there is very early rapid and often uniform enhancement with a rapid washout phase as the portal vein enhances. The enhancement washes out rapidly and the lesion becomes iso-intense during the parenchyma phase of enhancement.

If hepatocyte-specific contrast is used, the initial gadolinium effects of such contrast as primovist mimic these appearances; however, because of the proliferation of bile ducts within these lesions (the route of excretion of this type of contrast), there is concentration of contrast within the lesion which becomes a high signal on the delayed phase.

Further information can be derived from imaging with reticulo-endothelial specific contrast such as SPIO. Focal nodular hyperplasia often contain

125

variable numbers of Kupffer cells and these cells take up SPIO particles leading to a reduction in signal on T2-weighting.[11] Thus, if imaged post-SPIO, the lesion should take up a variable amount of SPIO. Some FNH will take up as much SPIO as the background liver becoming isodense on the post-contrast imaging while some FNHs have less Kupffer cells than the liver and take up less SPIO. The lesion can appear to have failed to take up any SPIO and to have maintained its pre-contrast signal mimicking a malignant lesion or adenoma, both of which fail to take up SPIO. It is vital, if there is a high clinical suspicion of an FNH, that pre-contrast imaging includes a comparable sequence to post-contrast examination. This allows both the signal from the lesion and the background lesion to be interrogated pre- and post-SPIO to demonstrate if there has been some partial uptake of SPIO (Figs 9–12).

Hepatic adenoma

Hepatocellular adenoma presents as a solitary large encapsulated tumour, which is hypervascular with prominent peripheral vascularity. This tumour was rare before the introduction of the contraceptive pill in the 1960s with only a handful of previously reported cases. The hepatic adenoma is composed of sheets of hepatocytes, which can produce bile, but no bile ductile, portal vein tracts or terminal hepatic arteries are present. These tumours are often large, out-growing their blood supply so become necrotic with evidence of internal haemorrhage. The tumour can rupture leading to a life-threatening bleed. Hepatic adenomas often also contain large amounts of fat and glycogen.

On ultrasonographic examination, hepatic adenomas, which often have a high lipid content, are often hyperechoic but the appearance can be rather non-specific. Colour Doppler examination can demonstrate large peripheral vessels: these are subcapsular and characteristic of adenoma.[12] As an adenoma derives blood from the hepatic artery, the post-contrast appearances detected on contrast-enhanced ultrasound mimic the early post-contrast of both dynamic CT and MR. There is strong homogeneous early enhancement, which is of short duration. Following this early arterial enhancement, there is prompt portal venous washout and an iso-intense appearance during both the portal and sinusoidal phases of contrast enhancement.[13]

Hepatic adenomas are rare but can be difficult to diagnose accurately. Because these lesions are a benign proliferation of hepatocytes, the imaging characteristics can be very similar to primary hepatocellular carcinoma with only subtle differences. It is vital to know if the patient has a cirrhotic liver or any history of background liver disease.

Hepatic adenomas often have a heterogeneous appearance on MRI. There are often areas of both high and low signal on T1–weighting corresponding to both fat deposition and necrosis. The use of in and out-of-phase T1 imaging is important to confirm the presence of any fat within the lesion. In approximately one-third of lesions, a peripheral capsule can be demonstrated; this is low signal on both T1 and T2 weighting.[12] A capsule is often found on a hepatocellular carcinoma; therefore, while the presence of a capsule helps to differentiate the lesion from an FNH, it does not help differentiate the lesion from a malignant tumour. As an adenoma derives blood from the hepatic artery, dynamic enhanced gadolinium imaging will produce an early enhancement with portal venous washout and an iso-intense appearance in the parenchymal phase. Rarely, the peripheral feeding vessels can be identified.[15]

If SPIO is used to differentiate adenomas from FNH, the absence of Kuppfer cells in adenoma will maintain signal post-SPIO. However, neither metastatic deposits nor primary hepatocellular carcinoma contain Kuppfer cells and will also maintain signal post SPIO. Again, whilst the use of SPIO will delineate an adenoma from FNH, this type of contrast will not delineate an adenoma from a malignancy.

Lesion in a cirrhotic liver

Hepatocellular carcinoma (HCC) is the fifth most common tumour in the world and is the third most common cause of cancer-related death after lung and stomach.[16] Cirrhosis is the strongest predisposing factor for HCC, with approximately 80% of cases of HCC developing in a cirrhotic liver.[17] The annual incidence of HCC is 2–6.6% in patients with cirrhosis compared with 0.4% in patients without cirrhosis. The primary cause of the liver disease varies depending on the ethnic and cultural background of the group. Risk factors include alcohol-induced cirrhosis, haemochromatosis and chronic hepatitis B and C infection. The presenting symptoms can vary greatly from an asymptomatic lesion identified at follow-up to rapidly deteriorating liver function tests. Alpha-fetoprotein is used as a biochemical marker in the context of chronic liver disease but can be within the normal range in up to 40% of cases of hepatoma.[18]

Cirrhosis is the end result of chronic liver disease and is characterised by the replacement of the normal hepatic architecture with fibrous septa[19] and the development of nodules. These nodules can vary from small micronodules < 3 mm to macronodules > 3 mm or a mixed picture[20] These nodules can also range from benign regenerative nodules to malignant HCC. An appreciation of the step-wise progression from regenerative to low-grade dysplasia, high-grade dysplasia and eventually HCC as key features of these nodules can help discriminate benign from malignant on MRI.

1. **Regenerative nodule** – defined as a hepatocellular nodule containing one or more portal tracts located in a liver that has evidence of cirrhosis. Regenerative nodules are present in all cirrhotic livers and are surrounded by fibrous septa. Regenerative nodules are composed of proliferating normal stroma surrounded by fibrous bands these nodules can be difficult to detect on unenhanced MRI as their signal is similar to background liver. Occasionally, regenerative nodules can be hyperintense on T1-weighting; this is thought due to the presence of lipid or protein in the nodule. The blood supply to these nodules is primarily from the portal vein with very little contribution from the hepatic artery and, because of this, there is no evidence of enhancement of these nodules in the arterial phase of contrast enhancement.[21]

2. **Dysplastic nodule** – defined as a nodule of hepatocytes of at least 1 mm in diameter with dysplasia of low- or high-grade but no histological criteria of malignancy, usually found in a cirrhotic liver.[22] Dysplastic nodules are found in up to 25% of cirrhotic livers. High-grade dysplasia is considered

pre-malignant. Dysplastic nodules are usually similar in signal intensity to regenerative nodules, in that they are iso-intense to the background and can be difficult to detect on unenhanced MRI. As with regenerative nodules, dysplastic nodules can occasionally be high signal on T1-weighting, as a result of copper retention within these nodules. Low-grade dysplastic nodules receive the majority of their blood supply via the portal vein and so do not enhance in the arterial phase. However, as the nodule develops high-grade dysplasia, more of the blood supply is via the hepatic artery and so early enhancement becomes a feature.

Hepatocellular carcinoma

Hepatocellular carcinoma can have an extremely variable range of signals on both T1- and T2-weighting. The majority of lesions are low-signal intensity on T1 and high-signal on T2. The increased signal is an important feature of malignancy and discriminates high-grade dysplasia from hepatocellular carcinoma. High-grade dysplastic nodules are usually iso-intense on T2-weighting.

Although a low signal on T1-weighting is the most common image finding in approximately one-third of cases, the opposite, high signal on T1-weighting can be detected.[23] Although this finding was originally thought to represent the presence of fat within the tumour, it can represent haemorrhagic necrosis or even intracellular glycogen. It is a useful observation, for there are very few benign lesions that produce a high signal on T1-weighting. High signal on T1 is usually a feature found in well-differentiated hepatoma.

Variable signal intensity has also been described on T2-weighting, with some researchers suggesting that this change in signal is related to the histological type of the tumour. Most poorly differentiated tumours have been shown to demonstrate high signal whereas well-differentiated tumours can be iso-intense with the surrounding liver on T2-weighting. These features mimic the appearance of a dysplastic nodule.

The presence of a tumour capsule is an indicator of malignant disease. The presence of a capsule is of major prognostic significance; the median survival

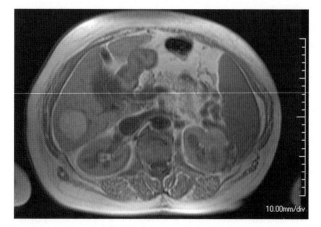

Fig. 13 Hepatocellular carcinoma. T1-weighted in-phase MR of the liver. There is a large, well-demarcated lesion within segment 6 of the liver. This lesion is high signal on T1-weighting whilst unusual in a background of cirrhosis is highly suspicious for a hepatocellular carcinoma.

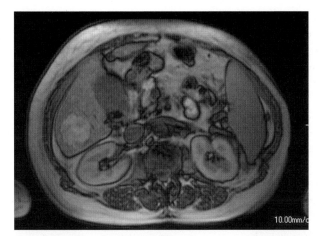

Fig. 14 Hepatocellular carcinoma. T1-weighted out-of-phase MR of the liver. The lesion maintains the majority of the high signal on the out-of-phase MR image. This suggests that these appearances are not due to the presence of fat but probably either glycogen or copper.

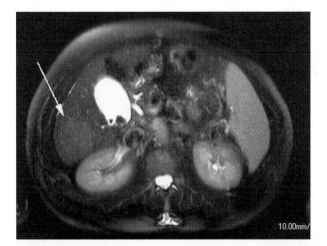

Fig. 15 Hepatocellular carcinoma. T2-weighted MR of the liver. The lesion shows a slight increase in signal on T2 weighting, this supports a malignant diagnosis.

time after diagnosis for an encapsulated hepatoma is 17.3 months compared to 4 months in patients where no capsule could be identified. The capsule often appears as a low-signal intensity rim on T1-weighted images and as a double layer on T2-weighting. The inner layer is of low-signal and the outer layer of high-signal intensity.

The presence of intratumoural septation often best visualised on T2-weighted imaging is noted in malignant disease.

However, the major feature of hepatocellular carcinoma is as a result of continued tumour neo-angiogenesis. As a dysplastic nodule becomes malignant, there is an increase in the recruitment of abnormal arterial supply, which produces rapid enhancement of the nodule in the arterial phase of contrast enhancement. Hepatocellular carcinoma then becomes iso-intense in

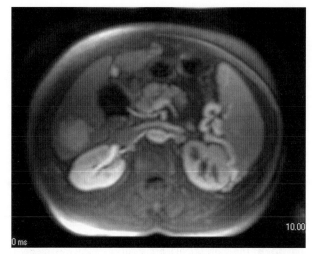

Fig. 16 Hepatocellular carcinoma. Post-gadolinium T1-weighted MR of the liver in the arterial phase. The lesion is hyperdense in the arterial phase, a typical feature of a hepatocellular carcinoma. There is radiological evidence of portal hypertension with recanalisation of the umbilical vein and multiple varices in the splenic hilum.

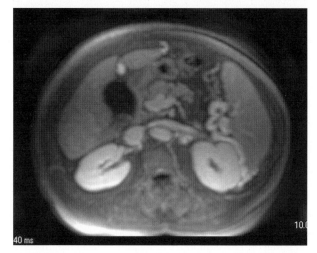

Fig. 17 Hepatocellular carcinoma. Post gadolinium T1 weighted MR of the liver in the portal phase. The lesion becomes isodense in the portal phase of enhancement. The varices are more prominent.

the portal venous phase, becoming hypo-intense in the parenchymal phase. This combination of features is highly specific for HCC with a reported sensitivity 86% and specificity 96%.[24]

Hepatocellular carcinomas do not contain reticulo-endothelial system cells and so do not take up iron oxide following the administration of SPIO, maintaining signal on the post contrast examination; conversely, both dysplastic and regenerative nodules do contain a variable number of Kupffer cells and take up SPIO. Thus, SPIO has an important role in differentiating benign from malignant nodules.

Portal vein invasion is another feature of HCC, this is thought to occur as a result of the venous return from the tumour into the vein and can occur in up

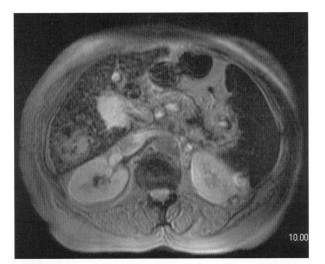

Fig. 18 Hepatocellular carcinoma. Post iron oxide T2-weighted MR of the liver. There has been patchy uptake of iron throughout the liver indicating wide-spread fibrosis. The lesion has failed to take up iron oxide maintaining its signal indicating this is a malignant focal lesion.

to 44% of cases, although portal venous thrombosis is a feature of cirrhosis; tumour thrombus usually expands the vein (Figs 13–18).

Sensitivity of MRI in the detection of HCC

Several series have suggested the sensitivity and specificity of gadolinium-enhanced MR and iron oxide MR for the detection of HCC is 81% and 85%, respectively. This compares favourably with a sensitivity and specificity for CT of 68% and 93%, respectively.[25] All imaging modalities are accurate at detecting lesions of greater than 2 cm in diameter, but the most accurate method of detecting tumours between 1–2 cm is dual contrast MRI; this is a combination of gadolinium to identify the vascularity within the lesion, and SPIO to exploit the absence of Kuppfer cells leading to maintenance of the signal post contrast.[26,27]

Liver metastasis

One of the most difficult questions to answer is: 'what is the most accurate method of identifying liver metastases?' This question is often compounded because of the difficulties in defining a reproducible 'gold standard'. The only true accurate assessment of the sensitivity and specificity of any imaging modality is direct clinical pathological correlation, but only a minority of research papers have made this comparison. Many authors use intra-operative ultrasound as the gold standard, but, while accurate, this is a comparison of one imaging modality with another. Many papers compare two imaging modalities (often CT or MR) to try and establish accuracy, but this methodology is limited. Another factor in determining sensitivity is the rapid development of technology where published data lag behind changes in practice. The need for direct, clinical, radiological comparison produces another problem; often the series are too small to allow recruitment in a

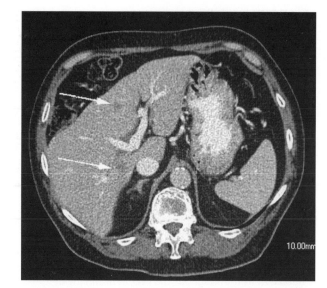

Fig. 19 Metastasis. Portal phase CT. Two low-attenuation lesions can be seen, one in segment 4 and one at the base of the caudate lobe. These are metastases (arrowed).

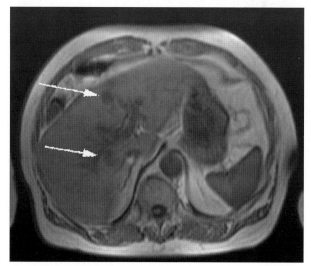

Fig. 20 Metastasis. T1-weighted MR of the liver. The two metastases are low-signal on this standard. T1-weighted MR image.

relatively short time before technology changes and, as such, this often means a single missed lesion has a large impact on any individual imaging modality's sensitivity and specificity.

Ultrasound is often the first-line imaging modality in patients with a history of cancer. The sensitivity of ultrasound in reported series is very wide and this reflects the variability associated with this modality. However, good-quality ultrasound in a suitable patient has a sensitivity approaching contrast-enhanced CT.

Computed tomography remains the mainstay of cancer imaging and the reported sensitivity of this method ranges from 73–85%.[28–32] Many studies

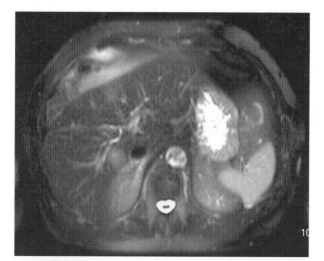

Fig. 21 Metastasis. T2-weighted MR of the liver. The two metastases are intermediate signal which suggests the lesions are malignant.

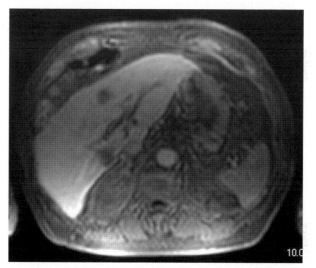

Fig. 22 Metastasis. Post gadolinium T1-weighted MR of the liver in the parenchymal phase. Both the focal lesions have 'washed out' of contrast on this phase of enhancement.

have demonstrated that iron oxide enhanced MR (SPIO-MR) is the most accurate non-invasive method of detecting liver metastases.[33–38] These studies have confirmed that this method is not only accurate at identifying the number of metastases but in the size of the smallest lesion detected. However, even this method is poor at detecting subcentimetre lesions.

Most lesions larger than 1 cm are detected with any of the current imaging methods, but the detection of smaller lesions is poor. Many recently published studies have produced conflicting results. One such study compared three state-of-the-art imaging techniques directly with surgical resection.

A recent meta-analysis tried to assess all available data to compose an evidence-based imaging strategy for the identification of metastatic colorectal

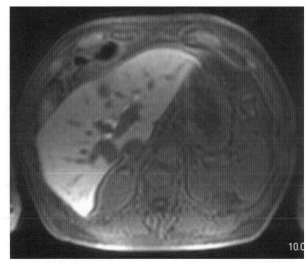

Fig. 23 Metastasis. Delayed phase of hepatocyte-specific contrast. The hepatocyte-specific contrast has been taken up on this delayed phase. Some contrast can be seen in the biliary tree. The metastases have not taken up any contrast.

disease. This study included only papers with histological correlation, intra-operative observation which included both manual palpation and intra-operative ultrasound and/or follow-up ultrasound as reference standards. The analysis was based on publications between 1990 and 2003. Initially, 165 articles were identified but, after review, only 61 were eligible for inclusion. The following sensitivities for the detection of colorectal metastases were reported.[39] For lesions over 1 cm, for helical CT, non-enhanced MRI, post-gadolinium MRI and post-SPIO MRI, the sensitivities were 74%, 66%, 69% and 90%, respectively. For lesions below 1 cm, these sensitivities dropped to 23%, 13%, 12% and 30%, respectively (Figs 19–23).

CONCLUSIONS

The versatility of MR in assessing the liver continues to increase, with accurate diagnosis of not only focal liver lesions but of diffuse liver disease. The use of different sequences and liver-specific contrast media can identify various cell types within a lesion and can produce important diagnostic information without the need to biopsy.

Key points for clinical practice

• In and out-of-phase T1-weighted magnetic resonance is very good at discriminating fat within the liver.

• Haemangioma, although a great mimic, has a characteristic appearance on both unenhanced and enhanced magnetic resonance imaging.

• Iron oxide contrast can be use to differentiate an area of focal nodular hyperplasia from an adenoma.

(continued)

Key points for clinical practice (continued)

- It can be very difficult to discriminate an adenoma from a malignant lesion.

- The appearance of hepatocellular carcinoma is very variable but enhancement in the arterial phase with wash out of contrast in the parenchymal phase is very sensitive for malignancy.

- Magnetic resonance imaging is the most accurate method of identifying liver metastasis using either iron oxide particulate agents (SPIO) or hepatocellular-specific contrast media.

References

1. Merkle EM, Nelson RC. Dual phase gradient – echo in-phase and opposed phase hepatic MR imaging: a useful tool for evaluating more than fatty infiltration or fatty sparing. *Radiographics* 2006; **26**: 1409–1418.
2. Grossholz M, Terrier F, Rubbia L *et al*. Focal sparing in the fatty liver as a sign of an adjacent space-occupying lesion. *AJR Am J Roentgenol* 1998; **171**: 1391–1395.
3. Karhunen PJ. Benign hepatic tumours and tumour like conditions in men. *J Clin Pathol* 1986; **39**: 183–188.
4. Craig GR, Peters RL, Edmonson HA. Tumours of the liver and intrahepatic bile ducts. In: *Atlas of Tumour Pathology*, 2nd series. Washington DC: Armed Forces Institute of Pathology, 1989.
5. McFarland EG, Mayo-Smith WW, Saini S *et al*. Hepatic haemangiomas and malignant tumours: improved differentiation with heavily T2-weighted conventional spin-echo MR imaging. *Radiology* 1994; **193**: 43–47.
6. Semelka RC, Brown ED, Ascher SM *et al*. Hepatic haemangioma: a multi-institutional study of appearance on T2-weighted and serial gadolinium-enhanced gradient-echo MR images. *Radiology* 1994; **192**: 401–406.
7. Karhunen PJ. Benign hepatic tumours and tumour like conditions in men. *J Clin Pathol* 1986; **39**: 183–188.
8. Wanless I, Mawdsley C, Adams R. On the pathogenesis of focal nodular hyperplasia of the liver. *Hepatology* 1985; **5**: 1194–1200.
9. Lee M, Hamm B, Saini S *et al*. Focal nodular hyperplasia of the liver: MR findings in 35 proved cases. *AJR Am J Roentgenol* 1991; **156**: 317–320.
10. Buetow PC, Pantongrag-Brown L, Buck JL, Ros PR, Goodman ZD. Focal nodular hyperplasia of the liver: imaging–pathologic correlation. *Radiographics* 1996; **16**: 369–388.
11. Grandin C, Van Beers BE, Robert A *et al*. Benign hepatocellular tumours: MRI after superparamagnetic iron oxide administration. *J Comput Assist Tomogr* 1995; **19**: 412–418.
12. Arrive L, Flejou J-F, Vigrain V *et al*. Hepatic adenoma: MR findings in 51 pathologically proved lesions. *Radiology* 1994; **193**: 507–512
13. Paulson EK, McClellan JS, Washington K *et al*. Hepatic adenoma: MR characteristics and correlation with pathologic findings. *AJR Am J Roentgenol* 1994; **163**: 113–116.
14. *Deleted at proof.*
15. Chung KY, Mayo-Smith WW, Saini S *et al*. Hepatocellular adenoma: MR imaging features with pathologic correlation. *AJR Am J Roentgenol* 1995; **165**: 303–308.
16. Parkin DM, Bray F, Ferlay J, Pisani P. Estimating the world cancer burden: Globocan 2000. *Int J Cancer* 2001; **94**: 153–156.
17. Llovet JM, Burroughs A, Bruix J. Hepatocellular carcinoma. *Lancet* 2003; **362**: 1907–1917.
18. Marrero JA, Lok AS. Newer markers for hepatocellular carcinoma. *Gastroenterology* 2004; **127**: S113–S119.
19. Baron RL, Peterson MS. Screening the cirrhotic liver for hepatocellular carcinoma with CT and MR imaging: opportunities and pitfalls. *Radiographics* 2001; **21**: s117–s132.
20. International Working Party. Terminology of nodular hepatocellular lesions. *Hepatology* 1995;

22: 983–993.

21. Willatt JM, Hussain HK, Adusumilli S, Marrero JA. MR imaging of hepatocellular carcinoma in the cirrhotic liver: Challenges and controversies. *Radiology* 2008; **247**: 311–330.

22. Theise ND, Schwartz M, Miller C, Thung SN. Macroregenerative nodules and hepatocellular carcinoma in forty four sequential adult liver explants with cirrhosis. *Hepatology* 1992; **16**: 949–955.

23. Earls JP, Theise ND, Weinreb JC *et al.* Dysplastic nodules and hepatocellular carcinoma: thin section MR imaging of explanted cirrhotic livers with pathologic correlation. *Radiology* 1996: **201**; 207–214.

24. Freeny PC, Grossholz M, Kaakaji K, Schmiedl UP. Significance of hyper attenuating and contrast-enhancing hepatic nodules detected in the cirrhotic liver during arterial phase helical CT in pre-liver transplant patients: radiologic-histopathologic correlation of explanted livers. *Abdom Imaging* 2003; **28**: 333–346.

25. Colli A, Fraquelli M, Casazza G *et al.* Accuracy of ultrasonography, spiral CT, magnetic resonance, and alpha-fetoprotein in diagnosing hepatocellular carcinoma: a systematic review. *Am J Gastroenterol* 2006; **101**: 513–523.

26. Bhartia B, Ward J, Guthrie JA, Robinson PJ. Hepatocellular carcinoma in cirrhotic livers: double-contrast thin-section MR imaging with pathologic correlation of explanted tissue. *AJR Am J Roentgenol* 2003; **180**: 577–584.

27. Ward J, Guthrie JA, Scott DJ *et al.* Hepatocellular carcinoma in the cirrhotic liver: double-contrast MR imaging for diagnosis. *Radiology* 2000; **216**: 154–162.

28. Kuszyk BS, Bluemke DA, Urban BA *et al.* Portal-phase contrast-enhanced helical CT for the detection of malignant hepatic tumors: sensitivity based on comparison with intra-operative and pathologic findings. *AJR Am J Roentgenol* 1996; **166**: 91–95.

29. Valls C, Lopez E, Guma A *et al.* Helical CT versus CT arterial portography in the detection of hepatic metastasis of colorectal carcinoma. *AJR Am J Roentgenol* 1998; **170**: 1341–1347.

30. Ward J, Naik KS, Guthrie JA, Wilson D, Robinson PJ. Hepatic lesion detection: comparison of MR imaging after the administration of superparamagnetic iron oxide with dual-phase CT by using alternative–free response receiver operating characteristic analysis. *Radiology* 1999; **210**: 459–466.

31. Scott DJ, Guthrie JA, Arnold P *et al.* Dual phase helical CT versus portal venous phase CT for the detection of colorectal liver metastases: correlation with intra-operative sonography, surgical and pathological findings. *Clin Radiol* 2001; **56**: 235–242.

32. Valls C, Andia E, Sánchez A *et al.* Hepatic metastases from colorectal cancer: preoperative detection and assessment of resectability with helical CT. *Radiology* 2001; **218**: 55–60.

33. Hagspiel KD, Neidl KF, Eichenberger AC, Weder W, Marincek B. Detection of liver metastases: comparison of superparamagnetic iron oxide-enhanced and unenhanced MR imaging at 1.5 T with dynamic CT, intraoperative US, and percutaneous US. *Radiology* 1995; **196**: 471–478.

34. Seneterre E, Taourel P, Bouvier Y *et al.* Detection of hepatic metastases: ferumoxides-enhanced MR imaging versus unenhanced MR imaging and CT during arterial portography. *Radiology* 1996; **200**: 785–792.

35. Van Beers BE, Lacrosse M, Jamart J *et al.* Detection and segmental location of malignant hepatic tumors: comparison of ferumoxides-enhanced gradient-echo and T2-weighted spin-echo MR imaging. *AJR Am J Roentgenol* 1997; **168**: 713–717.

36. Müller RD, Vogel K, Neumann K *et al.* SPIO-MR imaging versus double-phase spiral CT in detecting malignant lesions of the liver. *Acta Radiol* 1999; **40**: 628–635.

37. Ward J, Chen F, Guthrie JA *et al.* Hepatic lesion detection after superparamagnetic iron oxide enhancement: comparison of five T2-weighted sequences at 1.0 T by using alternative–free response receiver operating characteristic analysis. *Radiology* 2000; **214**: 159–166.

38. Vogl TJ, Schwarz W, Blume S *et al.* Preoperative evaluation of malignant liver tumors: comparison of unenhanced and SPIO (Resovist)-enhanced MR imaging with biphasic CTAP and intraoperative US. *Eur Radiol* 2003; **13**: 262–272.

39. Bipat S, van Leeuwen MS, Comans EF *et al.* Colorectal liver metastases: CT, MR imaging, and PET for diagnosis–meta-analysis. *Radiology* 2005; **237**: 123–131.

Fiona Gordon

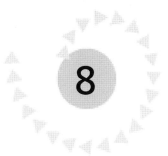

Hepatitis E – the new epidemiology

Hepatitis E virus (HEV) is transmitted enterically and causes an acute self-limiting disease in most patients. It was first recognised as a disease distinct from hepatitis A and B in India in 1980, when it was termed enterically transmitted non-A, non-B hepatitis (ET-NANB). HEV infection is the commonest cause of acute self-limiting hepatitis in adults in developing countries, due to genotypes 1 and 2, and is transmitted by contamination of water supplies and poor sanitation. In industrialised countries, the virus is much less prevalent, but becoming apparent as a cause of previously unexplained acute hepatitis. Its frequency is likely to increase with rising awareness. In these countries, genotypes 3 and 4 predominate in indigenous infections and may well be transmitted from swine reservoirs. A sub-unit vaccine has been developed with good efficacy in clinical trials.

STRUCTURE

HEV is a non-enveloped, spherical, single-stranded, positive-sense RNA virus approximately 27–34 nm in diameter. It has been classified recently as being the only member of the *Hepevirus* genus in the *Hepeviridae* family of viruses,[1] and bears some structural similarity to rubella. Identification by immune electron microscopy was first achieved by Balayan in 1983, following experimental self-ingestion of faecal material from Asian patients and imaging extracts from his own faeces.[2] The 7.2-kb hepatitis E viral genome was first cloned and sequenced in 1991[3] and comprises three large open reading frames (ORF). The largest ORF (1693 codons) codes for non-structural proteins which are responsible for the processing and replication of the virus. The second ORF (660 codons) codes for structural proteins and the third ORF (123 codons) is of uncertain function.

Fiona H. Gordon MA MD MBBChir FRCP
Consultant Hepatologist, Bristal Royal Infirmary, Marlborough Street, Bristol BS2 8HW, UK
E-mail: fiona.gordon@UHBristol.nhs.uk

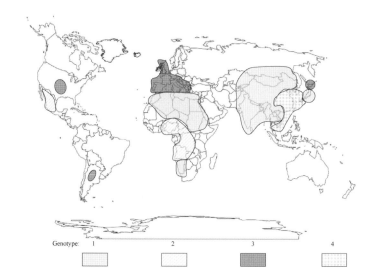

Fig. 1 Geographic distribution of HEV genotypes.

GENOTYPES

Four HEV genotypes are known to infect humans and a fifth has been proposed that infects birds alone.[4] Genotypes 1 and 2 are found almost exclusively in humans, whereas genotypes 3 and 4 are well-described in other mammals, notably swine. Genotype 1 is found in hyperendemic disease areas (Africa and Asia), genotype 2 in Mexico and Central Africa, genotype 3 in industrialised countries (North America, Europe and Japan) and genotype 4 in eastern Asia (China, Japan, Taiwan and Vietnam) as shown in Figure 1. Genotypes 1 and 2 are more virulent than other genotypes and account for human HEV infections in most developing countries, genotype 1 exclusively so in India.

EPIDEMIOLOGY

HISTORICAL PERSPECTIVE

Hepatitis E was first recognised as being distinct from hepatitis A in 1980,[5] although several large epidemics of waterborne hepatitis were reported prior to this, notably in Delhi in 1955,[6] affecting 29,300 people. A retrospective analysis of sera collected from this and 15 further hepatitis outbreaks in India (1955–1993) confirmed that all but one (Andaman Islands 1987) was likely to have been caused by HEV.[7]

Large epidemics of the newly-recognised HEV have been reported, mainly from poorly-resourced regions of South Asia, including Myanmar/Burma (1976–1977), Kashmir (1978) and 79,000 cases in Kanpur, India in 1991.[8] HEV outbreaks were first reported from the American subcontinent in 1986 in Mexico.[9] The largest epidemic reported to date affected over 100,000 individuals in the Xinjiang region of China between 1986 and 1988.[10]

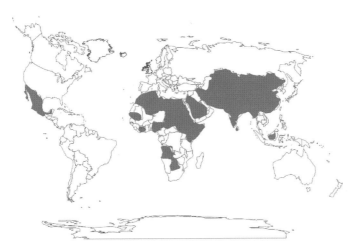

Fig. 2 Geographic distribution of HEV. Shaded areas denote regions where > 25% of sporadic non-ABC hepatitis is due to HEV.

CURRENT GLOBAL PREVALENCE

The cloning and sequencing of the HEV genome by Tam and colleagues[3] in 1991 was a huge technical advance, from which the diagnostic accuracy of HEV increased greatly. Consequently, HEV became recognised as being responsible for the majority of adult-acquired, acute-infective hepatitis in Central and Southeast Asia[11] and second only to hepatitis B as the major cause of acute hepatitis in parts of the Middle-East.[12] HEV continues to be endemic in areas in which sanitation and hygiene are poor, due to faecal contamination of water supplies. For example, large epidemics have occurred in refugee camps in Sudan and Chad in recent years.[13] A map illustrating countries with high endemic rates is shown in Figure 2. HEV genotype 1 or 2 accounts for infection in areas of high endemic rates and adults between the ages of 20–29 years form the largest group affected. In contrast, sero-epidemiological studies show that the prevalence of anti-HEV antibodies is low in children in these areas.[14]

INDUSTRIALISED COUNTRIES – EMERGING EPIDEMIOLOGY

The prevalence of HEV is very low in industrialised countries and was once considered to occur only in individuals who had travelled to endemic countries. Case-report frequency has increased considerably over the past 5 years and many studies have identified individuals with no travel history, giving rise to the hypothesis that indigenous or 'autochthonous' HEV exists in countries of low prevalence. For example, just 17 cases had been reported to the UK main public health reference laboratory during 1996–2003, but 329 cases were reported in 2005 alone, 100 of whom had no travel history.[15] Similar patterns have been reported from the US,[16] Australia,[17] Taiwan,[18] Japan[19] and at least six countries in Western Europe. Virtually all of these cases have been found to be caused by the less virulent genotypes 3 or 4. These genotypes seem to affect a much older age-group, peaking in those over 60 years of age in UK cases,[15] which contrasts with a peak age of attack of genotypes 1 and 2 in 20–29 year-olds, in high-prevalence countries. In England and Wales, most cases have been associated with estuarine or coastal habitat, although this association may be confounded by the known observation from census data that many elderly people in this country reside close to the sea.

POPULATION-BASED STUDIES IN INDUSTRIALISED COUNTRIES

A study of age-specific prevalence of HEV IgG from the US, demonstrated a much higher prevalence of anti-HEV antibodies in healthy blood-donors than expected, with an overall rate of 18.3% compared with just 11.3% for hepatitis A IgG.[20] Despite this finding, less than 12 cases of acute HEV infection were reported to US public health services at that time. The prevalence of anti-HEV was particularly high in states that were large producers of swine. A recent study in Devon and Cornwall has shown the sero-prevalence of HEV-IgG to be 16% in healthy blood donors, compared with 46% for hepatitis A virus.[21] An alternative approach to assessing HEV prevalence has been to examine multiple sewage specimens from 'non-endemic countries' for the presence of HEV RNA by PCR and to sequence the strains extracted for phylogenetic analysis. One such study conducted in Barcelona yielded 15 strains likely to be genotype 3, with 43.5% of 46 sewage samples testing positive for HEV.[22] Together, these findings have prompted the suggestion that HEV should be actively excluded in all UK patients with acute hepatitis of unknown aetiology.[15]

TRANSMISSION ROUTES IN INDUSTRIALISED COUNTRIES

Case-to-case spread of HEV is very rare.[23] Genotypes 1 and 2 survive in primates only;[24] strikingly, genotype 3 has been found to be present in 80% of UK domestic pigs.[25] An epidemiological study of all cases reported in the UK during 2003–2005 suggested that contact with pigs or consumption of pork is a risk factor for HEV and proposed that zoonotic spread of HEV may be the preferred route of transmission in the UK.[26] HEV sequences have been recovered from pigs' liver purchased in butchers in The Netherlands and the US.[27,28] Similarly, almost the entire HEV genotype 3 genome has been recovered from wild boar meat and venison in Japan.[29] Wild boar in Italy are thought to be another potential HEV reservoir, with sequences recovered bearing even closer genomic homology to human and domestic pig strains than those found in Japanese wild boar.[30] Occupational contact with pigs has also been associated with HEV infection in slaughterhouse workers,[31] veterinary surgeons[32] and surgical trainees,[33] who use pigs to practice surgical techniques. Despite the observed association of HEV infection with pigs and deer, many patients with documented HEV have no history of contact with pigs or pork ingestion,[15] raising the possibility that other food sources are responsible. An association with shellfish ingestion has been reported in a small number of cases in the UK[15] and Japan[34] and HEV antibodies have been found in cows and sheep but HEV itself has yet to be recovered. Rats, domestic cats and dogs are other potential mammalian reservoirs.

Finally, a small number of case-reports exist of blood-borne HEV.[35] Although this transmission route remains very rare, the number of such cases may increase with greater recognition of HEV infection as a cause of acute hepatitis.

CLINICAL PRESENTATION AND DIAGNOSTIC TESTS

HEV infection results in a self-limiting acute hepatitis in most patients, but a small subset of patients develop fulminant hepatitis, death occurring in 0.5–3% in endemic countries.[36] The incubation period ranges between 2–9 weeks, with a mean of approximately 6.5 weeks. Signs and symptoms parallel those of acute hepatitis A infection, namely malaise, anorexia, nausea, vomiting, fever with abdominal discomfort pruritic jaundice, pale stools and dark urine. Arthralgias, diarrhoea and rashes are also reported.

Serum alanine aminotransferase (ALT) levels remain elevated for 3 to 13 weeks from symptom onset, with HEV being detectable in blood and stool from about 3 weeks from exposure until normalisation of ALT in most patients. Viraemia can be more short-lived at just 7 days in some patients and may predate symptom onset. Faecal shedding of virus is variable, but has been reported to persist for at least 30 days from first symptoms.[37] Therefore, confirmation by detection of viral genomic RNA in serum and/or faeces by nested or real-time PCR may be of limited use and is not always commercially available.

The presence of HEV IgM in serum by ELISA confirms acute infection, IgG denoting previous infection.[38] Variable specificity, particularly of IgG ELISA in

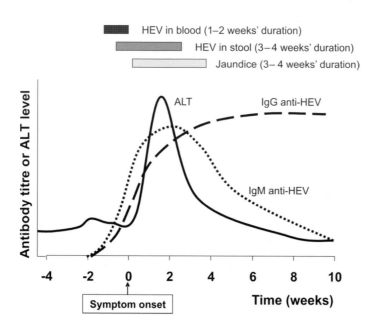

Fig. 3 Time course of HEV infection showing relationship between serum ALT, symptoms, HEV serological markers and HEV RNA. Adapted from the viral hepatitis slide-set published by the US Centers of Diseases Control and Prevention <http://www.cdc.gov/ncidod/diseases/hepatitis> April 2008.

genotype 3 infections, has been noted.[39] Furthermore, elevated IgG levels do not necessarily persist life-long, perhaps limiting the validity of such assays in epidemiological studies. The temporal relationship between symptom onset, serology and viraemia is shown in Figure 3.

Liver biopsy findings are very similar to those of acute hepatitis A, with a predominant lobular hepatitis, with spotty necrosis and balloon-degeneration of hepatocytes. Cholestatic features can predominate in some patients with cannalicular bile plugs and peri-portal inflammation, but relatively well-preserved lobular architecture.[6] These features resolve completely on recovery. In patients with fulminant hepatitis, bridging necrosis and sub-massive necrosis may be seen. Chronic HEV infection has been reported in organ recipients and is discussed below.

RISK FACTORS FOR POOR PROGNOSIS

HEPATITIS E AND PREGNANCY

If HEV is acquired in the third trimester of pregnancy, the mortality rate increases to 15–25%,[40] with a high incidence of fetal loss also. A recent study of pregnant women in a large refugee camp in western Darfur, Sudan reported an attack rate of 19.4% during a 6-month period of an epidemic, with a mortality rate of 31%.[41] This is a higher mortality rate than for other viral hepatitis infections occurring in pregnancy and the reasons for this are unclear. Most studies, to date, relate to genotype 1 and 2 infection acquired in endemic countries. Reports of severe hepatitis in pregnancy due to genotypes 3 or 4 in countries with low-endemic incidence are scarce, although those reported to date appear to have good outcome.[42,43]

CHRONIC LIVER DISEASE

A recent case-control study in India has illustrated that pre-existing cirrhosis is associated with both an increased HEV prevalence (28% versus 4.5% in healthy controls) and higher 1-year mortality rate of 70% compared with 30% in non-infected cirrhotics.[44] In this study, most patients' cirrhosis was due to chronic hepatitis B or C infection (64%). Similar observations have been made in the UK[45] and France,[46] albeit in much smaller numbers of patients. In these two series, mortality was associated with age and male sex.

Patients with chronic hepatitis B infection (69% non-cirrhotic) studied in China developed a more protracted course of HEV infection with prolonged jaundice and higher rates of decompensation and mortality amongst patients with cirrhosis.[47] This mirrors the higher observed morbidity and mortality rate with acute hepatitis A super-infection in patients with either chronic hepatitis B or C. Interestingly, hepatitis B viral load was transiently suppressed in 18% of patients during HEV infection.

CHRONIC HEPATITIS E IN ORGAN RECIPIENTS

To date, chronic, persistent, hepatitis E infection with histological evidence of cirrhosis has been reported only in recipients of either liver or renal transplants. In a recent French series of HEV infection in 14 transplant recipients (liver, renal and kidney and pancreas), low total lymphocyte counts and infection early in the post-transplant recovery phase appeared associated with a higher risk of chronicity.[48] HEV infection has also been proposed as being responsible for chronic hepatitis of 'unknown aetiology' in liver transplant recipients, following a study of retrospectively saved tissue samples from two such patients in The Netherlands.[49] One of these patients required re-transplantation due to cryptogenic cirrhosis, which was subsequently attributed to chronic HEV infection.

PREVENTION

In endemic countries, the spread of HEV infection can be limited by improving availability of clean water supplies. Travellers to endemic regions should avoid water or ice of uncertain origin, consumption of undercooked shellfish and should take care with uncooked fruit and vegetables which may have been washed in contaminated water.

A recombinant subunit HEV vaccine has been developed which has been evaluated in a large Phase II, randomised, double-blind, placebo-controlled trial in Nepal. Vaccine was given to 898 members of the Nepalese army in Kathmandu and efficacy was demonstrated in 95.5%, with just three cases in the vaccine group, compared with 66 in those who received placebo.[50] Resources are likely to limit its use in those countries with highest endemic rates, but widespread paediatric use in these countries could significantly reduce the world-wide morbidity of HEV.

Key points for clinical practice

- Hepatitis E (HEV) is a non-enveloped RNA virus with four main genotypic variants in humans. Genotypes 1 and 2 are exclusive to humans, whereas genotypes 3 and 4 also infect a variety of mammals, notably swine.

- HEV infection is transmitted enterically. It remains highly endemic in areas of poor sanitation where purified water supplies are often scarce.

- The majority of adult-acquired acute infective hepatitis in Central and South-east Asia is caused by HEV infection with genotypes 1 or 2. Conversely, HEV infection is of low endemic frequency in industrialised countries, such as the UK, where it is usually caused by genotype 3 or 4.

- The prevalence of HEV genotype 3 infection is high in domestic and wild pigs. These animals may well act as the main zoonotic reservoir for human infections in industrialised countries.

- Acute infection can be confirmed by the presence of HEV RNA in blood and/or stool, although the period of maximum viraemia may well have passed before symptoms and liver function test derangement emerge. Serum IgM is a more robust marker of acute infection.

(continued)

Key points for clinical practice *(continued)*

• Infection is self-limiting in most patients, but a fulminant course is more likely in pregnant females, immunosuppressed patients (*e.g.* transplant recipients) and those with pre-existing chronic liver disease. Persistent infection with progressive fibrosis has been reported in organ transplant recipients (liver or kidney) only.

• A recombinant sub-unit vaccine has shown efficacy in clinical trials but is not yet licensed.

References

1. Emerson SU, Anderson D, Arankalle A *et al*. Genus *Hepevirus*. In: Fauquet CM, Mayo MA, Maniloff J, Desselberger U, Ball LA. (eds) *Virus Taxonomy: Eighth Report of the International Committee on Taxonomy of Viruses*. London: Elsevier/Academic Press, 2004; 853–857.
2. Balayan MS, Andjaparidze AG, Savinskaya SS *et al*. Evidence for a virus in non-A, non-B hepatitis transmitted via the fecal-oral route. *Intervirology* 1983; **20**: 23–31.
3. Tam AW, Smith MM, Guerra ME *et al*. Hepatitis E virus (HEV): molecular cloning and sequencing of the full-length viral genome. *Virology* 1991; **185**: 120–131.
4. Huang FF, Sun ZF, Emerson SU *et al*. Determination and analysis of the complete genomic sequence of avian hepatitis E virus (avian HEV) and attempts to infect rhesus monkeys with avian HEV. *J Gen Virol* 2004; **85**: 1609–1618.
5. Khuroo MS. Study of non-A, non-B hepatitis. Possibility of another human hepatitis virus distinct from post-transfusion non-A, non-B type. *Am J Med* 1980; **68**: 818–824.
6. Gupta DN, Smetana HF. The histopathology of viral hepatitis as seen in the Delhi epidemic (1955–56). *Indian J Med Res* 1957; **45**: 101.
7. Arankalle VA, Chadha MS, Tsarev SA *et al*. Seroepidemiology of water-borne hepatitis in India and evidence for a third enterically-transmitted hepatitis agent. *Proc Natl Acad Sci USA* 1994; **91**: 3428–3432.
8. Naik SR, Aggarwal R, Salunke PN, Mehrotra NN. A large waterborne viral hepatitis E epidemic in Kanpur, India. *Bull World Health Org* 1992; **70**: 597–604.
9. Epidemiologic Notes and Reports Enterically Transmitted Non-A, Non-B Hepatitis – Mexico. *MMWR Morb Mortal Wkly Rep* 1987; **36** (36).
10. Zhuang, H. Hepatitis E and strategies for its control. Viral hepatitis in China: problems and control strategies. *Monogr Virol* 1992; **19**: 126.
11. Das K, Agarwal A, Andrew A, Frosner GG, Kar P. Role of hepatitis E and other hepatotrophic virus in aetiology of sporadic acute hepatitis: a hospital-based study from urban Delhi. *Eur J Epidemiol* 2000; **16**: 937–940.
12. Gomatos PJ, Monier MK, Arthur RR *et al*. Sporadic acute hepatitis caused by hepatitis E virus in Egyptian adults. *Clin Infect Dis* 1996; **23**: 195–196.
13. Nicand E, Armstrong GL, Enouf V *et al*. Genetic heterogeneity of hepatitis E virus in Darfur, Sudan, and neighboring Chad. *J Med Virol* 2005; **77**: 519.
14. Arankalle VA, Tsarev SA, Chadha MS *et al*. Age-specific prevalence of antibodies to hepatitis A and E viruses in Pune, India, 1982 and 1992. *J Infect Dis* 1995; **171**: 447–450.
15. Lewis HC, Boisson S, Ijaz S *et al*. Hepatitis E in England and Wales. *Emerg Infect Dis* 2008; **14**: 165–167.
16. Tsang TH, Denison EK, Williams HV *et al*. Acute hepatitis E infection acquired in California. *Clin Infect Dis* 2000; **30**: 618–619.
17. Heath TC, Burrow JN, Currie BJ *et al*. Locally acquired hepatitis E in the Northern Territory of Australia. *Med J Aust* 1995; **162**: 318–319.
18. Hsieh SY, Yang PY, Ho YP, Chu CM, Liaw YF. Identification of a novel strain of hepatitis E virus responsible for sporadic acute hepatitis in Taiwan. *J Med Virol* 1998; **55**: 300–304.

19. Suzuki K, Aikawa T, Okamoto H. Fulminant hepatitis E in Japan. *N Engl J Med* 2002; **347**: 1456.

20. Meng XJ, Wiseman B, Elvinger F *et al.* Prevalence of antibodies to hepatitis E virus in veterinarians working with swine and in normal blood donors in the United States and other countries. *J Clin Microbiol* 2002; **40**: 117–122.

21. Dalton HR, Stableforth W, Hazeldine S *et al.* Autochthonous hepatitis E in Southwest England: a comparison with hepatitis A. *Eur J Clin Microbiol Infect Dis* 2008; **27**: 579–585.

22. Clemente-Casares P, Pina S, Buti M et al. Hepatitis E Virus epidemiology in industrialized countries. *Emerg Infect Dis* 2003; **9**: 448–454.

23. Aggarwal R, Naik SR. Hepatitis E: infrafamiliar transmission versus waterborne spread. *J Hepatol* 1994; **21**: 718–723.

24. Meng XJ, Halbur PG, Haynes JS *et al.* Experimental infections of pigs with the newly-identified swine hepatitis E virus (swine HEV), but not with human strains of HEV. *Arch Virol* 1998; **143**: 1405–1415.

25. Banks M, Heath GS, Grierson SS *et al.* Evidence of the presence of hepatitis E virus in pigs in the United Kingdom. *Vet Rec* 2004; **154**: 223–227.

26. Ijaz S, Arnold E, Banks M *et al.* Non-travel-associated hepatitis E in England and Wales: demographic, clinical, and molecular epidemiological characteristics. *J Infect Dis* 2005; **192**: 1166–1172.

27. Bouwknegt M, Lodder-Verschoor F, van der Poel WHM, Rutjes SA, de Roda Husman AM. Hepatitis E virus RNA in commercial porcine livers in The Netherlands. *J Food Prot* 2007; **70**: 2889–2895.

28. Feagins AR, Opriessnig T, Guenette DK, Halbur PG, Meng XJ. Detection and characterization of infections hepatitis E virus from commercial pig livers sold in local grocery stores in the USA. *J Gen Virol* 2007; **88**: 912–917.

29. Martelli F, Caprioli A, Zengarini M *et al.* Detection of hepatitis E virus (HEV) in a demographic managed wild boar (*Susscrofa scrofa*) population in Italy. *Vet Microbiol* 2008; **126**: 74–81.

30. Takahashi K, Kitajima N, Abe N, Mishiro S. Complete or near-complete nucleotide sequences of hepatitis E virus genome recovered from a wild boar, a deer, and four patients who ate the deer. *Virology* 2004; **330**: 501–505.

31. Drobeniuc J, Favorov MO, Shapiro CN *et al.* Hepatitis E virus antibody prevalence among persons who work with swine. J *Infect Dis* 2001; **184**: 1594–1597.

32. Pérez-Gracia MT, Mateos ML, Galiana C *et al.* Autochthonous hepatitis E infection in a slaughterhouse worker. *Am J Trop Med Hygiene* 2007; **77**: 893–896.

33. Colson P, Kaba M, Bernit E, Motte A, Tamalet C. Hepatitis E associated with surgical training on pigs. *Lancet* 2007; **370**: 935.

34. Li TC, Miyamura T, Takeda N. Detection of hepatitis E virus RNA from the bivalve yamato-shijimi (*Corbicula japonica*) in Japan. *Am J Trop Med Hygiene* 2007; **76**: 170–172.

35. Colson P, Coze C, Gallian P *et al.* Transfusion-transmitted hepatitis E, France. *Emerging Infect Dis* 2007; **13**: 648–649.

36. Enterically transmitted non-A, non-B hepatitis – East Africa. *MMWR Morb Mortal Wkly Rep* 1987; **36**: 241.

37. Mast EE, Alter MJ, Holland PV, Purcell RH. Evaluation of assays for antibody to hepatitis E virus by a serum panel. Hepatitis E Virus Antibody Serum Panel Evaluation Group. *Hepatology* 1998; **27**: 857–861.

38. Aggarwal R, Kini D, Sofat S, Naik SR, Krawczynski K. Duration of viraemia and faecal viral excretion in acute hepatitis E. *Lancet* 2000; **356**: 1081–1082.

39. Herremans M, Bakker J, Duizer E, Vennema H, Koopmans MP. Use of serological assays for diagnosis of hepatitis E virus genotype 1 and 3 infections in a setting of low endemicity. *Clin Vaccine Immunol* 2007; **14**: 562–568.

40. Patra S, Kumar A, Trivedi SS, Puri M, Sarin SK. Maternal and fetal outcomes in pregnant women with acute hepatitis E virus infection. *Ann Intern Med* 2007; **147**: 28–33.

41. Boccia D, Guthmann J-P, Klovstad H *et al.* High mortality associated with an outbreak of hepatitis E among displaced persons in Darfur, Sudan. *Clin Infect Dis* 2006; **42**: 1679–1684.

42. Andersson MI, Hughes J, Gordon FH, Ijaz S, Donati M. Of pigs and pregnancy. *Lancet* 2008; **372**: 1192

43. Nagasaki F, Ueno Y, Mano Y *et al*. A patient with clinical features of acute hepatitis E viral infection and autoimmune hepatitis. *Tohoku J Exp Med* 2005; **206**: 173–179.

44. Kumar Acharya S, Kumar Sharma P, Singh R *et al*. Hepatitis E virus (HEV) infection in patients with cirrhosis is associated with rapid decompensation and death. *J Hepatol* 2007; **46**: 387–394.

45. Dalton HR, Hazeldine S, Banks M, Ijaz S, Bendall R. Locally acquired hepatitis E in chronic liver disease. *Lancet* 2007; **369**: 1260.

46. Peron JM, Bureau C, Poirson H *et al*. Fulminant liver failure from acute autochthonous hepatitis E in France: description of seven patients with acute hepatitis E and encephalopathy. *J Viral Hepat* 2007; **14**: 298–303.

47. Fan ZP, Lin SH, Cai SP *et al*. An analysis of the clinical characteristics of patients with chronic hepatitis B superinfected with acute hepatitis E. *Zhonghua Shi Yan He Lin Chuang Bing Du Xue Za Zhi* 2007; **21**: 325–327.

48. Kamar N, Selves J, Mansuy JM *et al*. Hepatitis E virus and chronic hepatitis in organ-transplant recipients. *N Engl J Med* 2008; **358**: 811–817.

49. Haagsma EB, van den Berg AP, Porte RJ *et al*. Chronic hepatitis E virus infection in liver transplant recipients. *Liver Transplant* 2008; **14**: 547–553.

50. Shrestha MP, Scott RM, Joshi DM *et al*. Safety and efficacy of a recombinant hepatitis E vaccine. *N Engl J Med* 2007; **356**: 895–903.

John E. Smithson Wolf W.W. Woltersdorf

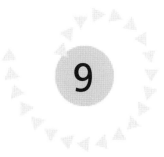

9

Chronic pancreatitis – how should we diagnose it?

The term 'chronic pancreatitis' does not imply a specific disease or pathological disorder. Instead, it is generally taken to mean an end point for a variety of different destructive processes, resulting in permanent and irreversible damage to the pancreas. An analogy could be made with cirrhosis in advanced liver disease. As glandular inflammation and fibrosis progress, clinical manifestations will develop, typically a variable combination of pain and failure of exocrine and endocrine function. The term 'exocrine pancreatic insufficiency' is sometimes used interchangeably with chronic pancreatitis, but this is misleading because the former may be short term, reversible or due to non-pancreatic pathology. The leading cause of chronic pancreatitis in many parts of the world, particularly in Westernised countries, is alcohol; a large number of other aetiologies are also recognised; however, in a significant, and perhaps unknown, proportion of cases the disorder remains idiopathic. The TIGAR-O system, devised in the US for classifying the various causes of chronic pancreatitis, is shown in Table 1. The alternative M-ANNHEIM classification has been proposed more recently by a European group from the city of the same name;[1] the elements are very similar but organised in a slightly different way. The precise pathogenic pathway leading to chronic pancreatitis will vary according to the specific cause; in some cases, it is the cumulative effect of recurrent or acute relapsing pancreatitis which leads, ultimately, to irreversible pancreatic damage rather than a steadily progressive process.

The detection and diagnosis of chronic pancreatitis rest on a combination of clinical history, pancreatic function testing, imaging and histology. However,

John E. Smithson MD FRCP (for correspondence)
Consultant Gastroenterologist, Department of Gastroenterology, University Hospitals Bristol, Bristol BS2 8HW, UK. E-mail: John.Smithson@UHBristol.nhs.uk

Wolf W.W. Woltersdorf MD MRCP FRCPath
Consultant Chemical Pathologist and Head of U-STAR Research Medical Director of Avon Diagnostic Laboratories Ltd, Department of Laboratory Medicine, University Hospitals Bristol, Bristol BS2 8HW, UK E-mail: www.woltersdorf@doctors.org.uk

Table 1 Classification and clinical evaluation of the causes of chronic pancreatitis

TIGAR-O category	Suggested evaluation
Toxic-metabolic	Alcohol, tobacco, drug and toxin history, renal function, serum estimation of triglycerides and calcium
Idiopathic	Social and travel history (tropical), exclusion of other factors
Genetic	Family history, consider genetic testing for PRSS1, SPINK1 and CFTR
Autoimmune	Obstructive pattern LFTs, raised serum IgG (especially IgG4), autoantibodies in some cases, characteristic histology, steroid responsive
Recurrent and acute severe-associated chronic pancreatitis	History, imaging for bile duct stones (EUS for microlithiasis) and congenital anomalies of pancreatic anatomy, manometry for suspected sphincter of Oddi dysfunction
Obstructive	Imaging to identify tumours, pancreatic stones and ductal strictures

The TIGAR-O system was devised by the Midwest Multicenter Pancreatic Study Group.[7]

there is often poor correlation between these different elements, and pathological confirmation of the disease is usually lacking. For example, it has long been known that up to 90% loss of exocrine function may need to occur before clinically important symptoms appear,[2] and the pancreas can be obviously disrupted or damaged on imaging and yet exocrine function may be relatively unaffected.[3] In other instances, function testing can be abnormal in the absence of detectable morphological changes in the gland. For these reasons, the definition of what constitutes chronic pancreatitis remains the subject of considerable debate. Over the years, a number of international symposia have attempted to produce a diagnostic classification of chronic pancreatitis that will prove both workable and generally acceptable to clinicians in this field. Perhaps the best known and longest established example arose from the Cambridge Symposium of 1983 shown in Table 2. This classification is based primarily on ductal appearances at endoscopic retrograde pancreatography (ERP), although ultrasound and computed tomography (CT) findings may also be incorporated. It is primarily a staging system and does not take into account aetiology. Now, 25 years on, the use of ERP as the method of choice for the diagnosis of chronic pancreatitis is diminishing given the risk that this procedure carries, the increasing refinement of ultrasound and CT, and the availability of newer non-invasive imaging techniques including magnetic resonance imaging (MRI) and endoscopic ultrasound (EUS). Alongside these technological developments have come a number of updated classifications for defining chronic pancreatitis (summarised by Schneider et al.[1]), but none has yet to gain universal acceptance, and the precise place for the newer imaging modalities in the diagnostic pathway remains to be determined. Tests of pancreatic function are also evolving, with increasing emphasis on non-invasive stool analysis rather than more laborious and error-prone techniques. Histology, perhaps the only true diagnostic 'gold standard' for chronic pancreatitis, is sought or available only in a minority of cases.

Table 2 The Cambridge classification of chronic pancreatitis according to appearances at endoscopic retrograde pancreatography (ERP)

Normal	Quality study visualising whole gland without abnormal features
Equivocal	Less than three abnormal branches
Mild	More than three abnormal branches
Moderate	Abnormal main duct and branches
Severe	As above with one or more of: Large cavities (> 10 mm) Gross gland enlargement (more than twice normal) Intraductal filling defects or calculi Duct obstruction, stricture or gross irregularity Contiguous organ invasion

This classification (Sarner and Cotton[41]) was published following an international symposium held in Cambridge, UK.

Difficulties with diagnosis have, in turn, resulted in uncertainty regarding the epidemiology of chronic pancreatitis. Classically, a key clinical feature of the condition is said to be persistent pain, and alcohol is held to be the key aetiological factor in the majority of cases. But emerging data based on faecal elastase, a relatively sensitive indirect measure of pancreatic function, challenge these long-held assumptions. They suggest that there may in fact be a 'hidden iceberg' of patients with chronic pancreatitis, which has a different clinical profile. For example, a recent study of patients in secondary care demonstrated that less than a third experienced chronic abdominal pain, and in only 15% was there a history of excess alcohol consumption.[4] Another population-based study[5] of older adults detected reduced faecal elastase in 11.5% whilst among an unselected group of diabetic patients, a surprisingly high proportion (23%) were found to have a faecal elastase level of <100 µg/g, indicative of severe pancreatic insufficiency.[6] Thus, the emergence of new diagnostic techniques may radically change our understanding of the epidemiology of chronic pancreatitis; the condition may, in fact, be much more common than suggested by previously cited prevalence figures of around 13 per 100,000 in adults (for further details see the comprehensive review of chronic pancreatitis by Etemad and Whitcomb[7]).

It is our intention to present a review of current diagnostic techniques for chronic pancreatitis. In particular, we will focus on recent developments in this field, especially with regard to pancreatic function testing and new types of radiological imaging.

PANCREAS FUNCTION TESTING

The diagnosis of chronic pancreatitis is hampered by the lack of specific symptoms and the absence of a biomarker that performs consistently well across the disease spectrum.[8] Whilst diagnosing established exocrine pancreatic insufficiency is usually straightforward, milder forms often represent an analytical challenge. Numerous types of biochemical tests exist, including blood and faecal test but their role in the diagnostic pathways is often confusing.

EXOCRINE FUNCTION TESTING

Exocrine function of the acinar cells can be assessed directly or indirectly.

Direct tests

Direct tests involve intravenous stimulation with secretagogues (*i.e.* secretin and/or cholecystokinin) and subsequent collection of pancreatic secretions by duodenal intubation. These tests have the advantage of measuring the functional exocrine reserve and secretory capacity, loss of which may precede structural abnormalities. However, there are a number of disadvantages that preclude the use of direct tube tests from routine use. First, it is an invasive procedure with inherent clinical risks. Second, they are complex and costly and not appropriate for routine assessments. Only few specialist centres now offer this service. Third, diagnostic sensitivity for mild-to-moderate exocrine loss is low due to the substantial functional reserve of the pancreas.

Indirect tests

Indirect pancreatic function tests are non-invasive. They can generally be subdivided into those that measure the result of exocrine failure (*i.e.* maldigestion and malabsorption) or analyse the presence or absence of pancreatic enzymes in faeces.

Blood tests

Blood tests seldom contribute to a diagnosis of chronic pancreatitis. The plasma activities of amylase, lipase or trypsin are usually normal except in cases with pseudocyst formation. Some patients with severe disease may have raised fasting blood glucose levels as a sign of global pancreatic insufficiency.

FAECAL FAT

Faecal fat estimation used to be a pillar in the assessment of steatorrhoea but is now rarely performed in the UK, largely due to its unpleasantness to patients and laboratory staff. In the era of automated assays and strict health and safety regulations, most laboratories no longer provide the infrastructure required for faecal fat quantification. Stool samples for faecal fat must be accurately timed, preferably over 3 or 5 days while the patient is on a defined diet and the entire collection is sent to the laboratory where it is homogenised. A small aliquot is then used for hydrolysis of the triglycerides to free fatty acids and glycerol and the free fatty acids are measured.

FAT GLOBULES

This is an alternative to the faecal fat collection and is still used in the assessment of children with failure to thrive and to monitor pancreatic enzyme supplementation therapy (*e.g.* in patients with cystic fibrosis).

A small, random, stool sample is mixed with a fat stain (*e.g.* Sudan Red) and examined microscopically for the presence of fat globules. This test only permits qualitative results and is, therefore, not suitable for routine diagnostic use in adult patients.

[^{14}C]-TRIOLEIN BREATH TEST

The [^{14}C]-triolein breath test is a tubeless test and does not require faecal collection. After ingestion of a test meal containing [^{14}C]-labelled triglycerides, fat metabolism results in the production of [^{14}C]-labelled CO_2, which is measured in breath. This test has not gained wide-spread acceptance because of its complex technical requirements and lack of sensitivity.[9,10]

PANCREOLAURYL TEST

This test is based on the enzymatic hydrolysis of orally administered fluorescein dilaurate by pancreatic esterases. Free fluorescein is absorbed by the gut, undergoes hepatic conjugation and is excreted in urine, where it is measured by simple spectrophotometry. The test is repeated on the following day using an equimolar amount of free fluorescein in place of fluorescein dilaurate in order to exclude impaired intestinal absorption.[11] The result is expressed as a ratio of excretion on both consecutive days.[12] This test is much simpler and more convenient to perform but is not sensitive enough in mild-to-moderate exocrine insufficiency. False positives can occur in a range of intestinal conditions.[13] Unfortunately, the test substances were withdrawn from the UK market by Pfizer in 2005 due to manufacturing and supply issues. However, there is a very similar test based on the hydrolysis of a synthetic peptide N-benzoyl-L-tyrosyl-p-aminobenzoic acid (NBT-PABA) by chymotrypsin. The tripeptide, variously called NBT-PABA, BTP or Bentiromide, is administered orally together with the test meal to stimulate pancreatic secretion.

FAECAL ELASTASE-1

A different indirect approach involves the measurement of proteolytic pancreatic enzymes in stool. Historically, faecal chymotrypsin used to be part of the routine repertoire of many laboratories,[14,15] but was withdrawn from the UK market in 2000. However, in the mid-1990s, a new monoclonal assay for human-specific faecal elastase-1 (ScheBo® Biotech AG) became widely available and currently represents the most convenient biomarker for chronic pancreatic insufficiency.[16]

The faecal elastase (FE-1) assay has a number of practical and analytical advantages. It is absolutely pancreas-specific and the monoclonal antibodies to the human enzyme do not cross react with elastases from the food chain. Thus, patients do not need to interrupt pancreatic enzyme replacement therapy, which is usually of porcine origin.[17]

The concentration of FE-1 in faeces is five times greater than in pancreatic juice. This means that the molecule is stable during intestinal transit and its faecal concentration solely reflects the secretory capacity of the pancreas. The intra-individual variation is low and FE-1 results correlate well with the gold standard direct secretin–cholecystokinin test.[18] Sample collection is easy to perform even in children. Patients are required to collect a single, pea-sized stool sample into a sterile tube. Due to the high stability of faecal elastase *in vivo* and *in vitro*, samples can be mailed or transported at ambient temperature.[19] The reader should be aware that watery diarrhoea might lead to a dilutional effect and a false positive result.[20] Ideally, the test should be repeated on a formed stool sample.

The assay is based on a sandwich ELISA with two monoclonal antibodies. Tests are run in duplicates on a standard 96-well plate. The cost ranges between £15–35 per result depending on batch size. Studies have found an overall sensitivity of 64–93% and specificity of 83–95% when compared to direct function studies.[16,19] Unfortunately, the sensitivity of FE-1 in patients with mild-to-moderate chronic pancreatitis is considerably lower at 50–85%.[16,21]

In recent years, a new polyclonal ELISA test for human faecal elastase has become available (BIOSERV® Diagnostics). This assay uses two polyclonal antisera that recognise different epitopes of FE-1. Head-to-head comparisons showed good correlation,[22,23] but the polyclonal assay is still under investigation for potential interference with oral pancreatic supplements.[24]

PANCREATIC IMAGING

The morphology of the pancreas can be imaged using all of the usual radiological modalities, and even plain radiography of the abdomen will detect calcification in around one-third of advanced cases of chronic pancreatitis.[25] Debate continues as to which is the best single radiological test and, to some extent, this will depend on local resources and expertise. The ideal test would be non-invasive, highly accurate, safe and inexpensive but none of the currently available imaging modalities fulfil all of these criteria. Determining the precise sensitivity and specificity of any of these tests is difficult given the absence of confirmatory histology in most cases.

TRANSABDOMINAL AND ENDOSCOPIC ULTRASOUND

Transabdominal ultrasound is often the first form of imaging employed in the diagnosis of suspected chronic pancreatitis. It is cheap, quick and widely available, and, in experienced, hands may have a sensitivity and specificity of

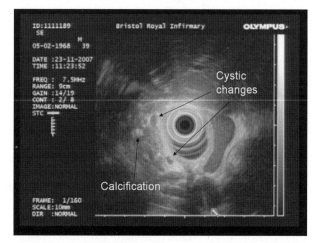

Fig. 1 EUS image of chronic pancreatitis. The abnormalities demonstrated here in the head of the gland are included in the accepted group of criteria for the diagnosis of chronic pancreatitis. Image reproduced courtesy of Ms S.A. Norton, Bristol, UK.

Table 3 Endosonographic criteria for the diagnosis of chronic pancreatitis

Parenchymal features	Ductal features
Hyperechoic strands	Stones/calcification
Hyperechoic foci	Main duct irregularity
Lobularity	Main duct dilatation
Cysts	Hyperechoic main duct
	Visible side branches

The presence of five or more criteria indicates that chronic pancreatitis is highly likely. The clinical significance of four positive features or less remains the subject of debate. For further details see Raimondo and Wallace.[42]

up to 70% and 90%, respectively.[26] The technique enables detection of gland irregularity, parenchymal heterogeneity, calcification and abnormalities of the main duct. However, its accuracy may be compromised by truncal obesity, overlying bowel gas and the skill of the operator.

Endoscopic ultrasound (EUS) offers clear advantages over transabdominal ultrasound because the whole pancreas can be reliably assessed by placing the transducer in the stomach and duodenum, and there is no intervening bowel gas or fat to degrade the images obtained. Although the procedure is more invasive, it is generally safe. The main limitations are operator expertise, lack of interobserver agreement for individual findings, and availability.[27] However, the technique is now widely practised beyond specialised tertiary centres, and it has come to form a standard, if optional, component of gastroenterology training programmes. Early studies[28,29] laid the foundation for a system of classification of chronic pancreatitis according to parenchymal and ductal appearances at endosonography (Table 3). There remains some uncertainty as to the number of abnormal criteria which must be present before chronic pancreatitis can be reliably diagnosed. The spatial resolution and resulting sensitivity of EUS is high and, therefore, it can be difficult to evaluate the significance of minor abnormalities which are not accompanied by measurable changes in pancreatic function, and where histology is not available for comparison. Therefore, debate continues as to the specificity of EUS; critics argue that it tends to overdiagnose disease and may, in some cases, detect normal variation or simple age-related changes rather than true signs of pancreatic pathology. On the other hand, the technique appears to demonstrate subtle abnormalities before any of the other radiological modalities. Consequently, it shows considerable promise for the detection of early or mild chronic pancreatitis. Equally, the absence of any abnormal signs on EUS is also clinically useful because it allows chronic pancreatitis to be excluded with confidence. Figure 1 illustrates an EUS image of chronic pancreatitis.

ENDOSCOPIC RETROGRADE PANCREATOGRAPHY (ERP)

ERP was established in the 1980s as the most accurate imaging modality for chronic pancreatitis, and formed the basis for the internationally agreed

Table 4 Comparison of the utility of different imaging modalities in chronic pancreatitis

	Advantages	Disadvantages
ERP	Sensitive and specific, especially in skilled hands, remains the radiological 'gold standard' with which other imaging modalities are compared	Invasive, risk of inducing acute pancreatitis, displays ductal anatomy only, difficult to access pancreas in some post-surgical patients or in presence of gastric or duodenal obstruction
CT	Widely available technique, rapid acquisition of images, ductal and parenchymal visualisation	Less sensitivity than other modalities, especially for early or mild disease
EUS	The most sensitive imaging modality, allows detection of mild disease, also useful for exclusion of chronic pancreatitis if no features present	Invasive, technically demanding, interobserver variation, not yet widely available, may tend to overdiagnose chronic pancreatitis
MRI	Non-invasive, comparable sensitivity to ERCP but not hampered by post-surgical anatomy, secretin enhancement permits functional as well as improved morphological assessment	Lacks sensitivity for calcification, significant extra cost of secretin

grading system shown in Table 1. The shortcomings of the technique include its invasive nature, risk of inducing acute pancreatitis (15% overall in a recent prospective multicentre study of ERCP for all indications[30]) and operator dependence in obtaining and interpreting satisfactory radiological images. Its sensitivity is limited in early or mild disease, or where there is parenchymal involvement but sparing of the main ductal system. Several prospective comparative studies have been undertaken to assess the relative value of ERP and EUS.[29,31,32] These have demonstrated close correlation between the two modalities although some discrepancy remains in cases where there are mild abnormalities on EUS but pancreatography appears normal. Overall, it appears that ERP may be supplanted by EUS in future because of its lower sensitivity and higher risk to the patient. Nevertheless, ERP remains the most reliable and accessible pancreatic ductal imaging technique for many clinicians (Table 4).

COMPUTED TOMOGRAPHY (CT)

CT may be the radiological modality of choice for evaluating pancreatic cancer. It is undoubtedly reliable for detecting calcification and other changes in advanced chronic pancreatitis, but it lacks sensitivity for milder parenchymal disease and subtle branch duct abnormalities.[33] However, the advent of higher resolution spiral CT machines may enhance sensitivity of the technique to the point where it becomes comparable to the best of the other techniques. Further advantages of CT are that it is non-invasive, widely available, unaffected by overlying bowel gas and abdominal wall fat, and good for excluding non-pancreatic pathology causing symptoms which are hard to distinguish from those of chronic pancreatitis. For this reason, it can be considered a good initial diagnostic imaging test.

MAGNETIC RESONANCE IMAGING (MRI)

The concept of MRI of the pancreas is attractive because it is non-invasive and avoids the use of ionising radiation and intravenous contrast. Early comparisons with ERP showed its performance to be inferior;[34,35] however, as with CT, its accuracy can be expected to improve with new generation machines which provide better spatial resolution (now of the order of 1 mm).

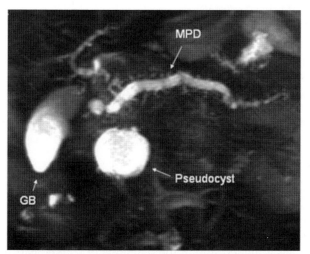

Fig. 2 MRI image of chronic pancreatitis. Several abnormalities are present including dilatation and irregularity of the main duct (MPD) and blunting of branch ducts. A pseudocyst is also shown. Image reproduced courtesy of Dr M. Callaway, Bristol, UK.

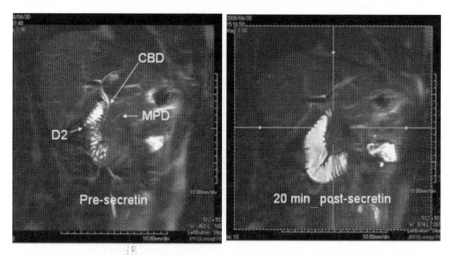

Fig. 3 MRI of the upper abdomen before and after secretin. The common bile duct (CBD) and main pancreatic duct (MPD) are clearly shown on the initial image. Following secretin injection, bicarbonate-rich juice is secreted into the duodenal lumen (D2). This can be quantitated by volumetric technique to permit an estimate of pancreatic exocrine function. Images courtesy of Dr M. Callaway, Bristol, UK.

Even so, it may not yet be sensitive enough to demonstrate reliably small duct changes and calcification. However, it does have an advantage over ERP when endoscopic access is difficult, for example, following Bilroth II gastrectomy or Roux-en-Y anastomosis. It has been shown that intravenous secretin injection prior to dynamic MRI improves the visualisation of ductal anatomy, and can also provide quantitative information regarding pancreatic functional reserve.[27,36,37] As yet, this technique for assessing pancreatic function requires further evaluation before it can be accepted as a standard part of clinical assessment. Figure 2 shows MRI of chronic pancreatitis and Figure 3 MRI before and after secretin injection.

POSITRON EMISSION TOMOGRAPHY (PET)

A clinical dilemma may occur in patients with a pancreatic mass, where other forms of imaging or histology have failed to differentiate between chronic pancreatitis and cancer. It has, therefore, been proposed that PET may be of value in such instances, because it should detect the biologically more active neoplastic lesions. However, this has not been borne out by research;[37] therefore, PET appears not to have a useful place in the diagnostic work-up of patients with chronic pancreatitis, and it should be reserved for cancer staging.

HISTOLOGY

Indications for biopsy and clinical use

Histology plays a limited role in the diagnosis of chronic pancreatitis when compared with diseases of the intestine or liver. The main reason for this is the relative inaccessibility of the gland, although it can be sampled reasonably safely by CT or ultrasound-guided needle biopsy. A more difficult problem is the potentially patchy nature of chronic pancreatitis, increasing the chance of a sampling error and incorrect staging of the disease. The characteristic features that can be expected in a diseased gland include loss of acini, fibrosis, inflammatory cell infiltrates and neuronal hyperplasia; there may be relative sparing of the islets and intralobular ducts.[38] Logically, pancreatic histology should be the gold standard by which all other diagnostic tests are measured. In practice, the usual clinical scenario is that biopsy is undertaken, not necessarily to prove the presence of chronic pancreatitis, but rather to exclude malignancy. Alternatively, tissue for histology is obtained at the time of surgical resection. Some authors consider that tissue biopsy remains a key step in the diagnosis of chronic pancreatitis,[7] and this may be attempted more widely in future as clinicians become more familiar and comfortable with an EUS-guided approach.

TESTING FOR SPECIFIC CAUSES OF CHRONIC PANCREATITIS

When faced with a patient who has proven chronic pancreatitis but without any clear aetiology, the question of further investigation arises in order to determine the precise cause of the disease. The rationale for this is that it may identify specific disorders, the treatment of which could, in turn, alleviate or prevent further pancreatic damage. A guide to the clinical evaluation of patients for aetiological causes is included in Table 1.

The differential diagnosis of chronic pancreatitis will vary according to the characteristics of the background population. Thus, in developing countries such as China and India, so-called 'tropical chronic pancreatitis' exceeds alcohol as the leading cause of the disorder.[39] The precise aetiology of this condition is not understood; toxic, nutritional, infectious and genetic factors have all been proposed but final proof for any of these is lacking. It differs from alcoholic chronic pancreatitis in having a younger age of onset, and greater frequency both of calcification and diabetes, which tends to be ketosis-resistant. Owing to its specific clinical profile, this condition has been subclassified by the American Diabetes Association and the World Health Organization as fibrocalculous pancreatic diabetes (FCPD).

The recognition that chronic pancreatitis may be familial or hereditary led to the discovery in 1996 of causative mutations in PRSS1, the cationic trypsinogen gene.[40] Inheritance is autosomal dominant with an estimated penetrance of approximately 50%, that is about half of those who inherit one of the common mutations will develop chronic pancreatitis.[7] Other genetic mutations which are associated with chronic pancreatitis include those of the cystic fibrosis transmembrane conductance regulator (CFTR) and pancreatic secretory trypsin inhibitor type 1 (SPINK1). Mutation testing for all of these genes is available in a small number of specialist laboratories. However, these tests should only be requested when they can be expected to benefit the management of the patient concerned, or where they will inform counselling of at-risk relatives. If in doubt, the gastroenterologist should involve the expertise of a clinical geneticist.

A small subset of patients with chronic pancreatitis have an autoimmune aetiology, a condition which is characterised by lymphocytic infiltration of the pancreas with resultant loss of exocrine function and extrahepatic biliary obstruction due to swelling of the pancreatic head. Certain serological markers have been described, notably elevated IgG_4 and a variety of autoantibodies, and the disease is steroid sensitive making it an important differential diagnosis to consider. Immunological mechanisms are also suspected where idiopathic chronic pancreatitis occurs in conjunction with other diseases with an immune basis, for example primary biliary cirrhosis, Sjögren's syndrome and inflammatory bowel disease.

There remains some debate as to whether certain causes of acute relapsing or recurrent pancreatitis such as sphincter of Oddi dysfunction can cause chronic pancreatitis. The same applies to gallstones, microlithiasis and pancreas divisum although, theoretically, any repeated insult to the pancreas which causes acute inflammation will ultimately lead to irreversible glandular destruction.

The importance of recognising obstructive causes of chronic pancreatitis is self evident; not only does this category include tumours, but timely therapy for stones or strictures could offset the later development of impaired function and chronic pain. Endoscopic techniques are steadily advancing, with the result that fewer patients should undergo pancreatic resection for symptom control in future.

SUMMARY AND FUTURE DIRECTIONS

The accurate and reliable detection and diagnosis of chronic pancreatitis is not straightforward, owing to the lack of non-invasive tests with both high sensitivity and specificity. There is a particular problem with early or mild disease. Furthermore, there may be discrepancies between the findings from different radiological modalities which, in turn, may disagree with the results of exocrine function testing. In addition, up to 90% of glandular function has to be lost before clinically important symptoms and signs develop. It is, therefore, not surprising that epidemiological data indicate that the condition is underdiagnosed, both in the hospital setting and in the community at large. For this reason, clinicians will need to lower their threshold of suspicion for the presence of chronic pancreatitis if more cases are to be detected and treated effectively. In the meantime, the classification of the condition remains problematic. It seems inevitable that there will be further co-operative international efforts in future to produce a consensus definition which embraces the newer imaging modalities and function tests. The field is rapidly evolving with the publication of new epidemiological data, and the advent of faecal elastase testing, secretin–MRI and endoscopic ultrasound.

We conclude with a suggested algorithm to direct the diagnosis of chronic pancreatitis (Fig. 4).

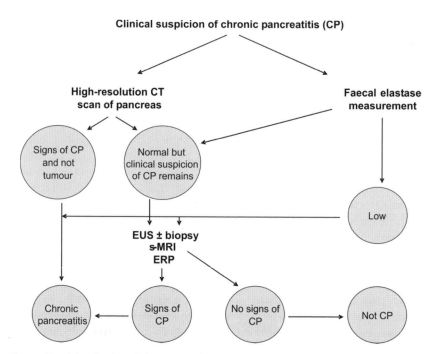

Fig. 4 Algorithm for initial diagnosis of chronic pancreatitis. In this system, CT scan and faecal elastase are suggested as initial screening tests. Because neither are highly sensitive for early or mild chronic pancreatitis, negative results do not rule it out; therefore, more sensitive tests should follow if clinical suspicion remains. A low faecal elastase-1 level alone is not diagnostic of chronic pancreatitis. Secretin-enhanced MRI (s-MRI) may be superior to standard MRI. The place of pancreatic biopsy in the diagnosis of chronic pancreatitis remains controversial. A normal EUS examination is useful for excluding chronic pancreatitis.

Key points for clinical practice

- It is likely that chronic pancreatitis is more common than was appreciated in the past, with an 'iceberg' of milder cases awaiting diagnosis.

- 'Classical' clinical features such as chronic pain, obvious steatorrhoea and a history of excess alcohol may be absent.

- Clinicians should have an increased index of suspicion for the presence of chronic pancreatitis if there is a history of persistent unexplained diarrhoea and particularly if there is co-existing diabetes mellitus.

- Faecal elastase-1 (FE-1) analysis is an easy, cheap and reproducible indirect method for assessing pancreatic exocrine function.

- It is highly sensitive for the detection of severe pancreatic exocrine insufficiency and has replaced more laborious and error-prone indirect tests.

- Only one random stool test is required for FE-1 measurement and digestive enzyme supplementation does not have to be stopped.

- Pancreatic imaging techniques are evolving rapidly. The long-established place of endoscopic retrograde pancreatography as the radiological test of choice is now being challenged by endoscopic ultrasound and MRI.

- Owing to its high sensitivity, EUS appears a particularly useful modality for the detection of early disease and for the exclusion of chronic pancreatitis.

- When combined with intravenous secretin, MRI has the additional advantage of allowing a quantitative functional assessment of pancreatic secretion.

- We can expect further efforts towards international consensus incorporating the newer diagnostic techniques in order to achieve a universal definition and classification of chronic pancreatitis.

References

1. Schneider A, Lohr JM, Singer MV. The M-ANNHEIM classification of chronic pancreatitis: introduction of a unifying classification system based on a review of previous classifications of the disease. *J Gastroenterol* 2007; **42**: 101–119.
2. DiMagno EP, Go VL, Summerskill WH. Relations between pancreatic enzyme outputs and malabsorption in severe pancreatic insufficiency. *N Engl J Med* 1973; **288**: 813–815.
3. Braganza JM, Hunt LP, Warwick F. Relationship between pancreatic exocrine function and ductal morphology in chronic pancreatitis. *Gastroenterology* 1982; **82**: 1341–1347.
4. Nowell E. Faecal elastase testing in secondary care: clinical evaluation in adult patients. Gut 2008; **57 (Suppl 1)**: A160.
5. Rothenbacher D, Low M, Hardt PD, Klor HU, Ziegler H, Brenner H. Prevalence and determinants of exocrine pancreatic insufficiency among older adults: results of a population-based study. *Scand J Gastroenterol* 2005; **40**: 697–704.
6. Hardt PD, Hauenschild A, Nalop J *et al*. High prevalence of exocrine pancreatic

insufficiency in diabetes mellitus. A multicenter study screening fecal elastase 1 concentrations in 1,021 diabetic patients. *Pancreatology* 2003; **3**: 395–402.

7. Etemad B, Whitcomb DC. Chronic pancreatitis: diagnosis, classification, and new genetic developments. *Gastroenterology* 2001; **120**: 682–707.

8. Siegmund E, Lohr JM, Schuff-Werner P. [The diagnostic validity of non-invasive pancreatic function tests – a meta-analysis]. *Z Gastroenterol* 2004; **42**: 1117–1128.

9. Duncan A, Cameron A, Stewart MJ, Russell RI. Limitations of the triolein breath test. *Clin Chim Acta* 1992; **205**: 51–64.

10. Pedersen NT, Jorgensen BB, Rannem T. The [^{14}C]-triolein breath test is not valid as a test of fat absorption. *Scand J Clin Lab Invest* 1991; **51**: 699–703.

11. Elphick DA, Kapur K. Comparing the urinary pancreolauryl ratio and faecal elastase-1 as indicators of pancreatic insufficiency in clinical practice. *Pancreatology* 2005; **5**: 196–200.

12. Dominguez-Munoz JE, Pieramico O, Buchler M, Malfertheiner P. Clinical utility of the serum pancreolauryl test in diagnosis and staging of chronic pancreatitis. *Am J Gastroenterol* 1993; **88**: 1237–1241.

13. Malfertheiner P, Buchler M, Muller A, Ditschuneit H. Influence of extrapancreatic digestive disorders on the indirect pancreatic function test with fluorescein dilaurate. *Clin Physiol Biochem* 1985; **3**: 166–173.

14. Cavallini G, Benini L, Brocco G *et al*. The fecal chymotrypsin photometric assay in the evaluation of exocrine pancreatic capacity. Comparison with other direct and indirect pancreatic function tests. *Pancreas* 1989; **4**: 300–304.

15. Walkowiak J, Herzig KH, Strzykala K, Przyslawski J, Krawczynski M. Fecal elastase-1 is superior to fecal chymotrypsin in the assessment of pancreatic involvement in cystic fibrosis. *Pediatrics* 2002; **110**: e7.

16. Loser C, Mollgaard A, Folsch UR. Faecal elastase 1: a novel, highly sensitive, and specific tubeless pancreatic function test. *Gut* 1996; **39**: 580–586.

17. Dominici R, Franzini C. Fecal elastase-1 as a test for pancreatic function: a review. *Clin Chem Lab Med* 2002; **40**: 325–332.

18. Walkowiak J, Cichy WK, Herzig KH. Comparison of fecal elastase-1 determination with the secretin-cholecystokinin test in patients with cystic fibrosis. *Scand J Gastroenterol* 1999; **34**: 202–207.

19. Stein J, Jung M, Sziegoleit A, Zeuzem S, Caspary WF, Lembcke B. Immunoreactive elastase I: clinical evaluation of a new noninvasive test of pancreatic function. *Clin Chem* 1996; **42**: 222–226.

20. Fischer B, Hoh S, Wehler M, Hahn EG, Schneider HT. Faecal elastase-1: lyophilization of stool samples prevents false low results in diarrhoea. *Scand J Gastroenterol* 2001; **36**: 771–774.

21. Gullo L, Ventrucci M, Tomassetti P, Migliori M, Pezzilli R. Fecal elastase 1 determination in chronic pancreatitis. *Dig Dis Sci* 1999; **44**: 210–213.

22. Borowitz D, Lin R, Baker SS. Comparison of monoclonal and polyclonal ELISAs for fecal elastase in patients with cystic fibrosis and pancreatic insufficiency. *J Pediatr Gastroenterol Nutr* 2007; **44**: 219–223.

23. Keim V, Teich N, Moessner J. Clinical value of a new fecal elastase test for detection of chronic pancreatitis. *Clin Lab* 2003; **49**: 209–215.

24. Schneider A, Funk B, Caspary W, Stein J. Monoclonal versus polyclonal ELISA for assessment of fecal elastase concentration: pitfalls of a new assay. *Clin Chem* 2005; **51**: 1052–1054.

25. Ammann RW, Akovbiantz A, Largiader F, Schueler G. Course and outcome of chronic pancreatitis. Longitudinal study of a mixed medical-surgical series of 245 patients. *Gastroenterology* 1984; **86**: 820–828.

26. Bolondi L, Li Bassi S, Gaiani S, Barbara L. Sonography of chronic pancreatitis. *Radiol Clin North Am* 1989; **27**: 815–833.

27. Wallace MB. Imaging the pancreas: into the deep. *Gastroenterology* 2007; **132**: 484–487.

28. Lees WR. Endoscopic ultrasonography of chronic pancreatitis and pancreatic pseudocysts. *Scand J Gastroenterol Suppl* 1986; **123**: 123–129.

29. Wiersema MJ, Hawes RH, Lehman GA, Kochman ML, Sherman S, Kopecky KK. Prospective evaluation of endoscopic ultrasonography and endoscopic retrograde

cholangiopancreatography in patients with chronic abdominal pain of suspected pancreatic origin. *Endoscopy* 1993; **25**: 555–564.

30. Cheng CL, Sherman S, Watkins JL *et al*. Risk factors for post-ERCP pancreatitis: a prospective multicenter study. *Am J Gastroenterol* 2006; **101**: 139–147.

31. Buscail L, Escourrou J, Moreau J *et al*. Endoscopic ultrasonography in chronic pancreatitis: a comparative prospective study with conventional ultrasonography, computed tomography, and ERCP. *Pancreas* 1995; **10**: 251–257.

32. Nattermann C, Goldschmidt AJ, Dancygier H. Endosonography in chronic pancreatitis – a comparison between endoscopic retrograde pancreatography and endoscopic ultrasonography. *Endoscopy* 1993; **25**: 565–570.

33. Luetmer PH, Stephens DH, Ward EM. Chronic pancreatitis: reassessment with current CT. *Radiology* 1989; **171**: 353–357.

34. Sica GT, Braver J, Cooney MJ, Miller FH, Chai JL, Adams DF. Comparison of endoscopic retrograde cholangiopancreatography with MR cholangiopancreatography in patients with pancreatitis. *Radiology* 1999; **210**: 605–610.

35. Takehara Y, Ichijo K, Tooyama N *et al*. Breath-hold MR cholangiopancreatography with a long-echo-train fast spin-echo sequence and a surface coil in chronic pancreatitis. *Radiology* 1994; **192**: 73–78.

36. Matos C, Bali MA, Delhaye M, Deviere J. Magnetic resonance imaging in the detection of pancreatitis and pancreatic neoplasms. *Best Pract Res Clin Gastroenterol* 2006; **20**: 157–178.

37. Nichols MT, Russ PD, Chen YK. Pancreatic imaging: current and emerging technologies. *Pancreas* 2006; **33**: 211–220.

38. Kloppel G, Maillet B. Pathology of acute and chronic pancreatitis. *Pancreas* 1993; **8**: 659–670.

39. Tandon RK. Tropical pancreatitis. *J Gastroenterol* 2007; **42 (Suppl 17)**: 141–147.

40. Whitcomb DC, Gorry MC, Preston RA *et al*. Hereditary pancreatitis is caused by a mutation in the cationic trypsinogen gene. *Nat Genet* 1996; **14**: 141–145.

41. Sarner M, Cotton PB. Classification of pancreatitis. *Gut* 1984; **25**: 756–759.

42. Raimondo M, Wallace MB. Diagnosis of early chronic pancreatitis by endoscopic ultrasound. Are we there yet? *JOP J Pancreas (Online)* 2004; **5**: 1–7.

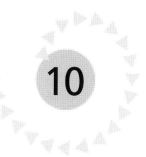

Robin Spiller

10

Targets for treatment in irritable bowel syndrome

The symptoms of irritable bowel syndrome (IBS), which include abdominal pain/discomfort, bloating and disordered bowel habit are within every human being's experience. Most self-manage their condition but recurrent symptoms sufficient to result in seeking medical help affect around 5% of the population. As a group, IBS patients are very heterogeneous and current management is often unsatisfactory, both to the patient and doctor. One problem for the consulting physician is the plethora of symptoms which some patients exhibit, making it difficult to know what the target for treatment really is. As Figure 1 shows, IBS symptoms can best be considered as being related to bowel habit, the severity of pain and the presence or absence of non-gastrointestinal symptoms. It is important to understand where any individual patient fits within the multiple dimensions of IBS, particularly whether the abnormality is predominantly central or peripheral in origin, since this will substantially influence the optimum approach to treatment.

IBS AND SOMATISATION

While, as a group, IBS patients have a higher incidence of prior psychiatric illness including anxiety, depression and panic disorders, these tend to aggregate in a small subgroup of patients who suffer from somatisation, characterised by multiple somatic complaints unexplained by known medical conditions.[1] A study in primary care in Bristol, UK indicated 46% of IBS patients were polysymptomatic compared with just 24% of those with organic gastrointestinal disease.[2] While true somatisation, meeting the Diagnostic and Statistical Manual for Mental Disorders IV (DSM IV) criteria, is rare, up to 10% of patients seen by doctors have a lesser disorder called 'physical symptom

Robin Spiller MD(Cantab) MSc(Lond) FRCP
Professor of Gastroenterology, Wolfson Digestive Diseases Centre, C Floor South Block, University Hospital, Nottingham NG7 2UH, UK
E-mail: robin.spiller@nottingham.ac.uk

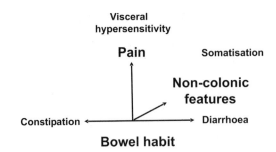

Fig. 1 Multiple dimensions to be considered when targeting therapy in an individual patient with IBS.

disorder' defined as one or more physical symptoms not fully explained by another medical or psychiatric disorder which has lasted more than 6 months.[3]

ABNORMALITIES IN PAIN PROCESSING IN SOMATISATION

Somatisation is an expression both of anxiety about the meaning of symptoms and abnormalities of pain processing. The underlying mechanism is likely to be similar in disorders such as fibromyalgia, temporomandibular joint dysfunction and chronic headaches in which excessive pain is seen in the absence of any obvious peripheral abnormality. Pain thresholds to deep pressure in fibromyalgia are significantly reduced compared with controls and, when equal amount of pressure are applied to both groups, fMRI of the brain indicates increased cerebral activation with spread of activation from the somatosensory cortex to multiple other brain areas.[4] This pattern of amplification of cortical pain signalling correlates with the subjective report.[4] Similar abnormalities are found in patients with idiopathic low back pain for which no abnormality can be found.

VISCERAL HYPERSENSITIVITY

This is one of the key features of IBS which usually has been assessed by distending the rectum with a balloon. This stimulus first induces a sensation of the desire to defecate, then discomfort and finally pain. Around half of all IBS patients report pain at pressures which are considered non-painful by healthy volunteers.[5] IBS patients also frequently show an abnormal cutaneous referral pattern, with pain perceived not only in the rectum as is normal, but also in the lower abdominal region.[5] This enhanced somatic referral suggests spinal sensitisation. This is a phenomenon seen in many painful conditions in which repeated pain stimuli lead to a facilitation of synaptic transmission within the dorsal horn pain pathways, a phenomenon know as 'central sensitisation'.[6] Pain signals then pass up the spinal cord with afferent branches to the brain-stem structures before reaching the thalamus for onward transmission to the cerebral cortex where conscious awareness occurs. Visceral stimuli activate not only the primary and secondary somatosensory cortex but also paralimbic and limbic structures. Stimulation of these areas mediates the affective and emotional response to visceral sensation.

DESCENDING MODULATION OF PAIN PERCEPTION

Pain transmission is not a one-way process and there are important descending influences on ascending pathways. Stimulation of the periaqueductal grey area in the brain stem can both facilitate and inhibit the response to noxious stimulation such as colorectal distension. The inhibitory process, termed 'diffuse noxious inhibitory control' (DNIC), which involves both serotonin and opioid pathways, probably mediates the analgesic effect of 'counter irritants' and appears defective in IBS patients.[7,8] Emotion has a strong influence on pain processing and one of the benefits of tricyclic antidepressants and cognitive behavioural therapy may be to inhibit stress- and anxiety-induced enhancement of pain transmission. Distraction can also reduce cerebral activation in response to painful stimuli, a phenomenon which cognitive behavioural therapy can exploit.

Extracolonic features are a key component of IBS, most strikingly lethargy, fatigue and poor sleep. These are unlikely to represent primary gut disorders but probably reflect central dysfunction and may respond to centrally acting agents such as tricyclic antidepressants.

IBS PATIENTS WHOSE SYMPTOMS ARISE PRIMARILY FROM DISORDERED GUT FUNCTION

Identifying patients with somatisation is useful because such patients largely account for the excess of psychiatric disease in IBS patients.[9] Excluding these leaves one with a group of patients in whom the predominant abnormality may lie within the bowel. The symptoms of either diarrhoea or constipation with or without bloating can then be addressed. This should start with a dietary assessment since dietary factors such as dietary fibre intake strongly influence gut function. Both constipation and diarrhoea can respond to dietary manipulation as will be discussed below. Another common and often most bothersome symptom is bloating. This describes an unpleasant sensation of distension which may, or may not, be associated with physical distension and a need to loosen the clothing. Those with physical distension are most commonly constipated and this may respond to treatment of constipation. However, those in whom the sensation is observed without visible distension are most likely to have visceral hypersensitivity as discussed above.

Animal experiments make it clear that stress stimulates colonic transit and delays gastric emptying, features which many patients will recognise. Experimental studies in IBS patients suggest that stress may also enhance visceral hypersensitivity which may account for the benefit of anxiolytics.

NEW TREATMENTS FOR IBS

As Figure 2 shows, the last few years has seen the appearance of many new products which, although largely still unavailable in Europe, may well appear shortly. Since they target specific mechanisms, studying the trial results increases our knowledge of the condition and these will be discussed according to their primary targets.

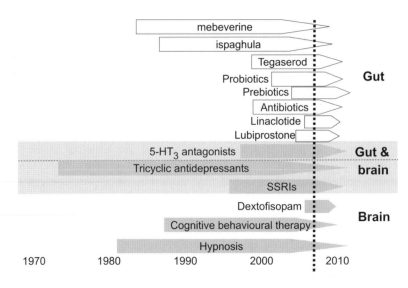

Fig. 2 Changing fashions in IBS treatment over the last 40 years: targeting the gut or the brain?

PERIPHERALLY ACTING TREATMENTS

Diet

The symptoms of many IBS patients are aggravated by eating and several open-label trials of exclusion diets have demonstrated that more than half of those agreeing to take part claimed to benefit.[10,11] The foods most commonly implicated were wheat and milk. However, there is undoubtedly a strong placebo element to these trials which in IBS can exceed 50%, so it is uncertain how much of the benefit is specific. In many cases, patients persisted on the diet for at least 1 year which argues that they did find some benefit. Earlier trials using double-blind dosing of substances patients were supposedly intolerant of were very limited and more suited to identification of true allergy. Most observers no longer believe that IBS patients are truly allergic to food since this usually manifests itself with clear-cut symptoms such as urticaria and asthma; such patients do not consult gastroenterologists but rather dermatologists and immunologists. Food intolerance seems more likely to be related to maldigestion, the best known example of which being lactose malabsorption, a condition with symptoms of abdominal pain, bloating and diarrhoea following lactose ingestion which closely mimic IBS.

Lactose intolerance

Most mammals, including human beings, cease to produce the lactase enzyme after weaning so that, world-wide, adult-acquired lactose intolerance is the norm. The gene for lactase persistence appears to have arisen in Northern European and is found in 90%. It has spread south and east so that the incidence of adult-acquired lactose intolerance increases steadily as one moves south east from 10% in north-western Europe to 40% in the Mediterranean and North African countries and 90% in the Far East. Malabsorbed lactose is osmotically active within the small bowel so that a 180-ml glass of water containing 50 g of lactose but no sodium increases in volume 10-fold as sodium and water pass down the electrochemical gradient across the permeable small bowel resulting in substantial ileo-colonic inflow. Once it enters the colon, lactose is rapidly fermented to short-chain fatty acids and gas which, together with the large fluid volume, stimulates acceleration of colonic transit with resulting diarrhoea. Excluding lactose can remove symptoms in lactose-intolerant subjects diagnosed with IBS.[12,13] However, the success or otherwise of lactose exclusion depends strongly on habitual lactose intake, since, even in those with lactose malabsorption, as much as 240 ml of milk can be taken without producing more symptoms than are observed after ingesting 240 ml of identical-looking, lactose-free, hydrolysed milk.[14] In clinical practice, many patients have already tried lactose exclusion before seeking medical help so this rarely helps.

Fermentable oligosaccharide, disaccharide, monosaccharide and polyols (FODMAPs)

More recently, it has been recognised that there are numerous other sources of poorly absorbed, osmotically active, dietary substances including fructose, the polyhydric alcohols sorbitol and mannitol, and oligofructans, polymers of fructose with a glucose-terminal molecule (*e.g.* inulin and raffinose). This has formed the basis of a low FODMAP diet.[15] To follow such a diet, it is important to recognise the common dietary items which include substantial (> 3 g) amounts of fructose per portion. These include the obvious sweet fruit (such as apples, pears, melons, cherries and leeches) as well as concentrated fruit juice and dried fruits (currants, sultanas, dates, figs and prunes) which have high concentrations. Further, less-well recognised sources include many soft drinks which are sweetened with high-fructose maize starch, a change in our diet which has occurred over the last decade without really being noticed. Another significant change is the increasing purchase of ready-made sauces which are often sweetened with fructose. Oligofructans are also found in significant amounts in wheat, pasta, wholemeal cereal, biscuits and, particularly, onions, leeks and asparagus, the highest content of all being found in Jerusalem artichokes which, in excess, are commonly associated with flatulence and diarrhoea (see Table 1).

Table 1 Sources of oligofructans in diet

Source	Serving size (g)	Fructan content (g)
White bread	65 (2 slices)	1.8
Pasta	165	2.5
Wholemeal cereal	60	1.9
Biscuit	40 (2 biscuits)	1.2
Onion	35	2.1
Leek	85	5.6
Asparagus	90 (6 spears)	2.6
Jerusalem artichoke	75	15

Adapted from Shepherd *et al.*[15]

Randomised, placebo-controlled trials of diet are difficult as they cannot be easily blinded. There is only one anecdotal report[15] in which 62 IBS patients, preselected because they had a positive breath hydrogen test after 35 g of fructose, were given advice on a low FODMAP diet and a 1-h education on the fructose and fructan content of foods. They were telephoned at a median of 14 months (range, 2–14 months) after the consultation and those who adhered to the diet reported an improvement compared to those who did not in a range of symptoms, particularly bloating, nausea and diarrhoea. Of course, this could all be placebo effect, though the same authors have recently undertaken a study on patients who had had colectomy and ileal pouch formation and showed that, in seven patients without pouchitis, median stool frequency fell from 8 to 4 on a low FODMAP diet.[16] They have also reported a randomised, placebo-controlled trial showing that a daily fructan/fructose drink (up to 19 g and 50 g, respectively) given over a 10-day period did indeed induce a significant increase symptoms in IBS patients when compared with a 20-g glucose drink.

The idea that food intolerance might somehow be related to an immune phenomenon persists. A recent study used the patient's serum IgG food antibodies to recommend an individualised exclusion diet. This showed, in a randomised control trial design, that the individualised food exclusion diet was better that a sham diet unrelated to the IgG antibodies with a number-needed-to-treat of 2.5 in those who adhered to the diet. However, the major defect in this study was that the majority of subjects had IgG antibodies to wheat and milk so that 49% of the treatment group had wheat excluded compared with just 8% in the sham group and 84% had milk excluded compared with 1.3% in the sham group in whom the major exclusion was potato and rice.[17] This non-random distribution of exclusions means that essentially this was a comparison of a wheat and milk exclusion diet compared with a rice and potato exclusion one and the difference observed could be unrelated to the IgG antibodies.

ROLE OF COLONIC MICROBIOTA

The gut microbiota are a vital component of colonic function and account for 70% of stool weight. Between 10–15% of dietary starch and a greater proportion of dietary non-starch polysaccharides enter the colon unchanged being resistant to human digestive enzymes. The complex colonic microbiota in the anaerobic colonic environment ferment these substances to short-chain fatty acids, predominately acetate, propionate and butyrate. These provide luminal nutrients for enterocytes and may account for as much as 15% of total energy absorption. Their absorption is sodium-linked and stimulates water absorption. There is extensive adaptation to dietary components as is shown by the increased fermentation capacity of the colon for lactulose when given repeatedly.[18] The importance of this function is seen when the microbiota are substantially diminished by antibiotic therapy. This leads to antibiotic-associated diarrhoea and the loss of colonic salvage of poorly absorbed carbohydrate.[19] Given the importance of colonic microbiota, it is logical to attempt to manipulate these for therapeutic benefit, an idea which has driven the current enthusiasm for probiotics.

Probiotics

These are live organisms which survive transit through the gut and are thought to provide health benefits. Typically, 1×10^{10} organisms are given daily some of which survive transit through the gut and can be detected in the stool. Their growth is limited though; when probiotics are stopped, they disappear from faecal cultures within about a week.[20] Within the colon, some probiotics including *Lactobacillus* spp. ferment unabsorbed, non-starch polysaccharides and oligo- and disaccharides lowering the pH, facilitating the growth of some bacteria such as *Bifidobacteria* spp. while inhibiting others.[21] Probiotics have a number of other desirable properties relevant to their use to reduce the duration of infectious diarrhoea including adherence to a range of human intestinal cell lines where they are able to inhibit the growth of enterotoxigenic *Escherichia coli* and to reduce the invasiveness and adherence of such organisms.[22] Similar findings have been reported for a range of *Lactobacillus* and *Bifidobacteria* spp. that are commonly found in fermented dairy products as well as others derived from healthy colons including *E. coli* Nissle 1917[23] and *Bifidobacterium infantis*. *E. coli* Nissle 1917 inhibits the adherence of adherent-invasive *E. coli* (AIEC),[23] which have been detected in ileal lesions of patients with Crohn's disease providing some logic for the development of probiotics as a treatment for Crohn's disease though, so far, without noted success. Recent evidence of low-grade inflammatory changes in IBS with altered gut permeability have increased interest in anti-inflammatory properties of probiotics which can enhance the barrier function of cultured cells[24] and inhibit the increase in colonic permeability induced in rats by stress.[25] In addition to these direct effects, colonic microbiota have an important immunomodulatory role and probiotics have been shown to inhibit the inflammatory response in many experimental colitis models.[26] Probiotics may stimulate regulatory T_{reg}-cells to exert their anti-inflammatory effects.[27,28] Recent evidence indicating immune activation in IBS patients and its correction by probiotic therapy suggests one possible mode of action in IBS.[29]

Clinical trials of probiotics in IBS

Recently, there have been numerous clinical trials with probiotics in IBS with variable results. One difficulty in evaluating these clinical trials is the different probiotics used and, in many cases, the rather small numbers of patients. One relatively consistent finding has been a reduction in flatulence seen with *Lactobacillus plantarum*[30] and *Lactobacillus reuteri*.[31] *Lactobacillus rhamnosus* was also shown to reduce distension in children with IBS.[32] However, mechanistic studies using *L. plantarum* in a small study of 12 IBS patients failed to show any effect on 24-h gas excretion or faecal weight.[33] Other studies have used composite scores making it difficult to ascertain exactly what the benefit is. One large, well-designed, randomised, double-blind, placebo-controlled trial in 362 unselected IBS patients showed a decrease in composite score and pain and discomfort with *B. infantis* 1×10^8 CFU/day.[34] A previous smaller study with *B. infantis* 1×10^{10} CFU/day in 25 IBS patients showed a reduction in pain and bloating and also an increased in peripheral blood mononuclear cell IL-10/IL-12 ratio suggesting a possible anti-inflammatory action.[35] Several studies from one research group using *L. rhamnosus* GG combined with *B. breve* and *Proprionobacterium freudenreichii* have shown an improvement in composite score, though from such a score it is impossible to calculate a number-needed-to-treat or to estimate how big an impact these will make in the clinic.[36]

Prebiotics

These comprise a range of poorly absorbed disaccharides (*e.g.* lactulose), non-starch polysaccharides and oligofructans (*e.g.* inulin, raffinose) which act as substrates for desirable bacteria. When combined with probiotics, the combination is known as a symbiotic. Since these poorly absorbed substances tend to exacerbate flatulence, they would not immediately appear a logical treatment for IBS. However, one randomised, controlled trial has shown a benefit of such a mixture[37] but this was only a 2-week trial and needs further confirmation.

Antibiotics

Broad-spectrum antibiotics markedly deplete the colonic flora, a phenomenon which is associated with overgrowth of resistant bacteria and may, in some cases, lead to life-threatening colitis including that due to *Clostridium difficile* and *Klebsiella oxytoca*.[38] Frequent use of antibiotics is associated with an increased risk for IBS.[39,40] Despite this, various groups have been treating IBS patients with antibiotics. One randomised, controlled trial used rifaximin 400 mg t.d.s. for 10 days and studied the response up to 10 weeks. Eighty-seven IBS patients were randomised and those receiving rifaximin reported an average improvement of 36% on a global symptom score (0–100) compared with just 21% on placebo at 10 weeks.[41] The original logic for such antibiotic treatment was a supposed demonstration of bacterial overgrowth using the discredited lactulose hydrogen breath test. Most authors have discounted this claim and it appears that the benefit reflects the effect of antibiotics on colonic flora with its inhibition of fermentation and hence gas production. However, as the current epidemic of *C. difficile* demonstrates, treating a not insubstantial proportion of the population with broad-spectrum antibiotics is fraught with hazard and cannot be recommended at present. Whether there is a role for non-absorbable, more selective antibiotics remains to be seen. Development of such products would require knowledge of which specific bacteria one wished to inhibit and we are, as yet, far from knowing this.

5-HYDROXYTRYPTAMINE (5-HT$_3$) ANTAGONISTS FOR IBS WITH DIARRHOEA

These were developed in the 1980s and proved highly successful treatments for nausea and vomiting associated with chemotherapy in which large amounts of serotonin are released into the circulation.[42,43] One noted side effect of such treatments was constipation. Ondansetron, a widely used anti-emetic medication, has been shown to delay transit through the distal colon.[44] Granisetron, a related 5-HT$_3$ receptor antagonist has been shown to reduced rectal sensitivity and post-prandial stimulation of colonic motility in IBS patients.[45] Alosetron was later developed with more specific action on the bowel though its initial development was as an anxiolytic.

Alosetron

This is one of the most extensively studied IBS treatments with six high-quality, randomised, placebo-controlled trials including 3118 patients, 75% with IBS-D.[46] These trials used 'satisfactory relief of IBS symptoms' as an endpoint for which alosetron achieved a 10–15% increase over the placebo response rate which averaged around 40%, giving a number-needed-to-treat of 7.[46] Other striking changes which occurred within a week of commencing treatment were an improvement in stool consistency and a reduction in urgency. There were also significant improvements in the relief of abdominal pain. One study made a direct comparison with mebeverine and showed a significant increase in those achieving adequate relief (58% versus 48%).[47] Alosetron was, however, withdrawn abruptly after it became apparent that there was a small increase in the incidence of ischaemic colitis. This affected approximately 1 in 700 patients and was associated with flare in abdominal pain and bloody diarrhoea. On discontinuing the drug, the symptoms rapidly ceased in all cases and caused no deaths. There were, however, deaths related to severe constipation, mostly in patients who were treated inappropriately, some on intensive care. Alosetron has been re-introduced as a result of patient pressure but under very strict control with many exclusions and is no longer being actively promoted. A related drug, cilansetron, which if anything showed somewhat greater potency than alosetron and was apparently beneficial in both males and females was withdrawn owing to suspected ischaemic colitis at a rate of around 4 per 1000 patient years of exposure.[48]

OPIOIDS FOR IBS WITH DIARRHOEA

Loperamide

This is a peripherally restricted μ-opioid agonist which slows bowel transit and increases anal tone without the sedating and nauseating effects of centrally acting opiates like codeine. It is widely used to control the symptoms of infectious diarrhoea and has been shown in small randomised, controlled trials to reduce stool frequency and urgency in IBS patients with diarrhoea.[49] It does not, however, control abdominal discomfort or pain and may cause an uncomfortable bloating sensation; therefore, patients often restrict its use to occasions when urgent defecation would be inconvenient, such as when they are travelling. However, it is valuable because it gives the patient a feeling of being in control.

5-HT$_4$ AGONISTS FOR IBS WITH CONSTIPATION

5-HT$_4$ activation acts presynaptically to enhance acetylcholine release.[50] 5-HT$_4$ receptors are coupled to G$_s$ proteins which increase cyclic AMP leading to decreased K$^+$ conductance, reducing resting cell membrane potential and increasing excitability thereby enhancing existing reflexes and peristalsis. 5-HT$_4$ agonists also have secretory effects.[51,52]

Tegaserod

Although recently withdrawn owing to a very slight excess of thrombotic events (1 per 1000 versus 0.1 per 1000 on placebo), related drugs are still under development, so understanding tegaserod's mode of action may yet be of value. Tegaserod is a 5-HT$_4$ partial agonist shown *in vitro* to stimulate release of CGRP, VIP and substance P from mucosal afferent nerves and enhance the peristaltic reflex.[53] When given by mouth to patients with constipation-predominant IBS, tegaserod accelerated colonic transit.[54] Large, well-designed, randomised, placebo-controlled trials in constipation-predominant IBS showed improvement of abdominal discomfort and pain and an increase in number of bowel movements compared to placebo. The beneficial effect of tegaserod was seen within the first week with an abrupt increase in defecation and a decrease in stool consistency. Subsequent studies confirmed these findings and also showed a reduction in bloating. A recent Cochrane review confirmed the benefit in constipation-predominant IBS but found the effect to be small, with a number-needed-to-treat of 17.[55]

Prucalopride

Prucalopride, another more potent and more selective 5-HT$_4$ agonist, is currently being evaluated for the treatment of both constipation and IBS-C. Prucalopride increases stool frequency and diminishes stool consistency in healthy volunteers while increasing the number of high-amplitude propagated contractions.[56] It has also been shown in several randomised, controlled trials to increase the number of bowel movements and decrease the percentage of bowel movements with hard and lumpy stools and straining in patients with chronic constipation.[57,58]

NOVEL SECRETAGOGUES FOR CONSTIPATED IBS

Lubiprostone

Lubiprostone is a prostaglandin E$_1$ derivative, which like its parent compound,[59] stimulates type 2 chloride channels located in the apical membranes of intestinal epithelial cells to stimulate secretion of sodium and water. Lubiprostone is highly gut selective with very low systemic bioavailability and virtually undetectable levels in blood.[60] Lubiprostone accelerates small bowel and colonic transit while retarding gastric emptying in healthy volunteers.[61] Randomised, controlled trials in patients with chronic constipation show a significant increase in spontaneous bowel movement frequency compared with placebo,[62] and a stimulation of defecation within 24 h of the first dose of the drug.[63] As might be predicted from the prostaglandin origin, the most commonly reported adverse event was mild-to-moderate nausea which resulted in treatment discontinuation in 5% of patients. The most recent dose-ranging study in IBS patients with constipation using 8–24 µg b.d. versus placebo showed significant benefit for abdominal pain and discomfort in the first month but, in common with other constipation trials, after 3 months there was no difference from placebo.[64]

Linaclotide

This 14-mer peptide is a structural analogue of the natural secretagogue, guanylin. This is the endogenous ligand of the guanylate cyclase receptor sub-type C (GC-C), which is mostly expressed on the luminal surface of intestinal epithelial cells. GC-C responds to both guanylin, uroguanylin and enteric bacterial peptides in the heat stable enterotoxin family (ST peptides).[65] Guanylin and uroguanylin are important natriuretic agents which enhance urinary excretion of oral ingested sodium.[66] Like the heat stable *E. coli* enterotoxin, linaclotide stimulates overall colonic transit in constipation-predominant IBS patients, associated with a softening of stool and facilitation of defecation.[67]

CENTRALLY ACTING TREATMENTS

Antidepressants

Tricyclic antidepressants (TCAs) have been used to treat IBS for many years. Meta-analyses suggest benefit, but the quality of older trials was poor.[49] A large recent, well-designed trial of 431 IBS patients compared desipramine 50–150 mg daily as tolerated with placebo, education versus cognitive behavioural therapy.[68] This showed a responder rate of 59.8% for desipramine compared with 47.4% for placebo, a non-significant difference on an intention-to-treat analysis. In contrast, the cognitive behavioural therapy responder rate was 70% compared to 37% education, a highly significant difference. However, many patients could not tolerate desipramine and 16% discontinued the drug while 9% of the remainder had no detectable drug in their blood. A per protocol analysis excluding these and other protocol violations showed 68.5% responded to desipramine versus 49.1% for the placebo group giving a number-needed-to-treat of 6.25. The benefit of TCAs does not appear to reside within their antidepressant properties, since the effect is, if anything, slightly greater in those who are not depressed.[68] However, as illustrated above, their use at effective antidepressant doses is limited by the frequent occurrence of side effects. As a result, many authors recommend low-dose amitriptyline 10–30 mg at night, a dose at which it acts more as a sedative than an anti-depressant.[69] However, given that amitriptyline has been off-patent for many years, there is no incentive to perform the expensive, but necessary, randomised control trials to prove the effectiveness of such regimens so the level of evidence for this treatment remains only that of clinical opinion.[69]

SELECTIVE SEROTONIN RE-UPTAKE INHIBITORS (SSRIS)

SSRIs are much better tolerated and have largely replaced TCAs as first-line treatment for depression. They block the re-uptake of serotonin at the synaptic level and enhance serotonergic effects within the brain. They also have effects peripherally, accelerating small bowel transit.[70] There are only a few, mostly small randomised, controlled trials in IBS but they do appear beneficial in some patients. One recent small mechanistic randomised, controlled trial showed citalopram significantly reduced the number of days per week with abdominal pain after both 3 weeks and 6 weeks of treatment compared with baseline while placebo had no effect.[71] There was also an improvement in abdominal pain and an increase in the proportion of patients who had a greater than 50% reduction in the number of days with pain. Effects were seen despite the fact that citalopram had no effect on colonic compliance nor did it reduce visceral hypersensitivity. A similar small mechanistic study using fluoxetine in non-depressed IBS patients again showed no effect on visceral hypersensitivity and this time no benefit on abdominal pain either. However, in a *post-hoc* subgroup analysis of just the hypersensitive patients, fluoxetine did reduce the number of patients reporting significant pain.[72] However, these results are based on very small numbers and need confirmation. A slightly larger study examined treatment with paroxetine of IBS patients who had failed a high-fibre diet. Paroxetine significantly improved overall well-being but had little effect on abdominal pain and bloating.[73] Interestingly, more paroxetine recipients than placebo recipients wanted to continue their study medication, confirming that patients felt better despite unchanged bowel symptoms. The largest and perhaps most convincing study randomised 257 patients to either psychotherapy, paroxetine or treatment as usual. Both paroxetine and psychotherapy were equally effective in improving quality of life though, again, IBS bowel symptoms were unchanged.[74] A subgroup analysis of the same study showed that the beneficial effect on quality of life was independent of changes in depression.[75] A smaller study of 45 cases of IBS from Tehran using fluoxetine 20 mg daily showed a significant improvement in both bloating and symptoms of constipation including hard stool and infrequent bowel movement.[76] It may be that, by selecting patients with constipation, the prokinetic action of SSRIs may give enhanced efficacy. No global assessment was made nor was any assessment made of psychological parameters though, compared with other studies, this was a very constipated group with over 64 having less than three bowel movements a week and 95% having hard stools and bloating. This study would support the idea that an SSRI should be tried in constipation-predominant IBS. There was no difference in adverse events between fluoxetine and placebo and none were severe enough to lead to discontinuation of medication confirming that, unlike TCAs, these drugs are well tolerated.

Dextofisopam

Dextofisopam is the D-enantiomer of tofisopam a benzodiazepine derivative with anxiolytic properties but lacking the anticonvulsant, sedative, and psychomotor retardation or amnesic effects of the older benzodiazepines.[77,78] It appears to act particularly on the autonomic centres and inhibits the autonomic response to stress including the acceleration of colonic transit.[79] Dextofisopam is used for the treatment of anxiety and alcohol withdrawal but does not cause dependency. A randomised, controlled trial of 200 mg b.d. dextofisopam versus placebo in 140 diarrhoea-predominant or alternating IBS patients showed dextofisopam to be superior to placebo during the first month of treatment with 73% versus 49% achieving adequate relief of symptoms. Unfortunately, there was evidence of tachyphylaxis and the difference between treatment groups declined during month 2 (56% versus 43%; $P = 0.084$) and month 3 (43% versus 38% difference; not significant). There was also an improvement in stool consistency but the reduction in stool frequency was seen only in women.[80] This might, however, still be a reasonable short-term treatment for flares in stress-related symptoms.

Pregabalin

Pregabalin is an anticonvulsant used in the treatment of neuropathic pain.[81] It has also been found beneficial for patients with generalised anxiety disorders and was the first medication approved by the US Food and Drug Administration specifically for the treatment of fibromyalgia with randomised, controlled trials showing a beneficial effect.[82,83] Like gabapentin, which pregabalin replaces, pregabalin binds to the $\alpha2\delta$-subunit of the voltage-dependent calcium channel. The $\alpha2\delta$-subunit is part of L-, P-, N- and R-type calcium channels and is widely distributed throughout the brain and muscle which may explain the frequent adverse reactions including drowsiness, visual disturbances, ataxia, constipation, confusion and, infrequently, depression. Drowsiness occurs in more than 10% of patients and may limit its use. There is one mechanistic study of pregabalin in IBS patients with visceral hypersensitivity who underwent a randomised, controlled trial receiving either 3 weeks of pregabalin titrated up to 150 mg t.d.s. as tolerated or placebo.[84] Pregabalin significantly inhibited visceral hypersensitivity compared with placebo and significantly increased rectal compliance. Mild dizziness and sleepiness was noted and the authors suggested that clinical trials in IBS might be warranted.

PSYCHOLOGICAL TREATMENTS

Patient education booklets

Patient support groups often claim that doctors are uninterested in IBS and provide little information to help the patients. A recent large randomised controlled trial with 420 patients in 54 primary care centres tested the concept that a comprehensive booklet outlining what is understood of the condition together with both dietary life-style advice as well as drug treatment would reduce consultations.[85]

At 1 year, there was a 60% reduction in annual primary healthcare consultations which fell from 3.7 (2.4) to 1.0 (1.6) whereas those who were managed in the normal way showed no change over the 1-year study period. Although symptom scores did not change significantly, patients did report a higher degree of perceived improvement in their symptoms. This same research group has shown a similar benefit in patients with ulcerative colitis; at 1 year following the intervention, patients who were encouraged to self-manage had made fewer hospital visits without any increase in the number of primary care visits.

Cognitive behavioural therapy

This usually involves 6–8 sessions of an hour each in which the therapist attempts to identify triggers for symptom exacerbation, particularly trying to understand how patients react to their symptoms aiming to teach them more effective ways of responding. The evidence for efficacy is uncertain and earlier meta-analyses concluded that many trials were too small and of an inadequate design to allow firm conclusions about any benefit.[86] More recently, there have been larger better designed studies and one study in primary care in which cognitive behavioural therapy was combined with mebeverine showed symptom improvement at 3 months and 6 months, though the effect had worn off by a year. However, at 1 year those treated with cognitive behavioural therapy showed significant benefit on work and social adjustment scales.[87] One large North American study (described above) enrolled 431 patients and randomised them to receive either cognitive behavioural therapy or education or desimipramine. On an intention-to-treat basis, cognitive behavioural therapy was significantly more effective than education and desimipramine.[68] However, it should be noted that there have also been contrary negative studies.[88]

Psychotherapy

Psychotherapy is usually reserved for more severe cases. In a recent study, 257 patients with severe IBS were randomised to 8 sessions of psychotherapy compared with 20 mg of fluoxetine or routine care.[74] Both psychotherapy and fluoxetine were superior to treatment as usual in improving health-related quality of life but there were no effects on IBS symptoms. However, despite this, psychotherapy was associated with a significant reduction in healthcare costs compared with routine care.[74]

Hypnosis

The first randomised, control trial showing benefit in IBS patients refractory to other treatments was in 1984.[89] The technique has slowly spread and there are now several other groups reporting similar findings. Hypnosis has been shown to reduce pain induced by rectal distension and also to improve somatisation and anxiety.[90] However, a recent Cochrane review described four studies including a total of 147 patients but concluded that the quality of trials was inadequate to make any definite conclusion as to efficacy.[91]

Key points for clinical practice

- Irritable bowel syndrome patients are highly heterogeneous and no one treatment will work in all cases.

- It is important to recognise a substantial subgroup of irritable bowel syndrome patients who suffer from 'somatisation' with multiple non-gastrointestinal complaints who do not respond to specific bowel directed therapy but do respond to centrally directed therapy.

- Once 'somatisers' have been identified and excluded, the substantial group remains in whom therapy should be directed to the predominant gastrointestinal symptoms.

- A careful dietary history may identify dietary excess or specific intolerance. Consideration should be given to lactose intolerance or excessive intake of FODMAPs (fermentable oligosaccharide, disaccharide, monosaccharide and polyols).

- There is much enthusiasm for probiotics but, so far, most trials have been too small and inconclusive. Antibiotics may have short-term benefit but the risks of wide-spread use means these cannot be recommended at present.

- Loperamide is useful to control urgency and frequent defecation but does little to control pain or discomfort.

Key points for clinical practice *(continued)*

- 5-HT$_3$ antagonists have been shown to be effective in treating irritable bowel syndrome with diarrhoea controlling urgency, loose stools and abdominal pain.

- 5-HT$_4$ agonists are efficacious in treating irritable bowel syndrome with constipation accelerating colonic transit, increasing stool frequency and relieving abdominal pain or discomfort.

- Tricyclic antidepressants are commonly used and may help by acting as mild anxiolytics to reduce pain perception.

- Psychological treatments including cognitive behavioural therapy, psychotherapy and hypnosis can be effective in selected patients but there is limited availability.

References

1. North CS, Downs D, Clouse RE *et al.* The presentation of irritable bowel syndrome in the context of somatization disorder. *Clin Gastroenterol Hepatol* 2004; **2**: 787–795.
2. Thompson WG, Heaton KW, Smyth GT, Smyth C. Irritable bowel syndrome in general practice: prevalence, characteristics, and referral. *Gut* 2000; **46**: 78–82.
3. Kroenke K. Physical symptom disorder: a simpler diagnostic category for somatization-spectrum conditions. *J Psychosom Res* 2006; **60**: 335–339.
4. Gracely RH, Geisser ME, Giesecke T *et al.* Pain catastrophizing and neural responses to pain among persons with fibromyalgia. *Brain* 2004; **127**: 835–843.
5. Mertz H, Naliboff B, Munakata J, Niazi N, Mayer EA. Altered rectal perception is a biological marker of patients with irritable bowel syndrome. *Gastroenterology* 1995; **109**: 40–52.
6. Knowles CH, Aziz Q. Visceral hypersensitivity in non erosive reflux disease (NERD). *Gut* 2008; **57**: 674–683.
7. Wilder-Smith CH, Schindler D, Lovblad K, Redmond SM, Nirkko A. Brain functional magnetic resonance imaging of rectal pain and activation of endogenous inhibitory mechanisms in irritable bowel syndrome patient subgroups and healthy controls. *Gut* 2004; **53**: 1595–1601.
8. Coffin B, Bouhassira D, Sabate JM, Barbe L, Jian R. Alteration of the spinal modulation of nociceptive processing in patients with irritable bowel syndrome. *Gut* 2004; **53**: 1465–1470.
9. Miller AR, North CS, Clouse RE, Wetzel RD, Spitznagel EL, Alpers DH. The association of irritable bowel syndrome and somatization disorder. *Ann Clin Psychiatry* 2001; **13**: 25–30.
10. Nanda R, James R, Smith H, Dudley CR, Jewell DP. Food intolerance and the irritable bowel syndrome. *Gut* 1989; **30**: 1099–1104.
11. Parker TJ, Naylor SJ, Riordan AM, Hunter JO. Management of patients with food intolerance in irritable bowel syndrome: The development and use of an exclusion diet. *J Hum Nutr Diet* 1995; **8**: 159–166.
12. Vernia P, Ricciardi MR, Frandina C, Bilotta T, Frieri G. Lactose malabsorption and irritable bowel syndrome. Effect of a long-term lactose-free diet. *It J Gastroenterol* 1995; **27**: 117–121.
13. Bohmer CJM, Tuynman HARE. The clinical relevance of lactose malabsorption in irritable bowel syndrome. *Eur J Gastroenterol Hepatol* 1996; **8**: 1013–1016.
14. Suarez FL, Savaiano DA, Levitt MD. A comparison of symptoms after the consumption of milk or lactose-hydrolyzed milk by people with self-reported severe lactose intolerance. *N Engl J Med* 1995; **333**: 1–4.

15. Shepherd SJ, Gibson PR. Fructose malabsorption and symptoms of irritable bowel syndrome: guidelines for effective dietary management. *J Am Diet Assoc* 2006; **106**: 1631–1639.

16. Croagh C, Shepherd SJ, Berryman M, Muir JG, Gibson PR. Pilot study on the effect of reducing dietary FODMAP intake on bowel function in patients without a colon. *Inflamm Bowel Dis* 2007; **13**: 1522–1528.

17. Atkinson W, Sheldon TA, Shaath N, Whorwell PJ. Food elimination based on IgG antibodies in irritable bowel syndrome: a randomised controlled trial. *Gut* 2004; **53**: 1459–1464.

18. Flourie B, Briet F, Florent C, Pellier P, Maurel M, Rambaud JC. Can diarrhea induced by lactulose be reduced by prolonged ingestion of lactulose? *Am J Clin Nutr* 1993; **58**: 369–375.

19. Rao SSC, Edwards CA, Austen CJ, Bruce C, Read NW. Impaired colonic fermentation of carbohydrate after ampicillin. *Gastroenterology* 1988; **94**: 928–932.

20. Alander M, Satokari R, Korpela R *et al*. Persistence of colonization of human colonic mucosa by a probiotic strain, *Lactobacillus rhamnosus* GG, after oral consumption. *Appl Environ Microbiol* 1999; **65**: 351–354.

21. Johansson ML, Nobaek S, Berggren A *et al*. Survival of *Lactobacillus plantarum* DSM 9843 (299v), and effect on the short-chain fatty acid content of faeces after ingestion of a rose-hip drink with fermented oats. *Int J Food Microbiol* 1998; **42**: 29–38.

22. Gopal PK, Prasad J, Smart J, Gill HS. *In vitro* adherence properties of *Lactobacillus rhamnosus* DR20 and *Bifidobacterium lactis* DR10 strains and their antagonistic activity against an enterotoxigenic *Escherichia coli*. *Int J Food Microbiol* 2001; **67**: 207–216.

23. Boudeau J, Glasser AL, Julien S, Colombel JF, Darfeuille-Michaud A. Inhibitory effect of probiotic *Escherichia coli* strain Nissle 1917 on adhesion to and invasion of intestinal epithelial cells by adherent-invasive *E. coli* strains isolated from patients with Crohn's disease. *Aliment Pharmacol Ther* 2003; **18**: 45–56.

24. Madsen K, Cornish A, Soper P *et al*. Probiotic bacteria enhance murine and human intestinal epithelial barrier function. *Gastroenterology* 2001; **121**: 580–591.

25. Ait-Belgnaoui A, Han W, Lamine F *et al*. *Lactobacillus farciminis* treatment suppresses stress induced visceral hypersensitivity: a possible action through interaction with epithelial cell cytoskeleton contraction. *Gut* 2006; **55**: 1090–1094.

26. Rachmilewitz D, Katakura K, Karmeli F *et al*. Toll-like receptor 9 signaling mediates the anti-inflammatory effects of probiotics in murine experimental colitis. *Gastroenterology* 2004; **126**: 520–528.

27. Schultz M, Linde HJ, Lehn N *et al*. Immunomodulatory consequences of oral administration of *Lactobacillus rhamnosus* strain GG in healthy volunteers. *J Dairy Res* 2003; **70**: 165–173.

28. Di GC, Marinaro M, Sanchez M, Strober W, Boirivant M. Probiotics ameliorate recurrent Th1-mediated murine colitis by inducing IL-10 and IL-10-dependent TGF-beta-bearing regulatory cells. *J Immunol* 2005; **174**: 3237–3246.

29. O'Mahony L, McCarthy J, Kelly P *et al*. Lactobacillus and bifidobacterium in irritable bowel syndrome: symptom responses and relationship to cytokine profiles. *Gastroenterology* 2005; **128**: 541–551.

30. Nobaek S, Johansson ML, Molin G, Ahrne S, Jeppsson B. Alteration of intestinal microflora is associated with reduction in abdominal bloating and pain in patients with irritable bowel syndrome. *Am J Gastroenterol* 2000; **95**: 1231–1238.

31. Niv E, Naftali T, Hallak R, Vaisman N. The efficacy of *Lactobacillus reuteri* ATCC 55730 in the treatment of patients with irritable bowel syndrome – a double blind, placebo-controlled, randomized study. *Clin Nutr* 2005; **24**: 925–931.

32. Bausserman M, Michail S. The use of *Lactobacillus* GG in irritable bowel syndrome in children: a double-blind randomized control trial. *J Pediatr* 2005; **147**: 197–201.

33. Sen S, Mullan MM, Parker TJ, Woolner JT, Tarry SA, Hunter JO. Effect of *Lactobacillus plantarum* 299v on colonic fermentation and symptoms of irritable bowel syndrome. *Dig Dis Sci* 2002; **47**: 2615–2620.

34. Whorwell PJ, Altringer L, Morel J *et al*. Efficacy of an encapsulated probiotic *Bifidobacterium infantis* 35624 in women with irritable bowel syndrome. *Am J Gastroenterol* 2006; **101**: 1581–1590.

35. O'Mahony L, McCarthy J, Kelly P et al. Lactobacillus and bifidobacterium in irritable bowel syndrome: symptom responses and relationship to cytokine profiles. Gastroenterology 2005; 128: 541–551.

36. Kajander K, Myllyluoma E, Rajilic-Stojanovic M et al. Clinical trial: multispecies probiotic supplementation alleviates the symptoms of irritable bowel syndrome and stabilizes intestinal microbiota. Aliment Pharmacol Ther 2008; 27: 48–57.

37. Bittner AC, Croffut RM, Stranahan MC. Prescript-Assist probiotic-prebiotic treatment for irritable bowel syndrome: a methodologically oriented, 2-week, randomized, placebo-controlled, double-blind clinical study. Clin Ther 2005; 27: 755–761.

38. Hogenauer C, Langner C, Beubler E et al. Klebsiella oxytoca as a causative organism of antibiotic-associated hemorrhagic colitis. N Engl J Med 2006; 355: 2418–2426.

39. Mendall MA, Kumar D. Antibiotic use, childhood affluence and irritable bowel syndrome (IBS). Eur J Gastroenterol Hepatol 1998; 10: 59–62.

40. Maxwell PR, Rink E, Kumar D, Mendall MA. Antibiotics increase functional abdominal symptoms. Am J Gastroenterol 2002; 97: 104–108.

41. Pimentel M, Park S, Mirocha J, Kane SV, Kong Y. The effect of a nonabsorbed oral antibiotic (rifaximin) on the symptoms of the irritable bowel syndrome: a randomized trial. Ann Intern Med 2006; 145: 557–563.

42. Cubeddu LX, Hoffmann IS, Fuenmayor NT, Malave JJ. Changes in serotonin metabolism in cancer patients: its relationship to nausea and vomiting induced by chemotherapeutic drugs. Br J Cancer 1992; 66: 198–203.

43. Castejon AM, Paez X, Hernandez L, Cubeddu LX. Use of intravenous microdialysis to monitor changes in serotonin release and metabolism induced by cisplatin in cancer patients: comparative effects of granisetron and ondansetron. J Pharmacol Exp Ther 1999; 291: 960–966.

44. Talley NJ, Phillips SF, Haddad A et al. GR 38032F (ondansetron), a selective 5HT$_3$ receptor antagonist, slows colonic transit in healthy man. Dig Dis Sci 1990; 35: 477–480.

45. Prior A, Read NW. Reduction of rectal sensitivity and post-prandial motility by granisetron, a 5-HT$_3$-receptor antagonist, in patients with irritable bowel syndrome. Aliment Pharmacol Ther 1993; 7: 175–180.

46. Cremonini F, Delgado-Aros S, Camilleri M. Efficacy of alosetron in irritable bowel syndrome: a meta-analysis of randomized controlled trials. Neurogastroenterol Motil 2003; 15: 79–86.

47. Jones RH, Holtmann G, Rodrigo L et al. Alosetron relieves pain and improves bowel function compared with mebeverine in female nonconstipated irritable bowel syndrome patients. Aliment Pharmacol Ther 1999; 13: 1419–1427.

48. Chey WD, Cash BD. Cilansetron: a new serotonergic agent for the irritable bowel syndrome with diarrhoea. Expert Opin Invest Drugs 2005; 14: 185–193.

49. Lesbros-Pantoflickova D, Michetti P, Fried M, Beglinger C, Blum AL. Meta-analysis: the treatment of irritable bowel syndrome. Aliment Pharmacol Ther 2004; 20: 1253–1269.

50. Taniyama K, Nakayama S, Takeda K et al. Cisapride stimulates motility of the intestine via the 5-hydroxytryptamine receptors. J Pharmacol Exp Ther 1991; 258: 1098–1104.

51. Kellum JM, Albuquerque FC, Stoner MC, Harris RP. Stroking human jejunal mucosa induces 5-HT release and Cl$^-$ secretion via afferent neurons and 5-HT$_4$ receptors. Am J Physiol 1999; 277: G515–G520.

52. McLean PG, Coupar IM. Investigation into the effect of 5-hydroxytryptamine on fluid transport in the rat small intestine. Gen Pharmacol 1998; 30: 227–231.

53. Grider JR, Foxx-Orenstein AE, Jin JG. 5-Hydroxytryptamine$_4$ receptor agonists initiate the peristaltic reflex in human, rat, and guinea pig intestine. Gastroenterology 1998; 115: 370–380.

54. Prather CM, Camilleri M, Zinsmeister AR, McKinzie S, Thomforde G. Tegaserod accelerates orocecal transit in patients with constipation-predominant irritable bowel syndrome. Gastroenterology 2000; 118: 463–468.

55. Evans BW, Clark WK, Moore DJ, Whorwell PJ. Tegaserod for the treatment of irritable bowel syndrome. Cochrane Database Syst Rev 2004; (1): CD003960.

56. De Schryver AM, Andriesse GI, Samsom M, Smout AJ, Gooszen HG, Akkermans LM. The effects of the specific 5HT(4) receptor agonist, prucalopride, on colonic motility in healthy volunteers. Aliment Pharmacol Ther 2002; 16: 603–612.

57. Emmanuel AV, Roy AJ, Nicholls TJ, Kamm MA. Prucalopride, a systemic enterokinetic, for the treatment of constipation. *Aliment Pharmacol Ther* 2002; **16**: 1347–1356.

58. Coremans G, Kerstens R, De PM, Stevens M. Prucalopride is effective in patients with severe chronic constipation in whom laxatives fail to provide adequate relief. Results of a double-blind, placebo-controlled clinical trial. *Digestion* 2003; **67**: 82–89.

59. Crowell MD, Harris LA, DiBaise JK, Olden KW. Activation of type-2 chloride channels: a novel therapeutic target for the treatment of chronic constipation. *Curr Opin Invest Drugs* 2007; **8**: 66–70.

60. Rivkin A, Chagan L. Lubiprostone: chloride channel activator for chronic constipation. *Clin Ther* 2006; **28**: 2008–2021.

61. Camilleri M, Bharucha AE, Ueno R *et al*. Effect of a selective chloride channel activator, lubiprostone, on gastrointestinal transit, gastric sensory, and motor functions in healthy volunteers. *Am J Physiol* 2006; **290**: G942–G947.

62. Johanson JF, Ueno R. Lubiprostone, a locally acting chloride channel activator, in adult patients with chronic constipation: a double-blind, placebo-controlled, dose-ranging study to evaluate efficacy and safety. *Aliment Pharmacol Ther* 2007; **25**: 1351–1361.

63. Johanson JF, Morton D, Geenen J, Ueno R. Multicenter, 4-week, double-blind, randomized, placebo-controlled trial of lubiprostone, a locally-acting type-2 chloride channel activator, in patients with chronic constipation. *Am J Gastroenterol* 2008; **103**: 170–177.

64. Johanson JF, Drossman DA, Panas R, Wahle A, Ueno R. Clinical trial: phase 2 study of lubiprostone for irritable bowel syndrome with constipation. *Aliment Pharmacol Ther* 2008; **27**: 685–696.

65. Giannella RA. Escherichia coli heat-stable enterotoxins, guanylins, and their receptors: what are they and what do they do? *J Lab Clin Med* 1995; **125**: 173–181.

66. Fonteles MC, Greenberg RN, Monteiro HS, Currie MG, Forte LR. Natriuretic and kaliuretic activities of guanylin and uroguanylin in the isolated perfused rat kidney. *Am J Physiol* 1998; **275**: F191–F197.

67. Andresen V, Camilleri M, Busciglio IA *et al*. Effect of 5 days linaclotide on transit and bowel function in females with constipation-predominant irritable bowel syndrome. *Gastroenterology* 2007; **133**: 761–768.

68. Drossman DA, Toner BB, Whitehead WE *et al*. Cognitive-behavioral therapy versus education and desipramine versus placebo for moderate to severe functional bowel disorders. *Gastroenterology* 2003; **125**: 19–31.

69. Spiller R, Aziz Q, Creed F *et al*. Guidelines on the irritable bowel syndrome: mechanisms and practical management. *Gut* 2007; **56**: 1770–1798.

70. Gorard DA, Libby GW, Farthing MJ. Influence of antidepressants on whole gut and orocaecal transit times in health and irritable bowel syndrome. *Aliment Pharmacol Ther* 1994; **8**: 159–166.

71. Tack J, Broekaert D, Fischler B, Van Oudenhove L, Gevers A, Janssens J. A controlled cross-over study of the selective serotonin reuptake inhibitor citalopram in irritable bowel syndrome. *Gut* 2006; **55**: 1095–1103.

72. Kuiken SD, Tytgat GN, Boeckxstaens GE. The selective serotonin reuptake inhibitor fluoxetine does not change rectal sensitivity and symptoms in patients with irritable bowel syndrome: a double blind, randomized, placebo-controlled study. *Clin Gastroenterol Hepatol* 2003; **1**: 219–228.

73. Tabas G, Beaves M, Wang J, Friday P, Mardini H, Arnold G. Paroxetine to treat irritable bowel syndrome not responding to high-fiber diet: a double-blind, placebo-controlled trial. *Am J Gastroenterol* 2004; **99**: 914–920.

74. Creed F, Fernandes L, Guthrie E *et al*. The cost-effectiveness of psychotherapy and paroxetine for severe irritable bowel syndrome. *Gastroenterology* 2003; **124**: 303–317.

75. Creed F, Guthrie E, Ratcliffe J *et al*. Does psychological treatment help only those patients with severe irritable bowel syndrome who also have a concurrent psychiatric disorder? *Aust NZ J Psychiatry* 2005; **39**: 807–815.

76. Vahedi H, Merat S, Rashidioon A, Ghoddoosi A, Malekzadeh R. The effect of fluoxetine in patients with pain and constipation-predominant irritable bowel syndrome: a double-blind randomized-controlled study. *Aliment Pharmacol Ther* 2005; **22**: 381–385.

77. Seppala T, Palva E, Mattila MJ, Korttila K, Shrotriya RC. Tofisopam, a novel 3,4-

benzodiazepine: multiple-dose effects on psychomotor skills and memory. Comparison with diazepam and interactions with ethanol. *Psychopharmacology (Berl)* 1980; **69**: 209–218.

78. Bond A, Lader M. A comparison of the psychotropic profiles of tofisopam and diazepam. *Eur J Clin Pharmacol* 1982; **22**: 137–142.

79. Yamaguchi K, Suzuki K, Niho T, Shimora M, Ito C, Ohnishi H. Tofisopam, a new 2,3-benzodiazepine. Inhibition of changes induced by stress loading and hypothalamic stimulation. *Can J Physiol Pharmacol* 1983; **61**: 619–625.

80. Leventer SM, Raudibaugh K, Frissora CL *et al*. Clinical trial: dextofisopam in the treatment of patients with diarrhoea-predominant or alternating irritable bowel syndrome. *Aliment Pharmacol Ther* 2008; **27**: 197–206.

81. Siddall PJ, Cousins MJ, Otte A, Griesing T, Chambers R, Murphy TK. Pregabalin in central neuropathic pain associated with spinal cord injury: a placebo-controlled trial. *Neurology* 2006; **67**: 1792–1800.

82. Crofford LJ, Rowbotham MC, Mease PJ *et al*. Pregabalin for the treatment of fibromyalgia syndrome: results of a randomized, double-blind, placebo-controlled trial. *Arthritis Rheum* 2005; **52**: 1264–1273.

83. Crofford LJ, Mease PJ, Simpson SL *et al*. Fibromyalgia relapse evaluation and efficacy for durability of meaningful relief (FREEDOM): a 6-month, double-blind, placebo-controlled trial with pregabalin. *Pain* 2008; **136**: 419–431.

84. Houghton LA, Fell C, Lea R *et al*. Pregabalin, a second generation alpha2 delta ligand reduces hypersensitivity to rectal distension in patients with irritable bowel syndrome. *Gastroenterology* 2005; **128**: A93.

85. Robinson A, Lee V, Kennedy A *et al*. A randomised controlled trial of self-help interventions in patients with a primary care diagnosis of irritable bowel syndrome. *Gut* 2006; **55**: 643–648.

86. Talley NJ, Owen BK, Boyce P, Paterson K. Psychological treatments for irritable bowel syndrome: a critique of controlled treatment trials. *Am J Gastroenterol* 1996; **91**: 277–283.

87. Kennedy T, Jones R, Darnley S, Seed P, Wessely S, Chalder T. Cognitive behaviour therapy in addition to antispasmodic treatment for irritable bowel syndrome in primary care: randomised controlled trial. *BMJ* 2005; **331**: 435.

88. Boyce PM, Talley NJ, Balaam B, Koloski NA, Truman G. A randomized controlled trial of cognitive behavior therapy, relaxation training, and routine clinical care for the irritable bowel syndrome. *Am J Gastroenterol* 2003; **98**: 2209–2218.

89. Whorwell PJ, Prior A, Faragher EB. Controlled trial of hypnotherapy in the treatment of severe refractory irritable-bowel syndrome. *Lancet* 1984; **2**: 1232–1234.

90. Palsson OS, Turner MJ, Johnson DA, Burnett CK, Whitehead WE. Hypnosis treatment for severe irritable bowel syndrome: investigation of mechanism and effects on symptoms. *Dig Dis Sci* 2002; **47**: 2605–2614.

91. Webb AN, Kukuruzovic RH, Catto-Smith AG, Sawyer SM. Hypnotherapy for treatment of irritable bowel syndrome. Cochrane Database Syst Rev 2007; (4): CD005110.

Chris Probert Tom J. Creed

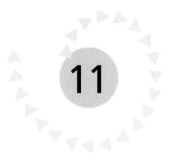

Recent advances in inflammatory bowel disease

Chronic inflammatory bowel disease, Crohn's disease and ulcerative colitis, afflicts 1 in 500 adults in the UK. The treatment is limited by the lack of understanding of the pathogenesis; however, research over the past decade has cast new light on the aetiology of both Crohn's disease and ulcerative colitis and is now offering new treatment strategies. In this chapter, we will review the most recent advances in aetiology and treatment of inflammatory bowel disease.

CROHN'S DISEASE

AETIOLOGY

Infection – or lack of it?

Epidemiological studies have reported that the highest incidence of Crohn's disease occurs in industrialised nations. Furthermore, it was noted that the incidence was greater in urban, rather than rural areas, although the development of dormitory villages has reduced this gradient. It was striking, then, that migrants studies found that when people moved from an area of low incidence to one of high incidence that the incidence of inflammatory bowel disease grew in the migrants. Furthermore, the change in disease pattern appears to occur in a predictable manner – initially there is a low incidence of inflammatory bowel disease, then the incidence in ulcerative colitis increases, followed by a rise in Crohn's disease. The change in pattern is often most noticeable in the second, and subsequent, generations. Such changes strongly

Chris Probert MD FRCP FHEA (for correspondence)
Professor of Gastroenterology, Clinical Science at South Bristol, University of Bristol and University Hospitals of Bristol, Bristol BS2 8HW, UK
E-mail: c.s.j.probert@bristol.ac.uk

Tom J. Creed MD MRCP
Consultant Gastroenterologist, University Hospitals of Bristol, Bristol BS2 8HW, UK
E-mail: t.j.creed@bristol.ac.uk

implicate an environmental factor; clearly genetic changes would not be seen over such a short interval.

There is a reciprocal relationship between the incidence of intestinal worms and that of Crohn's disease. In fact, there is a broader inverse relationship between infestations and atopic and/or autoimmune disorders leading to the suggestion that helminths may protect against such diseases. A series of studies led by Weinstock[1] implied that worms abrogate the immune response in inflammatory bowel disease; both shifting the Th1 (IL-12, IL-18 and IFN-γ)/Th2 (IL-4, IL-5, IL-9 and IL-13) ratio towards Th2 (which may benefit patients with Crohn's disease), and by subtly influencing the Th2 pathway (which may benefit those with ulcerative colitis).

Early clinical trial data appear to support a beneficial role for specific helminths (*Trichuris suis* and *Necator americanus*) in the treatment of Crohn's disease. In the former, 29 patients with moderately active Crohn's disease received eggs of the porcine worm three weekly; response was observed in 79% and remission achieved in 72%. It remains a challenging area of research and the results of large-scale clinical trials are eagerly awaited.

It has long been suggested that Crohn's disease is due to infection. The appearance of the disease resembles that of intestinal tuberculosis or Johne's disease of ruminants, a granulomatous enterocolitis caused by *Mycobacterium avium paratuberculosis* (MAP). Various species of *Mycobacteria*, including MAP, have been grown from the tissues of patients with Crohn's disease. However, the occurrence of MAP is inconsistent irrespective of the techniques used: not all Crohn's disease samples contain the organism and it is present in some control samples.[2] Consequently, *Mycobacteria* do not fulfil Koch's postulates.

Numerous treatment regimens targeting *Mycobacteria tuberculosis* have been investigated, without success.[3] Similarly, a well-designed, randomised, controlled trial (RCT) in which triple therapy (clarithromycin, rifabutin, and clofazimine) against MAP was administered to 213 patients for 2 years failed to show benefit.[4] Such studies have undermined the hypothesis that *Mycobacteria* cause Crohn's disease. However, as MAP is not found in all patients with Crohn's disease, it is possible that such therapy would only work in a subset of patients and so the debate continues, recently fuelled by the study of genes in Crohn's disease.

The small intestine is said to be sterile, but this is a relative term as recent data suggest that there are up to 10^5 organisms/ml in the proximal small intestine and up to a 1000-fold more in the ileum. It seems unlikely that the spatial relationship between sites of Crohn's disease and high bacterial load is a coincidence. The role for enteric organisms in the pathogenesis of Crohn's disease is strongly supported by the clinical response to faecal diversion. Remission often results from diversion of faeces from the colon, yet when the efflux was instilled into the colon disease recurrence occurred;[5] however, an ultrafiltrate of the efflux did not induce the same response.[5] Similar effects on the neoterminal ileum have recently been reported.[6] These studies suggest that intestinal flora itself may trigger Crohn's disease.

The flora of the distal ileum resembles that of the colon. In Crohn's disease, *Escherichia coli* species appear particularly common compared to healthy controls.[7] These *E. coli* species are, in fact, wide-spread within the intestine of individuals with Crohn's disease and are not specific to sites of disease. *E. coli* from patients with Crohn's disease also exhibit some unusual characteristics of adherence and invasion. Specifically, *E. coli* from patients with Crohn's disease show adhesion to mature epithelial cells and these adhesive strains are correlated with colonisation of the intestine.[7] The second unusual characteristic is invasion of epithelial cells. The LF82 strain has now been shown to invade a range of human epithelial cell lines efficiently. It is important to note that this invasion differs from that of conventional, pathogens such as *Shigella* spp., as LF82 requires the function of host-cell actin microfilaments and microtubules.[8] These two characteristics define the adherent invasive *E. coli* (AIEC).

The role of AIEC in the pathogenesis of Crohn's disease is supported by the finding that it can not only survive, but may also replicate, in macrophages and, in so-doing, leads to the secretion of TNF-α.[9]

Is it all in the genes?

Familial predisposition to Crohn's disease had been reported in numerous epidemiological studies. The same work, however, predicted that Crohn's disease has a complex inheritance in which numerous genes may play a part. Following the successful identification of HLA associations in various autoimmune disorders, such relationships were sought amongst patients with inflammatory bowel disease and, while the findings in ulcerative colitis were interesting, those in Crohn's disease were disappointing. Undeterred, studies continued and led to identification of the *NOD2* (*Card 15*) gene association with ileal and stenosing Crohn's disease.[10-12] The prevalence of *NOD2* mutations may be as high as 42% in early-onset ileal Crohn's disease.[13] Three mutations of *NOD2* have been described in association with Crohn's disease: Arg702Trp, Gly908Arg and Leu1007fsinsC. Each of these mutations is located close to, or in, the leucine-rich repeat domain (see below). Patients with Crohn's disease may have one, or multiple, mutations, or none at all. Meta-analysis suggests that having one mutation is associated with an odds ratio of having Crohn's disease of 2.4, having two abnormal alleles (whether homozygotic or compound heterozygotic) gives an odds ratio of 17.1.[12]

NOD2 protein is expressed in numerous cells of the innate immune response and the intestinal epithelium. It acts as a sensor for intracellular bacteria in response to muramyl dipeptide (MDP), a component of peptidoglycans, found in both Gram-positive and Gram-negative bacteria. Recognition by the leucine-rich repeat domain of NOD leads to activation of NF-κB which then triggers an inflammatory response by the production of cytokines, chemokines and acute phase proteins.[14]

Further evidence for the role of *NOD2* mutations comes from murine studies. NOD2-deficient mice have abnormally large Peyer's patches, raised levels of pro-inflammatory cytokines, abnormal mucosal permeability and increased bacterial translocation. While these are features of Crohn's disease in humans, the mice do not exhibit a Crohn's disease phenotype.[15]

Despite the compelling evidence for a role for the *NOD2* mutation in the development of Crohn's disease, it must be noted that most patients with Crohn's disease do not have a *NOD2* mutation, the association does not apply to non-ileal sites of Crohn's disease and most people with the *NOD2* mutation do not develop Crohn's disease at all.

To most gastroenterologists, autophagy is a new term, but suddenly it is everywhere. Autophagy is the process by which a cell recycles redundant organelles, but which also protects cells from intracellular pathogens. Given the evidence of intracellular bacteria, be they AIEC or MAP, the finding of a defect in autophagy is an exciting development. Mutations of two genes associated with autophagy have been reported that are strongly linked to Crohn's disease. The genes are *ATG16L1* and *IRGM*.[16]

ATG16L1 has been reported in three independent studies. A single nucleotide substitution occurs in a highly conserved domain in the gene. The gene is expressed by intestinal CD4 T-cells, clonal expansions of which are associated with Crohn's disease. *IRGM* variants have been reported in two studies. Neither gene has had the functional sequelae determined; however, defects in rodents are linked to invasion by *Salmonella typhimurium* and *Listeria monocytogenes*, respectively.[16]

Another topical gene is the IL-23 receptor. This gene is related to the activation of T-cells. Three studies have reported an uncommon variant in the receptor gene (Arg38Gln). Interestingly, the variant was associated in the reduction of risk of Crohn's disease and ulcerative colitis.[14,16] When taken in conjunction the potential association of a variant of the *IL-12B* gene (part of the p40 subunit that signals via IL-23R), the role of the IL-12/IL-23 pro-inflammatory pathway in the development of Crohn's disease requires urgent exploration.

TREATMENT

Antibodies to tumour necrosis factor

Infliximab is a chimeric antibody (75% human and 25% murine) against TNF-α. It is licensed for moderate-to-severe Crohn's disease not responsive to other therapies. TNF-α is a key mediator of inflammation in Crohn's disease. Infliximab reduces inflammation and may induce mucosal healing. Current UK practice is to give induction therapy (three infusions at 0, 2, and 8 weeks of 5 mg/kg infliximab). Responders may be considered for later therapy, non-responders should not be given further infliximab. Following the Accent 1 trial, response is anticipated in 65% of patients, with remission in 40%.[17] Scheduled maintenance therapy, in that trial, meant the remission was maintained to week 30 in 39% of patients receiving 5 mg/kg infliximab and 45% of those receiving 10 mg/kg infliximab. Steroid-free remission was achieved at 54 weeks in 31% and 37% of patients receiving scheduled 8-weekly infliximab therapy, at 5 mg/kg or 10 mg/kg, respectively. Quality of life measures were significantly improved in those patients who received scheduled therapy. Infusion reactions are rare. New guidance from the UK National Institute for Health and Clinical Excellence (NICE) is expected soon.

For patients with fistulating Crohn's disease, infliximab is also effective. NICE has approved its use, so long as there is active Crohn's disease as well as a fistula. Accent II[18] showed that infliximab reduced fistula drainage and maintained this response; 64% showed response to induction therapy. At 54 weeks, of those who responded and then had maintenance therapy, 36% had complete fistula closure. In a subgroup of 25 women with rectovaginal fistulas, closure was achieved in 61% and 45% of cases at weeks 10 and 14, respectively.

The second anti-TNF monoclonal antibody therapy to be licensed for Crohn's disease was adalimumab. This is a recombinant human IgG_1 monoclonal antibody designed to reduce the risk of antibody formation against the drug. It is given by subcutaneous injection. There have been four large studies of induction therapy with adalimumab in Crohn's disease – CLASSIC-I, CLASSIC-2, CHARM, and GAIN.[19–22]

CLASSIC-I[19] reported the outcome of therapy in 299 patients with moderate-to-severe Crohn's disease who were naïve to biological therapy. Patients were given a two-dose induction regimen and response or remission assessed at week 4. Of patients who received 160 mg then 80 mg dosing, 36% achieved remission while 50% responded with a fall in CDAI of > 100, compared with just 12% and 25% for these end-points in controls. In CLASSIC-2,[20] patients who had responded to therapy in CLASSIC-1 were re-randomised to maintenance with adalimumab or placebo. Overall, amongst responders who entered the CLASSIC-2, the remission rate at week 56 was 79% with adalimumab 40 mg every other week, 83% with 40 mg weekly, and 44% with placebo.

In CHARM,[21] patients with active Crohn's disease were recruited to a study with an open-label induction phase of 80 mg, then 40 mg, adalimumab, followed by randomisation to adalimumab 40 mg every other week or weekly, or placebo. After 56 weeks, remission was found in 36%, 41% and 12% for the three groups. CHARM also looked to peri-anal fistulas: 33% of patients receiving adalimumab achieved remission compared with just 13% who had placebo.

The final study to discuss is the GAIN trial.[22] This studied patients with active Crohn's disease, who had lost response or who were intolerant of infliximab. Induction was the same as CLASSIC-1. Remission, at week 4, was achieved in 21% of adalimumab-treated patients and 7% of controls.

The licensed regimen for adalimumab is 160 mg, followed by 80 mg two weeks later with a maintenance schedule of 40 mg every other week. NICE guidance is awaited.

There has been some concern about safety with anti-TNF antibodies. All patients should be screened for tuberculosis before these drugs are used. Heart failure is also a contra-indication. There have been several cases of fatal hepatosplenic T-cell lymphomas in young men with Crohn's disease treated with azathioprine and infliximab. Consequently, patients should be carefully selected and counselled before anti-TNF agents are used.

Originally, guidelines encouraged the co-prescription of immuno-suppressive agents alongside monoclonal therapies, in order to suppress the formation of antibodies against the monoclonal. Now, there is evidence that scheduled therapy with monoclonal antibodies is not associated with such antibody formation. The early use of 'top-down' therapy has been advocated.[23]

Granulocyte-macrophage colony stimulating factors

A Crohn's disease-like condition occurs in several immunodeficiency states. Treatment with granulocyte colony stimulating factor (G-CSF) and human granulocyte-macrophage colony stimulating factor (GM-CSF) improves such gastrointestinal complications. After promising open-label therapy in Crohn's disease, a large RCT has been performed. Although the study failed to reach its primary end-point, Sargramostim (GM-CSF) therapy was associated with a greater remission rate than placebo (40% versus 19%; $P = 0.01$).[24]

Leukopheresis

The Japanese have led the field of leukopheresis, a technique in which, it is claimed, subsets of white cells are selective removed from the circulation using a filter. In scheduled therapy, open studies have shown promise. For example, in a series of 44 patients with Crohn's disease treated with the Adacolumn, 41% achieved remission and a further 23% had a clinical response.[25] Side effects were few. Sham controlled studies have been performed and the results are expected soon.

Bone marrow and stem cell transplantation

Much evidence points to a genetic predisposition to Crohn's disease. Many of the newly recognised genetic associations are related to the immune response. In several patients with Crohn's disease, bone marrow transplantation has ameliorated the disease. It remains to be determined whether this is a result of the bone marrow or the drugs use. A large European trial is underway to determine the efficacy of bone marrow transplantation.

SUMMARY

These are exciting times in which some parasites may be useful to treat Crohn's disease and some bacteria may cause it. The role of bacteria may be determined by genes which may lead to a loss of intestinal defence or to a failure of killing of intracellular bacteria. Other genetic variants may protect against Crohn's disease. Migrant studies have shown that even if they have a role, genes are not the sole cause of Crohn's disease, then again microbes seem not to be solely responsible either. Regarding therapy, the anti-TNF agents have given renewed hope of long-term remission, albeit to a modest subset of patients. We are not entirely sure of the safest way to administer these drugs, yet. Finally, novel hypothesis and therapies remain under development: a cure for Crohn's disease may yet be found.

ULCERATIVE COLITIS

AETIOLOGY

Genetics

Our understanding of the contribution of genetics to the pathogenesis of inflammatory bowel disease has continued to accumulate with the work of large collaborative groups studying genome-wide associations. Whilst much of this work has centred upon Crohn's disease, pooling of the twin studies data in ulcerative colitis reveals concordance rates of 10% and 3% for monozygotic and dizygotic twins, respectively, suggesting a significant genetic component.[26–28]

A recent genome-wide association study identified a highly significant association between the *IL23R* gene on chromosome 1p31 and both Crohn's disease and ulcerative colitis.[29] The importance of this finding lies in the relationship between IL-12 and IL-23. IL-12 has been used as a model for the study of intestinal inflammation, and blockade of the IL-12 pathway has been shown to resolve intestinal inflammation. However, IL-12 has recently been shown to share a common p40 subunit with IL-23.[30] Therefore, some of the beneficial effects previously thought to be mediated by IL-12 blockade may more accurately represent IL-23 blockade.

IL-23 is thought to mediate effects through triggering the release of other pro-inflammatory cytokines. In addition, it is thought to promote a novel subset of IL-17-producing CD4[+] T-cells (termed Th17 cells) for which a precise role has yet to established, but they appear to have a prominent role as a regulatory cell.

There has been growing interest in the multidrug resistance 1 (MDR-1) gene and its product, P-glycoprotein 170, particularly in the setting of steroid-resistant ulcerative colitis. P-glycoprotein 170 is highly expressed in gut epithelial tissue and may play a role in mucosal protection. It has been shown that there is down-regulation of the MDR-1 gene and P-glycoprotein 170 in colonic inflammation, and it has been proposed that high levels of P-glycoprotein 170 in the colonic epithelium are protective for ulcerative colitis.[31] Supporting this hypothesis, MDR-1a knockout mice develop colonic inflammation when reared in a pathogen-free environment,[32] and a significantly reduced expression of MDR-1 mRNA has been demonstrated in ulcerative colitis but not Crohn's disease.[33] In addition, an association of the MDR-1 C3435T SNP with the development of ulcerative colitis has been demonstrated in a white Scottish population confirming the importance of the role of MDR-1 in disease pathogenesis in ulcerative colitis.[31]

The role of P-glycoprotein in steroid resistance may lie in its ability to transport glucocorticoids and other drugs actively out of cells, thereby reducing effective intracellular concentrations. Through this mechanism, effective delivery of glucocorticoids may be variable depending upon MDR-1 expression in an individual. Polymorphisms in the MDR-1 gene may, therefore, contribute to steroid resistance. The precise relationship of the MDR-1 gene and its product with glucocorticoid resistance remains unclear at present, but it is likely to be complex. This is because other factors may interact with constitutional expression. For example, a study of transcriptional regulation of MDR-1 following cytokine stimulation demonstrated that lymphocyte activation by IL-2 results in P-glycoprotein-mediated multidrug resistance.[34]

There are other recently described gene associations that have been implicated in both the pathogenesis and phenotype of ulcerative colitis including class I and II HLA associations (e.g. HLA DRB1*0103, DRB1*1502, DRB1*0401 and TNF promoter regions).[35] The study of such genetic associations is made more complex because of the influence of ethnicity and host interactions with environmental factors. There remains much more to be done in this area; in the future, gene arrays may identify those patients at greatest risk of colectomy, and enable bespoke treatment for an individual based upon their genetic profile.

Environment

In addition to the established environmental factors such as smoking and appendectomy upon the incidence of ulcerative colitis, evidence supporting the 'hygiene hypothesis' has grown.[36] This hypothesis proposed that raising children in an increasingly hygienic environment may negatively affect immune development, predisposing them to developing diseases with an autoimmune component. This was originally proposed in the context of asthma and atopy, but has since been implicated in the pathogenesis of many autoimmune diseases including both Crohn's disease and ulcerative colitis. Recent studies of helminth infection seem to support this hypothesis.

Helminth infections are rare in areas with a higher incidence of inflammatory bowel disease. Helminths stimulate a strong gut mucosal Th2 pattern of cytokine production, which may provide conditioning of the immune system to unrelated parasitic, bacterial or viral infections.[37] In the absence of this conditioning, there may be an aberrant immune response to pathogens. A recent study of the helminth *T. suis* in active ulcerative colitis has shown benefit over placebo.[38] The mechanism by which this exerts an effect in the adult (mature) immune system is not clear, but it adds weight to the possible conditioning effects of environmental agents.

Therefore, it is likely that a combination of differing genetic susceptibilities and a multitude of possible antigenic triggers are likely to account for the heterogeneity in both the disease phenotype and the response of individuals to treatment.

Clostridium difficile and ulcerative colitis

C. difficile associated diarrhoea is the most common nosocomial infection in the UK and represents a major challenge to the healthcare community.

Increasingly, patients with ulcerative colitis are becoming exposed to *C. difficile* with alarming results. One study has demonstrated that patients with *C. difficile* and inflammatory bowel disease have a four times greater mortality than patients admitted to hospital for inflammatory bowel disease alone or *C. difficile* alone, and median hospital stay is 3 days longer. In patients with *C. difficile* diarrhoea, significantly higher mortality and surgery rates were found in patients with ulcerative colitis compared with Crohn's disease.[39]

Prior treatment with antibiotics is not always necessary for developing *C. difficile* associated diarrhoea in ulcerative colitis, and the use of an immunosuppressant may be enough for this organism to colonise the gut. Careful exclusion of *C. difficile* is an important part of assessment of a flare of colitis. Analysis of volatile organic compounds from stool may be the future for rapid diagnosis of *C. difficile* and may eventually replace current microbiological techniques.[40]

MEDICAL TREATMENTS

5-Aminosalicylates

5-Aminosalicylates (5-ASAs) remain the mainstay of treatment for mild-to-moderate ulcerative colitis with proven benefit in the induction and maintenance of remission. They also bring the added benefits of reducing the risk of developing colorectal cancer. Despite these benefits, together with a good safety profile, non-adherence approaches 60% in some studies.[41] Factors associated with non-adherence include multiple concomitant medications, male gender, and single status.

In an attempt to increase adherence, once daily dosing of 5-ASAs has emerged. A novel release mechanism known as Multi Matrix System (MMX) has been developed which uses lipophilic and hydrophilic excipients enclosed within a pH-dependent film coating. Once daily dosing with this formulation of mesalazine has been explored in two Phase III studies. Combined analysis of these studies showed that, in mild-to-moderate ulcerative colitis, once daily treatment with MMX mesalazine at 2.4 g/day or 4.8 g/day demonstrated improvement in 58.1% and 62.1% (versus 32.7% for placebo), and remission in 37.2% and 35.1% (versus 17.5% for placebo), respectively.[42] Maintenance of remission with 2.4 g once daily MMX mesalazine was comparable to that achieved with the same dose given in divided doses (64.4% versus 68.5%, respectively).[43]

The PODIUM study approached the same problem in a slightly different manner. An existing mesalazine preparation (Pentasa granules) was used; the study looked at the maintenance of remission in patients with mild-to-moderate ulcerative colitis who had had a relapse within the last year. Mesalazine granules (2 g) were given to patients with ulcerative colitis either as a single daily dose or in two divided doses. Of the 362 patients studied, 73.8% of once-daily patients were in clinical and endoscopic remission compared with 63.6% in the twice-daily group ($P = 0.024$).[44]

Another approach has been to use higher doses of mesalazine such as in the ASCEND I and II trials,[45] and also to combine oral and rectal treatments. In the PINCE study,[46] 127 patients with extensive active ulcerative colitis received 4 g/day (twice-daily dosing) oral mesalazine for 8 weeks. During the initial 4 weeks, they additionally received an enema at bed-time containing 1 g of mesalazine or placebo. Remission was obtained in 64% of the mesalazine enema group and in 43% of the placebo enema group at 8 weeks ($P = 0.03$). This suggests that combined treatment is effective even in extensive ulcerative colitis.

Corticosteroids

Corticosteroids remain a major part of treatment but there are limitations to their use. In addition to their side-effect profile, they are not effective for maintenance of remission, and up to 30% of individuals demonstrate steroid resistance. Our understanding of steroid resistance is increasing. Our group have demonstrated the presence of a subgroup of activated CD4+ T-cells that continue to proliferate despite exposure to high-dose steroids. These CD4+CD25int cells are highly steroid resistant and may represent a target for future treatments in patients refractory to steroids. There is also interest in modifying steroid resistance with the use of IL-2 receptor antagonists.[47] A humanised anti-CD25 monoclonal antibody, daclizumab, was promising in a pilot study, but did not show efficacy in a randomised, placebo-controlled phase II trial.[48] Basiliximab, a chimeric monoclonal antibody directed against the IL-2 receptor, has been promising as a steroid sensitiser in an open-label study.[47] Results from a Phase IIb, randomised, controlled trial of basiliximab in moderate steroid refractory ulcerative colitis are awaited.

Treatment with biological agents

Infliximab

The ACT1 and ACT2 trials[49] demonstrated that infliximab is effective in achieving clinical response and remission for patients with moderately active ulcerative colitis failing alternative treatments. However, while over two-thirds of patients demonstrated a clinical response, only about one-third achieved the more important end-point of remission. In view of this, the use of infliximab in this group of patients has recently been rejected in the UK by NICE as it is not felt to be cost-effective.

However, infliximab is being increasingly used for the treatment of patients with severe ulcerative colitis who are failing other treatments. In a study of 45 patients with moderate-to-severe ulcerative colitis unresponsive to steroids, those receiving infliximab had a lower colectomy rate at 3 months compared to those receiving placebo.[50] However, for those patients with more severe disease there was no significant benefit. A retrospective study in Scottish patients with severe ulcerative colitis demonstrated a 66% response rate to infliximab, but a poor response in those with hypo-albuminaemia (a surrogate marker for severity of disease). There was one death and one systemic fungaemia in this series.

Therefore, infliximab is a useful addition to the armamentarium in ulcerative colitis, but may be less effective in those with very severe disease, and patients must be counselled carefully regarding potential side effects before its use.

Visilizumab

Visilizumab is a humanised monoclonal antibody directed against CD3. An uncontrolled pilot study suggested efficacy in ulcerative colitis, but a Phase III trial was stopped early because interim analysis showed a lack of efficacy and concerns about potential adverse events.

Growth factors

A number of studies have looked at the possibility of using growth factors to achieve mucosal repair. Of these, the most impressive data were seen for epidermal growth factor enemas used in combination with oral mesalazine.[51] The treatment group achieved an impressive 83% remission rate, but there remain concerns in using such agents because of the theoretical risk of dysplasia.

Probiotics

Probiotics are not classed as drugs and are a highly acceptable treatment to patients. Evidence for their efficacy in ulcerative colitis is accumulating. Their safety profile is generally very good, but they do have the potential to cause harm and are contra-indicated in the immunocompromised. Probiotics are a heterogeneous group of bacteria, each with differing properties; therefore, results from one preparation cannot be extrapolated to others. Those strains or preparations with evidence for an effect in ulcerative colitis are discussed below.

1. *E. coli* strain Nissle 1917 – Three RCTs have looked at this probiotic for maintenance of remission in ulcerative colitis.[52–54] These demonstrated

equivalence to 5-ASA treatment, although relapse rates were high in both 5-ASA and *E. coli* groups. The 2008 guidelines from the European Crohn's and Colitis Organisation (ECCO) on the management of ulcerative colitis suggest that *E. coli* Nissle should be considered as an alternative to 5-ASA as a maintenance treatment in ulcerative colitis.

2. VSL#3 – This has shown efficacy in pouchitis. In one study, 40 patients undergoing ileo-anal pouch anastomosis were randomised to treatment with VSL#3 or placebo in order to prevent pouchitis. At 12 months, only 10% of the VSL#3 group had had an episode of acute pouchitis compared to 40% in the placebo group.[55] In a further study of patients with chronic relapsing pouchitis randomised to either maintenance VSL#3 or placebo, relapse rates were 15% and 100%, respectively.[56] There have been several open-label studies suggesting efficacy of VSL#3 in both active ulcerative colitis and in the maintenance of remission of ulcerative colitis, but only one RCT. A study of balsalazide plus VSL#3 was superior to balsalazide alone or mesalazine alone in obtaining remission in mild-to-moderate active ulcerative colitis. The balsalazide/VSL#3 combination led to remission more quickly than balsalazide alone or mesalazine (4, 7.5, and 13 days, respectively) and also achieved greater rates of remission 80% versus 77% and 53.3%, respectively.[57]

With improvements in the composition and delivery of probiotics, in addition to the support of patients for such treatments, it is likely that we will see the use of probiotics increase.

SUMMARY

Our growing knowledge of the genetics of ulcerative colitis and some of the relevant environmental factors are enabling the development of new treatments. The latest biological treatments promise improvements in patient outcomes, although these powerful new drugs have potential side effects and should be used with care. Safer treatments are also being developed in the form of probiotics. These are highly acceptable to patients and will be used more commonly in the future. Finally, in addition to developing new treatments, we are learning how to use existing treatments, such as the 5-ASAs, more effectively.

Key points for clinical practice

Crohn's disease

- Certain bacteria, such as adherent invasive E. coli, are increasingly recognised as a factor in the pathogenesis of Crohn's disease.

- Individuals with mutations in the genes that deal with intracellular pathogens, such as those associated with autophagy, may be at risk of developing Crohn's disease.

- Modifying the immune response with the use of intestinal worms has shown promise in early clinical trials.   *(continued)*

Key points for clinical practice *(continued)*

- Concerns over the safety of anti-TNF-α treatments means that great care should be taken in selecting and counselling patients who may benefit from these treatments.

- Early 'top-down' treatment with anti-TNF-α preparations is advocated by some gastroenterologists but this approach is not currently licensed in the UK.

Ulcerative colitis

- Gene-wide association studies have identified a significant association of the IL-23R gene with both ulcerative colitis and Crohn's disease.

- The multidrug resistance 1 (MDR-1) gene and its product P-glycoprotein appear to be implicated in steroid resistance.

- The incidence of Clostridium difficile associated diarrhoea is increasing in patients with inflammatory bowel disease and has a poor outcome compared to the general population.

- 5-Aminosalicylate treatment is now available as once daily dosing. Higher doses and a combination of oral plus concurrent rectal treatments may be more effective.

- There is an increasing role for probiotics in the treatment of ulcerative colitis and pouchitis.

References

1. Weinstock JV. Helminths and mucosal immune modulation. *Ann NY Acad Sci* 2006; **1072**: 356–364.
2. Feller M, Huwiler K, Stephan R *et al*. *Mycobacterium avium* subspecies paratuberculosis and Crohn's disease: a systematic review and meta-analysis. *Lancet Infect Dis* 2007; **7**: 607–613.
3. Borgaonkar MR, MacIntosh DG, Fardy JM. A meta-analysis of antimycobacterial therapy for Crohn's disease. *Am J Gastroenterol* 2000; **95**: 725–729.
4. Selby W, Pavli P, Crotty B *et al*. Two-year combination antibiotic therapy with clarithromycin, rifabutin, and clofazimine for Crohn's disease. *Gastroenterology* 2007; **132**: 2313–2319.
5. Harper PH, Lee ECG, Kettlewell MGW, Bennett MK, Jewell DP. Role of faecal stream in the maintenance of Crohn's colitis. *Gut* 1985; **26**: 279–284.
6. D'Haens GR, Geboes K, Peeter M, Baert F, Penninckx F, Rutgeerts P. Early lesions of recurrent Crohn's disease caused by infusion of intestinal contents in excluded ileum. *Gastroenterology* 1998; **114**: 262–267.
7. Darfeuille-Michaud A, Neut C, Barnich N *et al*. Presence of adherent *Escherichia coli* strains in ileal mucosa of patients with Crohn's disease. *Gastroenterology* 1998; **115**: 1405–1413.
8. Barnich N, Dafeuille-Michaud A. Adherent-invasive *Escherichia coli* and Crohn's disease. *Curr Opin Gastroenterol* 2007; **23**: 16–20.
9. Glasser AL, Bringer MA, Claret L, Dafeuille-Michaud A. Adherent-invasive *Escherichia coli* strains from patients with Crohn's disease survive and replicate within macrophages without inducing host cell death. *Infect Immun* 2001; **69**: 5529–5537.
10. Ogura Y, Bonen DK, Inohara N *et al*. A frameshift mutation in *NOD2* associated with susceptibility to Crohn's disease. *Nature* 2001; **411**: 603–606.
11. Hugot JP, Chamaillard M, Zouali H *et al*. Association of *NOD2* leucine-rich repeat variants with susceptibility to Crohn's disease. *Nature* 2001; **411**: 599–603.
12. Economou M, Trikalinos TA, Loizou KT *et al*. Differential effects of *NOD2* variants on Crohn's

disease risk and phenotype in diverse populations: a meta-analysis. *Am J Gastroenterol* 2004; **99**: 2393–2404.

13. Kugathasan S, Collins N, Maresso K et al. *CARD15* gene mutations and risk for early surgery in pediatric-onset Crohn's disease. *Clin Gastroenterol Hepatol* 2004; **2**: 1003–1009.

14. Cho J. Inflammatory bowel disease: genetic and epidemiologic considerations. *World J Gastroenterol* 2008; **21**: 338–347.

15. Barreau F, Meiner U, Chareyre F et al. Card15/NOD2 is required for Peyer's patches homeostatic in mice. *PLoS ONE* 2007; **2**: e523.

16. Massey D, Parkes M. Common pathways in Crohn's disease and other inflammatory diseases revealed by genomics. *Gut* 2007; **56**: 1489–1492.

17. Hanauer SB, Feagan BG, Lichtenstein GR et al. Maintenance infliximab for Crohn's disease: The ACCENT I randomised trial. *Lancet* 2002; **359**: 1541–1549.

18. Sands BE, Anderson FH, Bernstein CN et al. Infliximab maintenance therapy for fistulizing Crohn's disease. *N Engl J Med* 2004; **350**: 876–885.

19. Hanauer SB, Sandborn WJ, Rutgeerts P et al. Human anti-tumor necrosis factor monoclonal antibody (adalimumab) in Crohn's disease: the CLASSIC-I trial. *Gastroenterology* 2006; **130**: 323–333.

20. Sandborn WJ, Hanauer SB, Rutgeerts P et al. Adalimumab for maintenance treatment of Crohn's disease: results of the CLASSIC II trial. *Gut* 2007; **56**: 1232–1239.

21. Colombel JF, Sandborn WJ, Rutgeerts P et al. Adalimumab for maintenance of clinical response and remission in patients with Crohn's disease: the CHARM trial. *Gastroenterology* 2007; **132**: 52–56.

22. Sandborn WJ, Rutgeerts P, Enns R et al. Adalimumab induction therapy for Crohn disease previously treated with infliximab. A randomized trial. *Ann Intern Med* 2007; **146**: 829–838.

23. D'Haens G, Baert F, van Assche G et al. Early combined immunosuppression or conventional management in patients with newly diagnosed Crohn's disease: an open randomised trial. *Lancet* 2008; **371**: 660–667.

24. Korzenik JR, Dieckgraefe BK, Valentine JF, Hausman DF, Gilbert MJ. Sargramostim for active Crohn's disease. *N Engl J Med* 2005; **352**: 2193–2201.

25. Ljung T, Thomsen OO, Vatn M et al. Granulocyte, monocyte/macrophage apheresis for inflammatory bowel disease: the first 100 patients treated in Scandinavia. *Scand J Gastroenterol* 2007; **42**: 221–227.

26. Subhani J, Montgomery S, Pounder RE, Wakefield A. Concordance rates of twins and siblings in inflammatory bowel disease [Abstract]. *Gut* 1998; **42**: A40.

27. Tysk C, Lindberg E, Jarnerot G, Floderus-Myrhed B. Ulcerative colitis and Crohn's disease in an unselected population of monozygotic and dizygotic twins. A study of heritability and the influence of smoking. *Gut* 1988; **29**: 990–996.

28. Orholm M, Binder M, Sørensen T, Rasmussen L, Kyvik K. Concordance of inflammatory bowel disease among Danish twins: results of a nationwide study. *Scand J Gastroenterol* 2000; **35**: 1075–1081.

29. Duerr RH, Taylor KD, Brant SR et al. A genome-wide association study identifies IL23R as an inflammatory bowel disease gene. *Science* 2006; **314**: 1461–1463.

30. Oppmann B, Lesley R, Blom B et al. Novel p19 protein engages IL-12p40 to form a cytokine, IL-23, with biological activities similar as well as distinct from IL-12. *Immunity* 2000; **13**: 715–725.

31. Ho G, Nimmo E, Tenesa A et al. Allellic variations of the multidrug resistance gene determine susceptibility and disease behaviour in ulcerative colitis. *Gastroenterology* 2005; **128**: 288–296.

32. Panwala CM, Jones JC, Viney JL. A novel model of inflammatory bowel disease: mice deficient for the multiple drug resistance gene, *mdr1a*, spontaneously develop colitis. *J Immunol* 1998; **161**: 5733–5744.

33. Langmann T, Moehle C, Mauerer R et al. Loss of detoxification in inflammatory bowel disease: dysregulation of pregnane X receptor target genes. *Gastroenterology* 2004; **127**: 26–40.

34. Tsujimura S, Saito K, Nakayamada S et al. Transcriptional regulation of multidrug resistance-1 gene by interleukin-2 in lymphocytes. *Genes Cells* 2004; **9**: 1265–1273.

35. Ahmad T, Armuzzi A, Neville M et al. The contribution of human leukocyte antigen complex genes to disease phenotype in ulcerative colitis. *Tissue Antigens* 2003; **62**: 527–535.

36. Strachan D. Hay fever, hygiene, and household size. *BMJ* 1989; **299**: 1259–1260.

37. Weinstock JV, Summers R, Elliott DE. Helminths and harmony. *Gut* 2004; **53**: 7–9.

38. Summers RW, Elliott DE, Urban JF, Thompson RA, Weinstock JV. *Trichuris suis* therapy for

active ulcerative colitis: a randomized controlled trial. *Gastroenterology* 2005; **128**: 825–832.

39. Ananthakrishnan AN, McGinley EL, Binion DG. Excess hospitalisation burden associated with *Clostridium difficile* in patients with inflammatory bowel disease. *Gut* 2008; **57**: 205–210.

40. Garner CE, Smith S, de Lacy Costello B *et al.* Volatile organic compounds from feces and their potential for diagnosis of gastrointestinal disease. *FASEB J* 2007; **21**: 1675–1688.

41. Kane S, Cohen R, Aikens J, Hanauer SB. Prevalence of nonadherence with maintenance mesalamine in quiescent ulcerative colitis. *Am J Gastroenterol* 2001; **96**: 2929–2933.

42. Sandborn WJ, Kamm MA, Lichtenstein GR, Lyne A, Butler T, Joseph R. MMX Multi Matrix System mesalazine for the induction of remission in patients with mild-to-moderate ulcerative colitis: a combined analysis of two randomized, double-blind, placebo-controlled trials. *Aliment Pharmacol Ther* 2008; **26**: 205–215.

43. Kamm MA, Lichtenstein GR, Sandborn WJ *et al.* Randomised trial of once- or twice-daily MMX mesalazine for maintenance of remission in ulcerative colitis. *Gut* 2008; **57**: 893–902.

44. Dignass A, Vermiere S, Adamek H *et al.* Improved remission rates from once versus twice daily mesalazine (Pentasa) granules for the maintenance of remission in ulcerative colitis: results from a multinational randomised controlled trial [Abstract]. *Endoscopy* 2007; **37**: A46–A47.

45. Hanauer SB, Sandborn WJ, Kornbluth A *et al.* Delayed-release oral mesalamine at 4.8 g/day (800 mg tablet) for the treatment of moderately active ulcerative colitis: The ASCEND II Trial. *Am J Gastroenterol* 2005; **100**: 2478–2485.

46. Marteau P, Probert CS, Lindgren S *et al.* Combined oral and enema treatment with Pentasa (mesalazine) is superior to oral therapy alone in patients with extensive mild/moderate active ulcerative colitis: a randomised, double blind, placebo controlled study. *Gut* 2005; **54**: 960–965.

47. Creed TJ, Probert CSJ, Norman MN *et al.* Basiliximab for the treatment of steroid-resistant ulcerative colitis: further experience in moderate and severe disease. *Aliment Pharmacol Ther* 2006; **23**: 1435–1442.

48. Van Assche G, Sandborn WJ, Feagan BG *et al.* Daclizumab, a humanized monoclonal antibody to the interleukin-2 receptor (CD25), for the treatment of moderately to severely active ulcerative colitis: a randomised, double-blind, placebo-controlled, dose-ranging trial. *Gut* 2006; **55**: 1568–1574.

49. Rutgeerts P, Sandborn WJ, Feagan BG *et al.* Infliximab for induction and maintenance therapy for ulcerative colitis. *N Engl J Med* 2005; **353**: 2462–2476.

50. Jarnerot G, Hertervig E, Friis-Liby I *et al.* Infliximab as rescue therapy in severe to moderately severe ulcerative colitis: a randomized, placebo-controlled study. *Gastroenterology* 2005; **128**: 1805–1811.

51. Sinha A, Nightingale JMD, West KP, Berlanga-Acosta J, Playford RJ. Epidermal growth factor enemas with oral mesalamine for mild-to-moderate left-sided ulcerative colitis or proctitis. *N Engl J Med* 2003; **349**: 350–357.

52. Rembacken B, Snelling A, Hawkey P, Chalmers D, Axon A. Non-pathogenic *Escherichia coli* versus mesalazine for the treatment of ulcerative colitis: a randomised trial. *Lancet* 1999; **354**: 635–639.

53. Kruis W, Schutz E, Frick P, Fixa B, Judmaier G, Stolte M. Double-blind comparison of an oral *Escherichia coli* preparation and mesalazine in maintaining remission of ulcerative colitis. *Aliment Pharmacol Ther* 1997; **11**: 853–858.

54. Kruis W, Fric P, Pokrotnieks J *et al.* Maintaining remission of ulcerative colitis with the probiotic *Escherichia coli* Nissle 1917 is as effective as with standard mesalazine. *Gut* 2004; **53**: 1617–1623.

55. Gionchetti P, Rizzello F, Helwig U *et al.* Prophylaxis of pouchitis onset with probiotic therapy: a double-blind, placebo-controlled trial. *Gastroenterology* 2003; **124**: 1202–1209.

56. Gionchetti P, Rizzello F, Venturi A *et al.* Oral bacteriotherapy as maintenance treatment in patients with chronic pouchitis: a double-blind, placebo-controlled trial. *Gastroenterology* 2000; **119**: 305–309.

57. Tursi A, Brandimarte G, Giorgetti G, Forti G, Modeo M, Gigliobianco A. Low-dose balsalazide plus a high-potency probiotic preparation is more effective than balsalazide alone or mesalazine in the treatment of acute mild-to-moderate ulcerative colitis. *Med Sci Monitor* 2004; **10**: 126–131.

Rachel Bradley

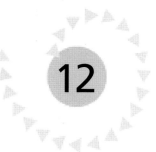

12

Disordered defaecation in the elderly

Disordered defaecation in the elderly is common and has important physical, psychosocial and financial consequences. It is difficult to determine the exact prevalence of constipation, due to reliance on self-reporting in many studies. However, it is estimated that 20% of community-dwelling elderly suffer with symptoms of constipation.[1,2] This rises to half of elderly patients admitted to hospital and two-thirds in nursing homes.[3] The reluctance to volunteer the symptom of faecal incontinence[4] means that its prevalence is even harder to determine. It is thought to be around 1% of adults in the community rising to 10% of patients in residential homes.[5,6] Disordered defaecation has a significant impact on quality of life.[4,7] Many elderly are obsessed with regular bowel habits due to strict toileting regimens in childhood. Disordered defaecation can cause depression and social isolation. Faecal incontinence, in particular, causes significant stress amongst carers and relatives, and may be the trigger for nursing home placement. Bowel care is also expensive in terms of district nurse and general practitioner time, containment products and laxative use (over £46 million per year in England[1,3]). Despite the prevalence of functional bowel problems in the elderly, there remains a lack of good evidence-based research on this subject. Many studies have been small, ill-defined, relied on self-reporting of symptoms and have had unclear outcome measures.[3] The aim of this chapter is to provide an overview of disordered defaecation in the elderly and practical advice for clinicians.

NORMAL DEFAECATION PHYSIOLOGY

In a normal gastrointestinal tract, stool passes through the ileocaecal valve in liquid form. The colon then absorbs water (and salts) as it is passed along by

Rachel Bradley MB ChB MRCP MSc
Consultant Physician & Geriatrician at University Hospitals Bristol, Upper Maudlin Street, Bristol BS2 8HW; and St Martins Continence Promotion Unit, Bath and Bristol General Hospital, UK
E-mail: rachel.bradley@UHBristol.nhs.uk

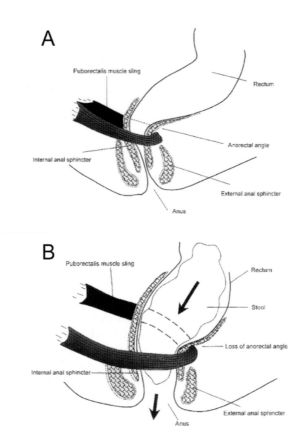

Fig. 1 The lateral view of the anal sphincter mechanism. (A) Continence is maintained by the tone in the puborectalis muscle creating an angle at the anorectal junction, by pulling the bowel forward. (B) During defaecation, the puborectalis muscle and external anal sphincter relaxes, opening up the anorectal angle. (Reproduced with permission from Getliffe and Dolman. *Promoting Continence*, 3rd Edn, p214 © 2007 Bailliere Tindall.)

persistalsis to arrive in a solid form at the rectum. Normal transit time is less than 3 days. The rectum acts as a reservoir for stool until such time that the 'call-to-stool' is made. There are two sphincters in the anus supplied by the pudendal nerve and hypogastric (autonomic) nerves, formed from the 2nd, 3rd and 4th sacral nerves. The internal anal sphincter consists of a ring of involuntary muscle that is the continuation of the circular rectal muscle coat and maintains a resting pressure. The external sphincter, consists of a ring of voluntary muscle fibres, and is attached to the coccyx posteriorly and perineal body anteriorly. Faecal continence is maintained by the puborectalis muscle (a sling of voluntary muscle which is the inner component of levator ani), which creates a 60—105° angle between the anal canal and the rectum by pulling the anorectal junction forward (Fig. 1A). In addition, the external sphincter can act to prevent leakage of flatus and diarrhoea.

When stool distends into the rectum, the sacral reflex arc is activated. This gives the sensation 'call-to-stool'. The sensory fibres in the rectum are able to distinguish between gas, liquid or solid. If defaecation is appropriate, the puborectalis and external sphincter relax, the anorectal angle opens up creating a funnel shape in the rectum allowing easy passage of stool (Fig. 1B). Strong waves of peristalsis, produced by the internal sphincter and upper part of the levator ani, also push the stool through the anal canal. This process is aided by raising the intra-abdominal pressure. If defaecation is deemed inappropriate, voluntary contraction of the external anal sphincter and puborectalis can occur, the stool is expelled back up into the rectum, and the sensation to defaecate dies down. There are many factors that affect the normal bowel function such as diet, exercise, and the central, mesenteric and autonomic nervous systems. A useful working definition of normal function is bowel opening 3 times a week up to 3 times a day, with the need to strain on less than 25% of occasions.[8]

THE AGEING BOWEL

There are age-related changes that occur in the bowel, such as reduction in the number of mesenteric neurones.[9] However, this has not been shown to reduce stool frequency in healthy elderly.[10,11] Common symptoms reported are straining and passing hard stool, implying more evacuation difficulties.[2] Women are more susceptible to constipation than men.[10] Elderly people with chronic disease may have slower gut transit times of 4–9 days and amongst immobile residents of nursing homes this can be up to 3 weeks.[12] This will increase the risk of constipation and overflow faecal incontinence (see below). The strength of the external sphincter decreases with age.[3] This is most noticeable in elderly women who have sustained an obstetric injury or strain chronically. The internal sphincter may thicken, but the mechanism appears unaffected by age. It may be affected by conditions such as diabetes mellitus, spinal cord injury or rectal prolapse. There is also a reduction in rectal sensation.[3]

CAUSES OF BOWEL DYSFUNCTION IN THE ELDERLY

The main causes of, and contributing factors for, constipation and faecal incontinence are listed in Tables 1–3.

Co-morbidities common in the elderly, such as arthritis and heart failure, compound the age-related changes in bowel function, resulting in functional problems. An unstable gait or reduced exercise tolerance may make it harder to reach the toilet in time (especially with faecal urgency) and worsen anxiety. Poor dexterity can impair the ability to undress and attend to personal hygiene. Immobility is associated with constipation and faecal incontinence in elderly living at home[2] and in care homes, where many people depend on carers for toileting. Immobility also suppresses the gastrocolic reflex, weakens abdominal and pelvic muscles. Depression is associated with constipation[2] and anxiety about faecal incontinence can lead to social isolation.

Unconscious patients will lose voluntary control of their bowels leading to faecal incontinence. This is the case for early severe stroke. However, less severe, but disabling, strokes may cause constipation exacerbated by reduced mobility. Many patients with advanced dementia have disordered defaecation, in particular faecal incontinence but also constipation.[5] The causes are multifactorial. Cognitive impairment means that they are less aware of the 'call-to-stool' and rectal contractions may be uninhibited. Confusion about the environment and communication difficulties may lead to defaecating in inappropriate places, and behavioural problems can cause faecal smearing and coprophagia.

CONSTIPATION

Diagnostic criteria for functional constipation have been developed.[8] Symptoms should have persisted for at least 3 of at least the last 12 months. Loose stools (without the use of laxatives) should not be present and there must be insufficient criteria to make a diagnosis of irritable bowel syndrome. Symptoms must include two of the following:

1. Straining in more than 1 in 4 defaecations.

2. Lumpy or hard stools in more than 1 in 4 defaecations.

3. Sensation of incomplete evacuation in more than 1 in 4 defaecations.

4. Sensation of anorectal obstruction/blockade in more than 1 in 4 defaecations.

5. Manual manoeuvres to facilitate more than 1 in 4 defaecations (*e.g.* digital evacuation, support of the pelvic floor).

6. Less than 3 defaecations per week.

Constipation may be categorised as either primary or secondary to a variety of illnesses, medications and other predisposing factors (see Tables 1 and 2). Primary constipation (sometimes called 'idiopathic') can be further sub-divided

Table 1 Contributing factors and causes of faecal incontinence and constipation in the elderly

Functional disability due to age-related co-morbidities and environment (common)
Immobility and frailty causing weak abdominal and pelvic muscles
Psychological disorders such as depression and anxiety
Behavioural • Lack of privacy and dignity • Ignoring the 'call-to-stool' • Learning disabilities
Dietary factors such as irregular meals, fibre content and fluids
Irritable bowel syndrome
Colorectal disease • Diverticulosis • Carcinoma
Chronic neurological conditions • Dementia (and frontal lobe injury) • Stroke and cerebrovascular disease • Parkinson's disease (primarily constipation) • Spinal cord disease such as cauda equina syndrome, disc prolapse, spina bifida • Multiple sclerosis

Table 2 Contributing factors and causes of constipation in the elderly

Normal colonic transit (common)

Slow colonic transit
- Megacolon/rectum
- Hirshsprung's syndrome (rare)

Anorectal disorders
- Rectal prolapse
- Rectocoele
- Post surgical abnormalities
- Anal fissures and haemorrhoids

Metabolic disorders
- Diabetes mellitus (causing diabetic autonomic neuropathy)
- Chronic kidney disease
- Hypothyroidism
- Hyperparathyroidism
- Addison's disease
- Electrolyte disturbances: hypercalcaemia, hypokalaemia and hypermagnesaemia

Polypharmacy and drug side effects, in particular:
- Anticholinergic agents: tricyclic antidepressants, antipsychotics, oxybutinin
- Analgesics: opiates, tramadol, codeine phosphate
- Non-steroidal anti-inflammatory drugs
- Diuretics: furosemide
- Iron and calcium supplements
- Calcium-channel blockers: verapamil
- Aluminium-containing antacids
- Anti-parkinsonian drugs
- Anti-histamines

into normal or slow colonic transit and defaecation disorders. There is often overlap of symptoms.[13]

Normal colonic transit constipation is the most common subtype. The stool frequency may be in the normal range, but patients complain of constipation, bloating, and pain (which differs from irritable bowel syndrome). Slow colonic transit constipation is more common in frail elderly and is characterised by a slow mouth to anus intestinal transit time.[13] Some of these patients develop a megacolon or megarectum, which is similar to Hirshsprung's disease. This is a very rare condition (usually present from birth) where there is an abnormality of the intramural plexus, colonic dilatation and failure of internal sphincter relaxation.

Disordered defaecation is particularly common in elderly women as a result of child-birth trauma and spinal cord disease. Pelvic floor dyssynergia may be present (also called 'anismus' or outlet obstruction). This is where poor co-ordination causes inappropriate contraction of the puborectalis muscle and failure of relaxation of the external sphincter, leading to delayed defaecation. The pathogenesis is often multifactorial and poorly understood. Rectal dyschezia may occur in the very elderly. This is the combination of reduced rectal tone, increased compliance and impaired sensation. Therefore, the 'call-to-stool' is not initiated until a greater degree of rectal distension has occurred,[3,13] which may result in recurrent impaction.

Table 3 Contributing factors and causes of faecal incontinence in the elderly

Constipation causing faecal loading with overflow (common)

Obstetric injury (pudendal nerve and sphincter damage)

Inflammatory bowel disease such as ulcerative colitis and Crohn's disease

Ischaemic colitis

Infective and antibiotic associated diarrhoea: *C. difficile*

Malabsorpion: coeliac disease

Lactose intolerance

Anorectal disease (anal sphincter damage)
- Third degree haemorrhoids
- Post surgical
- Rectal prolapse

Metabolic disorders
- Diabetes mellitus (autonomic neuropathy)
- Hyperthyroidism

Drug side effects, in particular:
- Excessive laxative use
- Antibiotics
- Gastrointestinal medications: antacids, misoprostol
- Cardiovascular medications: ace inhibitors, β-blockers, nifedipine, digoxin
- Others: bisphosphonates, strontium, colchicines, levodopa, carbamazepine, SSRIs

Constipation may result in faecal loading or impaction in the rectum and or colon. The term impaction is often used to describe hard stool, but this can occur with soft stool, especially if osmotic or bulk laxatives are being used. Faecal incontinence due to impaction with overflow of more proximal loose stool is very common.

Patients with Parkinson's disease are prone to slow transit constipation and disordered defaecating, because of the disease process which affects the enteric nervous system,[14] reduced mobility and side-effects of anti-parkinsonian medications. A rectocoele is the protrusion of anterior rectal and posterior vaginal wall into the vagina, whereas a rectal prolapse is the descent of the rectum. These both cause evacuation disorders, often accompanied with faecal incontinence.

FAECAL INCONTINENCE

Faecal incontinence is defined as the involuntary loss of stool. This can be loose or formed stool. The causes of chronic faecal incontinence are multifactorial (as listed in Tables 1 and 3). By far the commonest is constipation causing faecal impaction and overflow ('spurious diarrhoea'). In women, the post-menopausal pelvic muscle weakness may be complicated by child-birth trauma and pudendal nerve damage. Risk factors for faecal incontinence include prolonged second stage labour, forceps delivery, large babies over 4 kg and third degree tears.[15] This often presents in older age. Co-morbidities, such as diabetes mellitus and spinal cord disease may cause weakness of the internal sphincter due to neuropathies. Anorectal cancer may cause local damage to sphincter mechanisms.

Any increase in colonic motility (or shortened transit time) will result in less water being absorbed in the colon producing a loose stool or diarrhoea. This may overwhelm even a normal functioning external sphincter causing faecal incontinence. This is often the case in acute infective diarrhoea, such as *Clostridium difficile*, which is a particular problem amongst the elderly in hospitals and institutions. It is important to remember that faecal incontinence due to diarrhoea may be the presenting symptom of inflammatory bowel disease. Timed attacks of explosive diarrhoea may be due to diabetic autonomic dysfunction, especially at night. Malabsorption or lactose intolerance can cause loose stool and may be mistaken for faecal incontinence.

IRRITABLE BOWEL SYNDROME

Irritable bowel syndrome (IBS) is a group of functional disorders where abdominal pain or discomfort is associated with defaecation or a change in bowel habit. It may have symptoms that are constipation (IBS-C) or diarrhoea (IBS-D) predominant. It is, therefore, important to distinguish irritable bowel syndrome from chronic constipation and faecal incontinence, both for research and management purposes. This led to the development of criteria in 1992, which were updated in 2006 (ROME III).[8,16,17]

Symptoms must have occurred for at least 3 days per month and persisted for at least 3 of the last 6 months. The recurrent abdominal pain or discomfort should be associated with two of the following: (i) improvement with defaecation; and/or (ii) onset associated with a change in frequency of stool; and/or (iii) onset associated with a change in form (appearance) of stool.

Other general supportive symptoms of irritable bowel syndrome include feeling of incomplete bowel movement, passing mucus (white material) during a bowel movement and abdominal fullness, bloating or swelling. However, these symptoms can overlap with constipation and are not diagnostic of irritable bowel syndrome.

ASSESSMENT OF SYMPTOMS

History
When assessing bowel dysfunction in older people, a detailed history is required that includes the duration of symptoms, severity, associated pain, straining, anismus, prolapse, passive soiling, or requirement for digital stimulation. Many elderly people with chronic constipation lose rectal sensation and can no longer distinguish between wind and solid stool. Insensible loss of formed stool may be associated with external sphincter weakness or damage. Straining correlates well with colonic faecal loading.[2] It is also useful to know about co-existing urinary symptoms. A 1—2-week diary using the Bristol Stool Form Scale provides a useful objective measurement of stool frequency consistency (Fig. 2). Stool colour, the presence of blood and mucous should also be noted.

Any unexplained changes in bowel habit or 'red flag' symptoms require further exploration to exclude cancer and inflammatory bowel disease. The

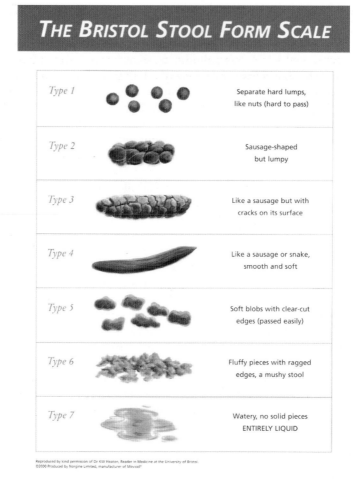

THE BRISTOL STOOL FORM SCALE

Type 1		Separate hard lumps, like nuts (hard to pass)
Type 2		Sausage-shaped but lumpy
Type 3		Like a sausage but with cracks on its surface
Type 4		Like a sausage or snake, smooth and soft
Type 5		Soft blobs with clear-cut edges (passed easily)
Type 6		Fluffy pieces with ragged edges, a mushy stool
Type 7		Watery, no solid pieces ENTIRELY LIQUID

Reproduced by kind permission of Dr KW Heaton, Reader in Medicine at the University of Bristol.
©2000 Produced by Norgine Limited, manufacturer of Movicol®

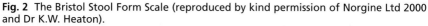

Fig. 2 The Bristol Stool Form Scale (reproduced by kind permission of Norgine Ltd 2000 and Dr K.W. Heaton).

'red flag' symptoms include: (i) rectal bleeding; (ii) weight loss; (iii) nocturnal abdominal pain or diarrhoea; (iv) anaemia; and (v) fever.

A detailed drug history, including past use of laxatives and anti-diarrhoea agents (including over-the-counter and herbal preparations) is essential. Duration, dose and frequency, compliance and the reason for discontinuation of bowel medications recorded. Note that excessive laxative use in younger life may result in slower bowel transit later on. The potential side effects and drug interactions from polypharmacy of regular medications should be considered. A past medical history will identify contributing co-morbidities, relevant surgery (and radiotherapy to the pelvis) and a detailed obstetric history.

Dietary habits (such as vegetarianism), any recent changes, soluble and insoluble fibre intake, fluid quantity and type (such as caffeine which is a bowel stimulant) are useful. A food and fluid diary recorded for 2–4 weeks allows this to be calculated in more detail. Other issues may be identified leading to functional difficulties, which include environmental factors (such as the toilet height) and co-morbidities (such as poor eye-sight, dexterity and mobility issues).

What is the impact on life-style or bothersome factor? There are very few validated quality-of-life assessment tools available for faecal incontinence.[7,18] Other psychosocial considerations include strict toileting regimens in childhood, ignoring the 'call-to-stool' and, in some cases, sexual abuse may have occurred. If there is a history of dementia or learning disability, a formal cognitive assessment may be appropriate. Finally, what are the patient's expectations of treatment?

Examination

A general physical examination should include nutritional status and a neurological examination if indicated (checking sacral sensation at S3/4 dermatomes, cutaneous anal reflex). This is followed by an abdominal, perineal and digital rectal examination. It is recommended that all specialist nurses undertaking digital rectal examination should undergo formal training.[19] Assessment of the perineal area should include looking for conditions such as rectal prolapse, haemorrhoids, skin tags, and atrophic vaginitis externally. Perineal movement can be observed and examination performed to assess resting anal tone, squeeze and recruitment of muscles (such as puborectalis), which may be slow. The anal squeeze strength can also be determined. A gap may be palpable in the sphincters in women who have had episiotomies or third degree tears. Tenderness should be noted, scarring from fissures, fistulas or surgery and any rectal masses (such as an enlarged prostate or tumour). A digital rectal examination also allows detection of faecal loading or impaction with soft or hard stool. A speculum, proctoscopy and rigid sigmoidoscopy may be indicated in certain circumstances but provides little additional information in functional bowel disorders.

MANAGEMENT

Investigations

Bloods tests are useful in excluding secondary causes of constipation or diarrhoea. These include: a full blood count, urea, electrolytes, liver function tests, thyroid function, serum albumin, calcium, C-reactive protein and tissue transglutaminase. A stool sample should be sent for microscopy and culture if infective diarrhoea is suspected. *C. difficile* toxin should be tested for in institutional or care home patients.

Treatment of functional bowel disorders should only occur after underlying pathological bowel disease has been excluded. If 'red flag' symptoms are detected, a referral should be made for a flexible sigmoidoscopy or colonoscopy. This may detect inflammatory bowel disease, cancer, possible ischaemia and observe melanosis coli (associated with prolonged anthraquinone laxative use). *C. difficile* should be treated early with appropriate antibiotics.

A plain abdominal X-ray is not required routinely, but is useful if high faecal impaction is suspected with an empty rectum on examination.[2] Normally, stool is soft until the mid transverse colon and produces opaque shadows filled with translucent 'bubbles' of air on a radiograph. In comparison, the descending colon normally contains more discrete, airless, rounded shapes of hard stool.[20] It may also reveal a megacolon, megarectum, intussusception or sigmoid volvulus.

All other investigations should be carried out in specialist units. They are generally not well tolerated and are unlikely to provide additional information that will alter management unless targeted to look for specific conditions or where surgery is being considered.[21] For example, colonic transit time studies using radio-opaque markers can confirm severe slow colonic transit constipation. Barium studies (without bowel cleansing preparation) may be useful if Hirschsprung's disease is suspected, illustrating the classical proximal colonic dilatation. Defaecating proctograms reveal a mixed neuromuscular deficiency. Neurophysiological studies using an electromyographic (EMG) needle assess anal sphincter strength and efficiency, integrity of nerve the supply (detecting pudendal nerve damage), and demonstrate nerve reflexes. Anorectal manometry can measure pressures and compliance in faecal incontinence. Endo-anal ultrasonography is one of the more useful investigations. It can demonstrate a 360° view and the extent of damage or loss of anal sphincters. It should be considered where intensive physiotherapy and other measures have failed to improved faecal incontinence sufficiently and surgery might be indicated.[22]

General management and life-style advice

It is essential to agree on realistic goals of treatment when managing disordered defaecation in the elderly, by means of a clear bowel management programme. Treatment is aimed at producing more predictable bowel motions, which require less straining (in constipation), and less frequent stools or continence (in faecal incontinence). For most people, this means achieving a 'Goldilock stool', which is 'not too hard or too soft' but just right (Bristol stool type 3/4).[23] Serial stool diaries, using the Bristol Stool Form Scale (Fig. 2), can provide helpful objective measures of the response to treatment. There are only three things that can be manipulated in conservative bowel management: (i) oral intake of diet and fluids; (ii) gut motility; and (iii) the consistency of the stool that comes out.[20]

It should be made clear that it may take several months to see the full benefits of life-style advice modifications. The thirst sensation is impaired with ageing. Therefore, ensuring appropriate fluid intake to improve general health and avoid constipation seems sensible, especially if patients are dehydrated. Five to 7 mugs per day or 1.5—2 l is recommended, but there are no studies to show it improves bowel function.[24] In faecal incontinence, avoiding gastric stimulants such as caffeine, alcohol and spicy foods may help. The recommended daily fibre intake is 20—35 g, but many elderly fail to achieve this. In constipation, a gradual intake in non-soluble fibre is recommended, such as cereals, wholemeal bread, fruit and vegetables. A sudden increase may cause bloating or, cramps. One small, nursing-home study reported a significant reduction in the use of laxatives by introducing a bran.[25] Other studies have looked at yoghurt, prunes, kiwi fruit, disaccharides, linseed oil and *Lactobacillus* spp. with variable results. It should be noted that for some patients, especially those with megacolon or severe slow colonic transit constipation, fibre could worsen symptoms as the stools become too bulky. Referral to a dietician may be warranted for advice regarding constipation or a trial of an exclusion diet. The latter may be helpful for irritable bowel syndrome, or conditions such as lactose intolerance where loose stools may exacerbate faecal incontinence. It is known that a lack of exercise can slow colonic transit time in healthy elderly.[26] However, exercise-intervention studies in nursing homes to improve constipation have been disappointing.[24,27] Counselling or referral to a clinical psychologist is useful for some patients with severe depression and anxiety.

Physiotherapy, pelvic floor exercises and biofeedback

Patients with constipation due to pelvic floor dyssynergia or faecal incontinence may benefit from referral to specialist physiotherapists for a targeted pelvic floor exercise programme and/or biofeedback techniques. There are three different methods of biofeedback; these involve sensory training (such as simulating defaecation using water filled balloons), electromyographic (relaying electromyographic activity from the pelvic floor via a visual display to the patient) and manometry feedback (looking at anal canal pressures). These techniques are aimed at improving muscle strength and aiding relaxation to enable better control during defaecation.

Recent studies in biofeedback for pelvic dyssynergia report benefit in more than half of patients.[28] In selective patients with faecal incontinence pelvic floor, biofeedback may also be beneficial. However, large, well-constructed, randomised, controlled trials with long-term follow-up are lacking for both pelvic floor exercises and biofeedback techniques. Consensus opinion and anecdotal evidence means that both are recommended by the UK National Institute for Health and Clinical Excellence (NICE) for faecal incontinence as second-line treatment.[6] Clearly, more research is needed in this area. Cognitive impairment and poor compliance may limit its use in the elderly.

Toilet access, position and toileting regimens

Improving toilet access is important to avoid functional incontinence. This may require the use of toileting aids such as a commode. However, a person's privacy and dignity must be respected otherwise the 'call-to-stool' may be suppressed. The 2003 national campaign *Behind Closed Doors* aimed to raise awareness amongst healthcare workers and carers about this issue.

Effective defaecation requires rectal support, anal outlet release and an effective expulsive pressure. The most effective position for defaecation is sitting, with the knees higher than the bottom. The lower the position, the more powerful the effect, (as is the norm in many less developed countries). A lower toilet seat, or a footstool to raise the knees, may be required to obtain this optimal position. The intra-abdominal pressure can be raised by contraction of the abdominal muscle wall against a closed glottis. However, this can lead to straining, which should be avoided as it may exacerbate haemorrhoids and rectal prolapse.

The 'brace and bulge' technique was developed by physiotherapists to enable evacuation without straining.[30] This can be taught to patients. It involves gentle breathing, slowly widening the waist (bracing) and then, when fully braced, pushing or propelling the waist backwards and downwards towards the back passage at an angle to improve defaecation. A constant pressure should be maintained, without straining. As the diaphragm moves to its lowest position, eccentric rectus abdominal muscle activity causes lower abdominal 'bulging' and anal release. This process can then be repeated after bracing outwards again.

Patients and carers are also advised to take advantage of the natural gastrocolic reflex when planning toileting regimens. This is often strongest in the morning after a hot drink or exercise.

Drugs treatment for constipation

In some patients, long-term use of laxatives is required to obtain the correct stool type. There have been several reviews looking at the use of laxatives in adults, but they contain very few studies in the elderly and most are in institutional settings.[1,31,32] Treatment should be tailored to the individual taking into consideration the mechanism of action. Several drug or dose adjustments may be required until the desired result is reached. Combination therapies, such as bulk laxatives and a stimulant, may be more successful than monotherapy.

Bulk-forming laxatives, such as bran, ispaghula (fybogel), methylcellulose (which also acts as a faecal softener) and sterculia (normacol), work by increasing faecal mass which stimulates peristalsis. They take several days to work and must be taken with plenty of water or else hard stools and intestinal obstruction may result. They are relatively well-tolerated in the elderly and most useful first-line for patients with small hard stools and normal colonic transit constipation.

Stimulant laxatives increase motility by stimulating colonic nerves. These include anthraquinones, (such as senna and danthron). Senna is the most powerful stimulant and is effective within 6—12 h. It is useful for short-term treatment of acute constipation. The use of dantron is now limited to palliative care as it is a potential carcinogen. The other available stimulant laxatives are diphenylmethane cathartics (such as bisacodyl and sodium docusate). Castor oil is no longer used. Side-effects of stimulant laxatives include abdominal cramp, diarrhoea, hypokalaemia and urine discolouration with anthraquinones. They should be reserved for second-line treatment and avoided in intestinal obstruction.

Faecal softeners (such as sodium docusate, which is also a stimulant) act by lowering surface tension, allowing penetration of hard faeces by water and fats. Liquid paraffin is no longer recommended because of its unpleasant side effects, which include anal seepage and lipoid pneumonia (rarely). However, it is still available over-the-counter. Softeners are useful if haemorrhoids or anal fissures are present.

Osmotic laxatives include sugars (such as lactulose, sorbitol), purgatives (such as magnesium hydroxide) and macragols (such as movicol). They draw water into the stool by osmosis, increasing stool bulk and stimulating colonic motility. They need to be given with plenty of water. Lactulose is effective, but takes 2–3 days to work and may be limited by its side effects of bloating, flatulence, nausea and cramps. The newer macrogols containing polyethylene glycol have electrolytes added to produce more balanced solutions (PEG+E). These appear to be safe in the treatment of chronic constipation. Movicol is also the only oral laxative recommended for faecal impaction (at a dose of 8 sachets daily in 1 l of water for up to 3 days, half if cardiovascular function is impaired). Osmotic laxatives are useful in megacolon or megarectum, where bulk laxatives may worsen symptoms. Magnesium hydroxide is also an osmotic laxative; it is useful for rapid bowel clearance, but not recommended for long-term use. The cautious addition of low-dose stimulants may be needed if bowels do not open for several days.

Rectal medications can be administered as suppositories or enemas. They are absorbed well by the mucosa and provide both local and systemic effects. There has been a move away from the use of regular phosphate enemas because of electrolyte disturbances. These include hyperphosphataemia, hypocalcaemia, hypernatraemia and metabolic acidosis, especially in older people with chronic renal failure.[33] Other osmotic micro-enemas (such as Microlax) are preferable or stimulant suppositories (such as glycerol). Arachis oil enema (ground nut, peanut oil) is a useful softener for anal strictures, but it must be warmed to body temperature and avoided in people with peanut allergies.

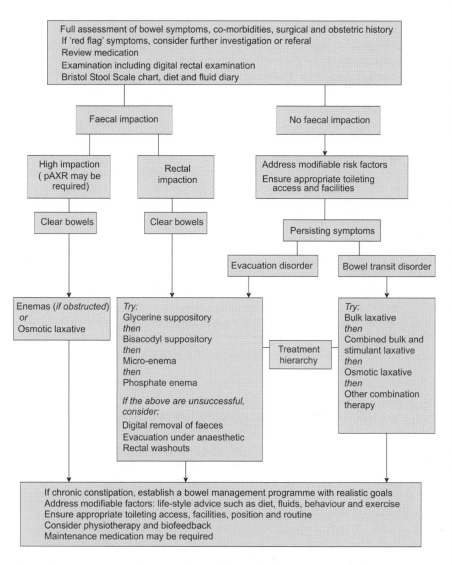

Fig. 3 The management of constipation in the elderly.

Other useful treatments include topical diltiazem cream for anal fissures.[34] Newer therapies, such as gut pro-kinetics (serotonin agonists and antagonists), misoprostol, colchicines, neurotrophin-3 (NT3) are yet to be tested fully in an elderly population.[3,13]

Acute constipation may present on the background of chronic constipation. Initial management should involve clearing the bowel followed by establishing a long-term bowel management programme to prevent recurrence. A useful algorithm is shown in Figure 3, adapted from the Royal College of Physicians working party on bowel care in the older person.[3]

Digital removal of faeces

Digital removal of faeces should no longer be part of routine clinical practice as there are recognised complications. Other measures of managing constipation should be considered first. The exceptions are patients with chronic neurological conditions, such as spinal cord injury, cauda equina, spina bifida and multiple sclerosis, where it may be part of their routine bowel management. It is important that this routine continues if they are admitted to hospital.

Digital removal of faeces should only be carried out in controlled conditions by a competent trained individual. Potential complications can range from pain, local mucosal damage, anal sphincter damage, vagal stimulation causing slowing of the heart rate to autonomic dysreflexia, (an exaggerated autonomic response particularly in spinal injury patients T6 or above). If it is not possible to remove or break up the rectal faecal mass easily (either because it is too hard or larger than 4 cm across), removal under general anaesthetic may be required to avoid considerable pain and anal sphincter damage. New guidelines have been developed to ensure consistency in approach.[19]

Drug treatment for faecal incontinence

Drugs used for the treatment of faecal incontinence are either aimed at slowing down gut transit time, (loperamide or codeine phosphate) or mopping up loose stool (bulk laxatives). The challenge is getting the balance right and not ending up with constipation instead. Loperamide syrup (not tablets) is useful as this can be titrated up from very low doses (2.5 ml). In some cases, a constipating agent with a stimulant (oral or rectal) may be required to achieve a predictable bowel action.

Drug treatment for irritable bowel syndrome

Drugs for irritable bowel syndrome are directed towards the predominant subtype: laxatives for constipation (except lactulose because of its side effects) and anti-motility drugs for diarrhoea (such as loperamide). Antispasmodics and low-dose tricyclic antidepressants may be helpful in some individuals. NICE has recently produced a clinical guideline on this topic.[17]

Rectal irrigation systems and anal plugs

The use of rectal irrigation systems is becoming increasingly popular in preference to surgical management.[35] Spinal injury patients have traditionally used these systems for faecal incontinence. The process involves inserting a catheter rectally and then inflating a balloon to block off the anus. Using a system of irrigation tubes, water fills the rectum, the lower colon then empties its contents. Cardiomed has been around for some time. A newer system (Peristeen) is now available on prescription. It is not cheap, but the cost can be offset against medication, containment products and nursing time. Patients do need to be dextrous enough to use the equipment and sit on a toilet or commode, but, if selected appropriately, it can vastly improve their quality of life. An anal plug can be used in between irrigations.

Surgery and sacral nerve stimulation

Surgery should only be considered after conservative measures have been tried. There are numerous different procedures available for intractable faecal incontinence. However, the failure rate can be up to 50% in some cases with a significant number worse off. The evidence base in the elderly is lacking[36] and co-morbidities often restrict this as a viable option. The management of rectal prolapse remains a challenge, but newer, less invasive, surgical techniques are being developed. A total colectomy with a stoma may be a drastic, but preferable, option for some individuals with severe constipation. Careful patient selection and counselling is essential.

Sacral nerve stimulation is a new minimally invasive technique, which may provide a viable treatment for faecal incontinence and constipation in the elderly. Initial trials in younger adults are encouraging[37] and it has the support of NICE. However, it is still expensive and only performed in specialist centres.

Other considerations

For some people, it may be appropriate to advise on odour control, sacral skin care, containment products (and provide a formal pads assessment), digitation techniques to aid bowel emptying, and adjustments of enteral tube feeding to reduce diarrhoea. Other therapies include abdominal massage and acupuncture.

The NICE faecal incontinence clinical guideline[6] is a useful reference that covers many of the management principles discussed.

Finally, prevention of disordered defaecation starts in childhood with appropriate toilet training and promotion of a healthy and active life-style. More research is needed looking at strategies to avoid post obstetric bowel complications, management of rectal prolapse, the impact of life-style modification, pelvic floor exercises, biofeedback and laxative regimens in the elderly. In hospitals (and institutions), it is important to be pro-active and not reactive by identifying at-risk patients. A risk assessment tool for constipation may be useful.[38] Reducing the risk of developing *C. difficile* infection requires adherence to strict antibiotic protocols and hand washing. Healthcare workers have a duty of care to identify people with bowel problems, assess, treat, and establish a bowel management programme or refer on to a specialist.[39]

A MULTIDISCIPLINARY APPROACH

The symptoms of the majority people with disordered defaecation can be improved or cured with treatment. The causes of bowel dysfunction in the elderly are usually multifactorial and require a multidisciplinary approach. In order to deliver appropriate care, a fully integrated service is required with clear referral pathways across primary, secondary and specialist care.[39,40] This should include access to specialist nurses, gastroenterologists, colorectal surgeons, geriatricians, neurologists, gynaecologists, radiology, anorectal physiology, physiotherapists, occupational therapists, dieticians and a clinical psychologist. Management and further research could be co-ordinated through a bowel dysfunction clinic.[20]

Key points for clinical practice

- Disordered defaecation is common in the elderly with co-morbidities.

- Constipation and faecal incontinence are symptoms not diagnoses, the causes of which are often multifactorial.

- The majority of symptoms can be cured or improved with a bowel management programme.

- Digital rectal examination is required as part of a full assessment.

- A stool diary, using the Bristol Stool Form Scale, provides a useful objective assessment of stool type and response to treatment.

- 'Red flag' symptoms require further gastrointestinal investigations or referral.

- It is important to address life-style factors and functional problems using a multidisciplinary approach.

- If medication is required, this should be tailored towards the individual.

- Other techniques such as physiotherapy biofeedback, rectal irrigation and sacral nerve stimulation may be helpful.

- Further research into disordered defaecation in the elderly is needed to clarify the best management strategies.

References

1. Health Technology Assessment (HTA). *Systemic review of the effectiveness of laxatives in the elderly.* 1997; 1: No.13.
2. Donald IP, Smith RG, Cruikshank JG, Elton RA, Stoddart ME. A study of constipation in the elderly living at home. *Gerontology* 1985; **31**: 112–118.
3. Royal College of Physicians. Bowel Care in Older People: Research into practice. *Clinical Effectiveness & Evaluation Unit.* London: Royal College of Physicians, 2002.
4. Stenzelius K, Westergren A, Hallberg IR. Bowel function among people 75+ reporting faecal incontinence in relation to help seeking, dependency and quality of life. *J Clin Nurs* 2007; **16**: 458–468.
5. Tobin GW, Brocklehurst JC. Faecal incontinence in residential homes for the elderly: prevalence, aetiology and management. *Age Ageing* 1986; **15**: 41–46.
6. National Institute for Health and Clinical Excellence. *Faecal incontinence. Clinical guidance 49.* London: NICE, 2007.
7. O'Keefe EA, Talley NJ, Zinsmeister AR, Jacobsen SJ. Bowel disorders impair functional status and quality of life in the elderly: a population-based study. *J Gerontol* 1995; **50**: M184—M189.
8. Thompson WG, Longstreth GF, Drossman DA, Heaton KW, Irvine EJ, Muller-Lissner SA. Functional bowel disorders and functional abdominal pain. *Gut* 1999; **45 (Suppl II)**: II43–II47.
9. Salles N. Basic mechanisms of the aging gastrointestinal tract. *Dig Dis* 2007; **25**: 112–117.
10. Leoning-Baucke V, Anurus S. Sigmoidal and rectal motility in healthy elderly. *J Am Geriatr Soc* 1984; **32**: 887–891.
11. Connell AM, Hilton C, Irvine G, Lennard-Jones JE, Misiewicz JJ. Variation of bowel habits in to

population samples. *BMJ* 1965; **2**: 1095–1099.

12. Brocklehurst JC, Kirkland JL, Martin J. Constipation in long-stay elderly patients: its treatment and prevention by lactulose, poloxalkol-dihydroxyanthroquinolone and phosphate enemas. *Gerontology* 1983; **29**: 181–184.

13. Bosshard W, Dreher R, Schnegg JF, Bula CJ. The treatment of chronic constipation in elderly people – an update. *Drugs Aging* 2004; **21**: 911–930.

14. Singaram C, Ashraf W, Gaumnitz EA *et al*. Dopaminergic defect of enteric nervous system in Parkinson's disease patients with chronic constipation. *Lancet* 1995; **346**: 861–864.

15. *Bowel Continence Nursing*. Bucks: Beaconsfield, 2004.

16. Drossman DA. The functional gastrointestinal disorders and the Rome III process. *Gastroenterology* 2006; **130**: 1377–1390.

17. National Institute for Health and Clinical Excellence. *Irritable bowel syndrome in adults. Clinical guideline* **61**. London: NICE, 2008.

18. Rockwood TH, Church JM, Fleshman JW et al. Fecal incontinence quality of life scale (FIQLS). Quality of life instrument for patients with fecal incontinence. *Dis Colon Rectum* 2000; **43**: 9–17.

19. Royal College of Nursing and Association for Continence Advice. *The procedure for the digital removal of faeces*. Guidelines. London: RCN, 2003.

20. Bubna-Kasteliz B. Faecal incontinence in older age – the use of a bowel dysfunction clinic. *CME Geriatr Med* 2000; 2: 56–60.

21. Wald A. Colonic and anorectal motility testing in clinical practice. *Am J Gastroenterol* 1994; **89**: 2109–2115.

22. Rieger NA, Sweeney JL, Hoffman DC, Young JF, Hunter A. Investigation of fecal incontinence with endoanal ultrasound. *Dis Colon Rectum* 1996; **39**: 860–864.

23. Barrett J. Faecal incontinence and constipation in the older adult. *British Geriatric Society* 2002 <www.bgs.org.uk>.

24. Stefan A, Muller-Lissner MD, Michael A, Kamm MD, Carmelo Scarpignato MD, Wald A. Myths and misconceptions about chronic constipation. *Am J Gastroenterol* 2005; **100**: 232–242.

25. Sturtzel B, Elmadfa I. Intervention with dietary fibre to treat constipation and reduce laxative use in residents of nursing homes. *Ann Nutr Metab* 2008; **52 (Suppl 1)**: 54–56.

26. Liu F, Kondo T, Toda Y. Brief physical inactivity prolongs colonia transit time in elderly, active men. *Int J Sports Med* 1993; **14**: 465–467.

27. Simmons SF, Schnelle JF. Effects of an exercise and scheduled-toileting intervention on appetite and constipation in nursing home residents. *J Nutr Health Aging* 2004; **8**: 116–121.

28. Bassotti G, Chistolini F, Sietchiping-Nzepa F, de Roberto G, Morelli A, Chiarioni G. Biofeedback for pelvic floor dysfunction in constipation. *BMJ* 2004; **328**: 393–396.

29. The Cochrane Collaboration. *Biofeedback and/or sphincter exercises for the treatment of faecal incontinence in adults*. London: Wiley, 2006.

30. Markwell S, Sapford R. Physiotherapy management of obstructed defaecation. *Aust J Physiother* 1995; **41**: 29–83.

31. Tramonte SM, Brand MB, Mulrow CD, Amato MG, O'Keefe E, Ramirez G. The treatment of chronic constipation in adults. A systemic review. *J Gen Intern Med* 1997; **12**: 15–24.

32. NHS Centre for Reviews and Dissemination. Effective Health Care. *Effectiveness of laxatives in adults*. 2001; vol **7**. no1. ISSN: 0965-0288.

33. Mendoza J, Legido J, Rubio S, Gisbert JP. Systemic review: the adverse effects of sodium phosphate enema. *Aliment Pharmacol Ther* 2007; **26 (Suppl 1)**: 9–20.

34. Sajid MS, Rimple E, Cheek E, Baig MK. The efficiency of diltiazem and glyceryltrinitrate for the medical management of chronic anal fissures. *Int J Colorectal Dis* 2008; **23**: 1–6.

35. Christensen P, Bazzocchi G, Coggrave M et al. A randomised, controlled trial of transanal irrigation versus conservative bowel management in spinal cord injured patients. *Gastroenterology* 2006; **131**: 738–747.

36. Norgine Pharmaceuticals. *Norgine risk assessment tool for constipation*. Norgine Pharmaceuticals, 2006.

37. The Cochrane Collaboration. *Surgery for faecal incontinence in adults*. London: Wiley, 2007.

38. The Cochrane Collaboration. *Sacral nerve stimulation for faecal incontinence and constipation*. London: Wiley, 2007.

39. Department of Health. *The National Service Framework for Older People*. London: DH, 2001; 37–38.

40. Department of Health. *Good Practice in Continence Services*. London: DH, 2000.

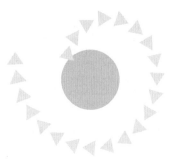

Index

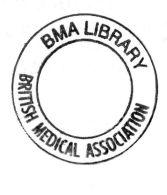